Health and Work
under Capitalism:

AN INTERNATIONAL PERSPECTIVE

Edited by Vicente Navarro and Daniel M. Berman

**POLICY,
POLITICS,
HEALTH AND
MEDICINE**
Series

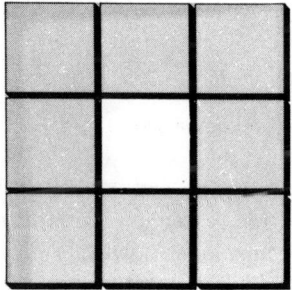

Baywood Publishing Company, Inc.

Farmingdale, N.Y.   11735

Library of Congress Catalog Card Number: 82-8715

ISBN: 0-89503-035-7

© 1983, Baywood Publishing Company, Inc.

Library of Congress Cataloging in Publication Data

Main entry under title:

Health and work under capitalism.

(Policy, politics, health, and medicine ; 5)
Includes bibliographical references.
1. Medicine, Industrial. 2. Labor and laboring classes—Medical care. 3. Capitalism. I. Navarro, Vicente. II. Berman, Daniel M. III. Series. [DNLM: 1. Occupational medicine—Collected works. 2. Cross-Cultural comparison—Collected works. WA 400 H4345]
RC963.3.H4   1982   616.9'803   82-8715
ISBN 0-89503-035-7

THE NATURE OF WORK UNDER CAPITALISM
AND ITS IMPLICATIONS IN HEALTH

A main characteristic of the dominant ideologies in western capitalist societies has been to perceive workers primarily as wage earners, i.e., consumers endowed with specific attributes such as income, education, and status, all defined in the spheres of exchange, distribution and consumption rather than in the world of production. In those ideological scenarios, work is seen primarily as a source of income enabling the worker to meet his needs and expectations. Citizens, in consumer societies, are defined as consumers rather than workers. Work as an activity and as a social relation does not appear in those theoretical scenarios.

This interpretation of our realities explains the overabundance of studies aimed at understanding the health of the people by looking at their diet, consumption, levels of expectations, life styles, utilization of medical services and so forth. Nowhere does this ideological bias of the consumer society appear more clearly than in medicine. The reality that the majority of citizens in the western capitalist world are workers is rarely noticed in medical textbooks. In the United States, for example, of more than one hundred medical schools, only twelve include occupational health in their curriculum, and even in those twelve, the overall time dedicated to the subject is extremely low (1). Very few U.S. physicians and other medical care professionals know how to take and interpret the work history of their patients or potential patients.

Thus, within the dominant ideological scenarios in consumer societies, work remains an unproblematic area, a mere source of income. For the most part, workers are perceived as being satisfied with their work. That picture is constantly and continuously presented by the establishment's media. The reality, however, is dramatically different. Many contributors to this volume show that there is indeed a great deal of dissatisfaction, resistance and struggle at the work place of the western capitalist countries, reflecting a rebellion by the workers against their conditions of work. That conflict and struggle has reached a point where great alarm has been expressed in the corridors of power. For example, one of the major recommendations of the powerful Trilateral Commission—which includes representatives of major corporate interests in the western capitalist world—is that something should be done about the conditions of work in western societies, since the rebellion of the workers against those conditions has reached such proportions that it seriously hinders the productivity and overall process of capital accumulation (2). In response, a whole cadre of "experts in human relations" has been called upon to make work less unbearable either by "humanizing" the work environment or by asking workers to participate in the spoils of their own sweat. In all these reforms, one thing has to be made clear: that these

3

reforms have to take place within the iron boundaries of a well-established set of power relations where the capitalist class or bourgeoisie is the dominant class. But it is precisely these social power relations which determine the nature of work in capitalist societies, making work not an instrument of joy, creativity and self-expression but, rather, an instrument of harm and oppression. The controllers of the process of work—the capitalist class—shape the nature of work to increase control over the workers in order to extract as much work from them as possible. In order to do this, they force upon the workers a set of relations where the owners and controllers of the process of work are the dominant class in society, and the subjects of that control—the workers—are the dominated class. A dominant/dominated type of relationship is thus established in all areas and spheres of society with its most unadultered form appearing at the work place. Democracy—wherever it exists—stops at the office door and the factory gate. As Mark Twain once indicated, nowhere does the dictatorship of those he called "the soft-handed and idle capitalists and superintendents" appear more clearly than at the sites of work where wealth is being produced. The application of that dictum today appears clearly in a recent declaration of a business leader in the United States who, in a moment of unguarded candor, exclaimed, "How long can our political democracy stand the seventy million who live the majority of their working hours in an atmosphere that is totalitarian?" (3) V. Navarro, B. Ellen Smith, and T. D. Sterling, in Section 1 of this volume, show how those capitalist social relations are being reproduced at the work place and their consequences and implications for health, for medicine and for medical knowledge.

The reality of damage at the work place is increasingly clear for all to see. Nowhere does the oppressive brutality of capitalism and the immense human suffering created by it appear more clearly than in the places of work of the majority of our working population. Day after day, workers are killed and physically and psychologically maimed where they work. More U.S. citizens die every year as a result of their employment than were killed in battle during over a decade of war in Vietnam (4). But while the casualties of that imperialist war appeared on the airwaves and in the pages of the national media, the casualties of the other war—the one fought in work places in the United States—are rarely mentioned. There is, indeed, a deafening silence—only occasionally broken by some news report of a "major" accident— regarding the carnage that is imposed for the benefit and glory of Capital on our working population. But the reality, a revolting reality, of that slaughter is over- whelming. In Section 2 of this volume, D. Coburn and D. Baker show the nature of some of the damage imposed on the workers at the work place; B. Castleman and M. J. Vera Vera show that the damage does not stop at the place of work but also occurs in the places where workers and their families live, study and enjoy themselves. The reality shown by the contributors to this volume is that work under capitalism kills workers or maims their lives. As a popular U.S. folk song says, "You don't just get money from your job, you also get sadness, sickness and frustration."

The class dominance which appears at the work place also appears and is repro- duced in all spheres of society including the political and ideological. Contrary to formal discourse, in western democracies, citizens are not equal. Their political and economic power depends on whether they are the controllers of the means and the process of work or whether they are the workers, subject to that control. The Henry upon in political debate—than do any workers. That situation explains the very limited protection of workers and the clear bias of existing legislation in all capitalist countries favoring the right of capital to accumulate profits over the rights of life and freedom from harm of the working population. Of course, workers are not powerless, and competition for power does exist. Occasional defeats for powerful capitalist interests do occur. After all, David did overcome Goliath. But the point of the story is that David was smaller than Goliath and that the odds were heavily against him. The imbalance in that Capital/Labor power relationship in favor of Capital is overwhelming indeed. The consequences of that reality for the health of workers and for the nature of occupational health and medicine in developed capitalist countries is presented in Section 3 by R. C. Clutterbuck (for the UK), G. Assennato and V. Navarro (for Italy); D. M. Berman (for the US); and H. U. Deppe (for West Germany).

Needless to say, the reality of class domination and its harmful consequences for the health of the laboring population is even clearer in the world of underdevelopment where the majority of the human and laboring population live. A. C. Laurell and J. V. Vilanilam show elements of that reality in their contributions in Section 4. In those parts of the world, the domination of capital over labor is further facilitated by capital's articulation within a set of international power relations—imperialism— that allows unhindered forms of exploitation, frequently facilitated by military muscle and sheer force. It is worth stressing in this section that capital is increasingly international. Capital from the core countries, in its search for higher profits and lower wages, crosses borders looking for other parts of the world where labor is less organized and where corporations can operate with little control. B. Castleman, in his concluding article, shows how the international mobility of capital also means the international mobility of harm and death.

Before ending this introduction, several points need to be stressed. One is that the essays published in this volume do not provide a homogeneity in terms of ideological position nor in terms of style. Nor are they presented as definitive pieces but, rather, as exploratory positions that, indeed, may require further elaboration. They have been chosen as representative of the different positions and concerns that have appeared in the pages of the *International Journal of Health Services* during the last few years. For reasons of space, many articles also relevant to the topic of this volume have not been included.

Also, many other subjects such as the articulation of class exploitation with other forms of exploitation such as race and gender exploitation need further discussion and elaboration.

Another point that needs to be made is that the focus of this volume has been on capitalist societies defining as such those social formations in which a class—the capitalist class or bourgeoisie—has a hegemonic dominance over the means of production, consumption and legitimation. It has not included the analysis of the relationship between work and health in post revolutionary or socialist societies. We are conscious of that important gap. We are indeed aware of the great urgency also to analyze those experiences. The workers' rebellion in Poland, protesting their conditions of work and the limited power and control over their own work and lives show how similar—although not identical—relations of oppression may be reproduced in post capitalist societies. The existence in some of these societies of such realities does not but, rather, the possibility in transitional societies of reproducing dominated/dominant types of relationships that hinder and may eventually determine the failure of their socialist projects. Socialism is, after all, not merely a project of redistribution of goods and services but, far more important, a project of redefinition of the production relations of which relations at work are key ones. The non-inclusion, in our analysis, of post capitalist societies does not indicate lack of awareness of the need to subject those experiences to rigorous analysis, but, rather, it reflects our position that the relationship between work and health in those societies responds to different forces—still poorly understood—than those operating under capitalism.

It is also worth stressing that it is not the intention of this volume to present "models" for changing the conditions of oppression at the work place. Suffice it to say that while we believe that the transformation of work—from an activity and a social relation that determines death and disease to another form of activity and social relation that determines health, joy, and happinesss—will require the transformation and end of capitalism, still, we believe that much needs to be done—and can be done—under capitalism to diminish that pathologic reality generated at the work place. Because of this perception, we have included some of the advances achieved by the working class and labor movements of capitalist countries, not to present them as "models" to be followed but, rather, as interesting experiences that merit attention in the international struggle for workers' liberation. As many contributors in this volume show, the realities presented in each country share some similarities and respond to similar forces. Capitalism is not a national but an international or transnational system. The international mobility and nature of capital requires not only a national but also an international answer. It is difficult to imagine a more compelling call for international solidarity and cooperation among workers' movements than the one to stop harm, disease and death. Part of the strategy for liberation is to learn from the enormously rich body of experiences embodied in the practice of the workers' movements in today's world. It is the intention of this volume to contribute to that learning and to that liberation.

REFERENCES

1. Mazzochi, A., Training occupational physicians. *Health Policy Advisory Center Bulletin (Health/PAC)*, 75: 7, March/April 1977.
2. Trilateral Task Force on the Governability of Democracies. *The Governability of Democracies.* Trilateral Commission, New York, 1975.
3. Quoted from Doye, R. J., *Management Accounting, 1970.*
4. The *President's Report on Occupational Safety and Health, 1972,* estimated the 100,000 deaths a year in the United States were caused by occupational disease (see esp. pp. 111 and 128). National Safety Council estimates for the total deaths caused by work accidents every year between 1963 and 1971 oscillate between 14,100 and 14,500 (see *Accident Facts*, National Safety Council, Chicago, 1972) p. 25. For more information, see "A Critical Review of Estimates of the Fraction of Cancer in the United States Related to Occupational Factors," a Report presented by the National Cancer Institute, National Institute of Environmental Health Sciences, National Institute for Occupational Safety and Health, critiques prepared by Dr. Reuel A. Stallones, Dr. Thomas Downs, 1978, mimeo. For more on this question, see Daniel M. Berman's *Death on the Job* (Monthly Review Press, New York, 1978) Chapter 2. According to the U.S. Department of Defense, there were 47,072 battle deaths and 10,390 other deaths in the Vietnam war from 1961 through 1975. *The 1980 Hammond Almanac,* Martin A. Bacheller, Editor in Chief (Hammond Almanac, Inc., Maplewood, N.J., 1980), p. 728.

Vicente Navarro

TABLE OF CONTENTS

PART 4: Occupational Health in Underdeveloped Capitalist Countries

PART 1

Ideology in Occupational Medicine

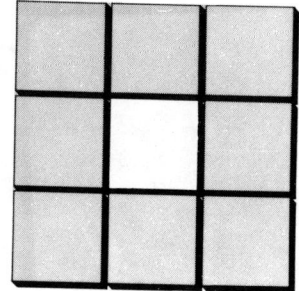

CHAPTER 1

Work, Ideology, and Science: The Case of Medicine

Vicente Navarro

"The docs keep telling me there's nothing wrong with the place where I work. I guess they're supposed to know it all because they've had a lot of education and everything. I'm no expert like they are, but I sure as hell know there's something wrong in that mill and the other guys are saying the same thing. One thing I know for sure—that place is killing us."

Cancer patient and steelworker from the Bethlehem Steel
Corporation mills, Sparrows Point, Maryland, 1978

INTRODUCTION
CLASS STRUGGLE AND HEALTH

There is a concern among the centers of power in the Western capitalist world that something is going wrong with the nature of work in that world. Editorials in the daily press, articles in scholarly papers, reports of powerful foundations, exposé programs on television, and—even more recently—some commercial films have focused on different dimensions and components of what has been called the "crisis at the workplace" in contemporary society. Part of this crisis is the rebellion of the working populations against their conditions of work, rebellions which appear in different

This article is an expanded version of one published under the same title in *Social Science & Medicine*, Summer 1980 issue.

forms such as absenteeism, turnover, or just plain sabotage. These have reached such proportions as to become a cause for major alarm by the establishments of those societies. An example of this concern and alarm is one of the reports of the powerful Trilateral Commission (1). A major recommendation of that Commission, which includes representatives of the power structure of the top capitalist developed societies, is that "a major intervention is required in the area of work in our societies" to attack workers' discontent and alienation at its roots, since, otherwise, those rebellions can threaten the very survival of the Western economic system—a euphemistic term which is used to define Western capitalism. The representatives of the bourgeoisie or capitalist class—or, to use a more American term, the corporate class—as the most class conscious of all classes, tend to perceive quite clearly from where they sit where trouble may come from, i.e. from the working class's rebellion against the main column on which the entire capitalist system is built: *the nature and the conditions on which basis work is extracted from the workers* (2).

On the other side of the ideological fence, progressive forces in the United States have only recently begun seeing signs of that potential storm. Many, however, still seem to be stuck in that scenario so widely emphasized by ideologists of capitalism and radicals alike that the working class has practically disappeared as an agent of change and, instead, has been absorbed into society, becoming part of the larger consuming and undifferentiated masses. According to some radical theorists, other groups are supposed to have taken over that task of carrying on the much needed struggle for change, while the working class has been "lost" and has become part of a one-dimensional society (3). Witness, for example, a recent publication edited by a leading radical in this country (4) who, in covering the changes in the cultural meaning of medicine, refers in his introduction to the impact of black's and women's struggles in the redefinition of health and medicine, but not once does he refer to the struggles which are taking place at the sites of work in the Western capitalist societies, struggles which I believe are among the most important ones in changing the nature of our society, including the definition of health and medicine. Just in the United States alone, millions of workers were involved in strikes last year which had to do primarily with work conditions and health. From the wildcat strikes among steelworkers in Ohio who asked to change conditions of work and medical regulations which applied in their working places, to the coal miners who struck for three months—threatening, as President Carter indicated, the stability of the economy, i.e. U.S. capitalism— for the right to strike for health and safety conditions and for the right to retain some form of control over their health plans, there are signs that major struggles are taking place at the workplace questioning the meaning of work under capitalism and its effects on the health and well-being of our working populations. Health-related issues have been triggering points in many of those struggles, and health-related movements have had an important impact on changing the nature of political and social institutions, including labor's own institutions. A most recent example is the key role played by the black lung movement in creating Miners for Democracy. That movement rallied the majority of coal miners around the issue of democratizing their union, the United Mine Workers, and overthrowing the corrupt Boyle leadership (5). A very important issue—a key one—in that fight was a health-related issue: the need to recognize and compensate black lung as an occupation-related condition, and the right to strike for safety conditions. The miners fought a tough battle to redefine health and medicine, showing—against the verdict of coal companies, state and federal legislative bodies and agencies, and even large sectors of the academic community—that coal mining is indeed a very unhealthy occupation in our society.

It would be erroneous to consider those struggles as new or limited only to the United States. The long struggle which the working class carried out in the 19th and 20th centuries in the United States and many other countries as well to limit the daily working hours to eight already had as its goal a redefining of the meaning of work and health. As an Italian folk song of the 19th century (6) put it:

> We want to change the social order
> We are fed up with work without meaning
> We want to enjoy life and health, sun, and flowers
> We want eight hours for work, eight hours to rest, and
> eight hours to live, to have joy, and to dream.

This history of the working class in the United States, and other countries as well, is punctuated by a continuous struggle to redefine the nature of work and health. And these struggles have heightened to such an extent that, as the Trilateral Commission indicates, they are threatening the current international capitalist order. Most of the strikes in the Western developed capitalist world in the last two decades have had to do with working conditions and how those working conditions affect the well-being and health of the laboring populations (7). Actually, a key characteristic of the current international capitalist crisis is the conflict which appears between the demand by the representatives of capital for higher productivity at the workplace (extracting as much work as possible from each worker) and the resistance by the workers (although not always by their unions) to that demand for higher productivity. The workers know quite well the meaning and impact which higher productivity—with higher speeds of work, longer number of working hours, night shifts of workers, and the like—has on their health and lives. Economic successes that have been presented as "miracles," highly applauded in established centers of power, have concealed the enormous sacrifices which they have implied for the working populations. Just one example among many is the economic "miracle" in the 1960s in Italy. Even in the land of the Vatican, that economic "miracle" did not have much of a spiritual intervention. The spiritual had a bloody, earthy touch. Just in terms of cost of major occupational injuries at the workplace, the figures speak for themselves: 440,000 in 1946, 950,000 in 1956, and 1,400,000 in 1970 (8). There was a clear relationship between higher productivity and higher damage at the workplace in the 1950s and '60s (the period of the "miracles"), not to speak of the immense suffering in disease, stress, malaise, and ruined personal and family lives. Actually, the social unrest and final explosion which took place in Italy in the late '60s, and in particular in the "hot autumn" of 1969 when workers and communities took over factories and other economic and social institutions, represented a rebellion against those working and living conditions. In those rebellions, the control of work, the meaning and purpose of that work, and its consequences in workers' lives were the focus of the struggle. As a group of workers indicated in the slogan they hung on the door of the factory they had taken over: "We want a society where workers will sing while working." (9)

Needless to say, these struggles against the nature of work under capitalism occur not only because of the actual damage imposed on the worker at the workplace, but also because of the harm created to the workers both within and outside the working place and in all dimensions of their lives. Two recent examples show how work under capitalism affects the most profound and intimate aspects of workers' lives, including their sexuality, and how workers rebel against that damage. One occurred recently at the British Leyland factory in the United Kingdom when management wanted to establish a night shift. The workers rebelled and struck because they perceived that that change would affect their sexual relations with their partners. Their slogan, "Make love, not night work," put it quite clearly. Similarly, the workers of Pesaro in Italy noticed that when using machines which have a high frequency of wave lengths, they felt their sexual appetite diminish. When they approached the occupational doctors of the factory, they were told that something was wrong with them or their lovers. Consequently, they were advised to change lovers. But the workers felt that their change in sexuality did not have anything to do with their lovers but with the bosses' machines, and in what has been called the first "strike for love" in Italy, they struck and forced management to change those machines (10).

In summary, the fight for the realization of health is very much at the center of the conflict between capital and labor which takes place at the workplace and heightens in moments of crisis like the current one. The struggle which occurs at the places of work in our Western societies is a most important one, since it questions the very basic social power relations of capitalism (11).

The Nature of Work Under Capitalism

Let us analyze the conditions of work of the working class, that class by whose sweat and pain the goods and services in our society are produced. A primary characteristic of work is that its controllers increasingly shape the nature of work to optimize their pattern of control over the productive process, the individual producers, and the collectivity of producers—the working class (12). By means of this process, the workers are: (a) compartmentalized into increasingly narrower tasks; (b) hierarchicalized by a division of labor which reproduces the class relations in society; and (c) expropriated from all possibility of controlling, influencing, or having a say in the design or development of the work process or of the products they create.

The outcome of this process is a set of relations which cannot be defined as less than totalitarian. Democracy, the capacity of individuals to control their own lives, stops at the gates of the working places. This set of authoritarian relations, where one class—the bourgeoisie—controls that process of production and work and the other—the working class—doesn't, is what Marx called the *dictatorship of the bourgeoisie,* understanding as such not a specific political form of government but rather an overwhelming dominance and control which the bourgeoisie has over the means and processes of production. Nowhere for the millions of workers does that dictatorship appear more clearly than at the place of work. Michael Bosquet (13), in his usual vivid way, puts this quite clearly when he invites the reader to:

> Try putting 13 little pins in 13 little holes 60 times an hour, eight hours a day. Spot-weld 67 steel plates an hour, then find yourself one day facing a new assembly-line needing 110 an hour. Fit 100 coils to 100 cars every hour; tighten seven bolts three times a minute. Do your work in noise "at the safety limit," in a fine mist of oil, solvent and metal dust. Negotiate for the right to take a piss—or relieve yourself furtively behind a big press so that you don't break the rhythm and lose your bonus. Speed up to gain the time to blow your nose or get a bit of grit out of your eye. Bolt your sandwich sitting in a pool of grease because the canteen is 10 minutes away and you've only got 40 for your lunch-break. As you cross the factory threshold, lose the freedom of opinion, the freedom of speech, the right to meet and associate supposedly guaranteed under the constitution. Obey without arguing, suffer punishment without the right of appeal, get the worst jobs if the manager doesn't like your face. Try being an assembly-line worker.

There is a popular movie in the United States—"Blue Collar"—which shows the inside of a factory, i.e. how people work, a theme very rarely treated by the media in the United States. And in spite of its many serious political and ideological flaws, it shows what the inside of a factory looks like. It shows in essence the Gulags of Capitalism. Actually, this movie understates the conditions of work, since it was filmed in a small car factory rather than in a more typical large one where the speed of work is much higher. The managers of those more typical car manufacturing industries did not want to show the inside of their factories (14).

But these characteristics of assembly line work are not unique to workers in the automobile industry or workers in manufacturing alone. Many other studies have been done showing how assembly line work, where the individual worker is carrying out *predetermined tasks* over which he or she does not have much control, is also the most frequent type of work among sales, clerical, and large sectors of public service workers. Indeed, that expansion of the atomized hierarchical and authoritarian division of labor is growing rather than diminishing in most areas of work in society, and is being presented as needed to increase the efficiency and productivity of the worker, i.e to extract as much work as possible from the worker. But that demand by representatives of the capitalist class is not made without misgiving about how long the working class will tolerate those conditions of work. As a leading exponent of the establishment put it, "How long can our political system stand the seventy million who live the majority of their working hours in an atmosphere which is totalitarian?" (15)

In the following pages of this article, I will explain how *bourgeois ideology reproduces these dominant/dominated relations* in the sphere of production (Section I), in the arena of politics (Section II), and in the area of science, including medicine (Section III).[1] Needless to say, dominance does not mean complete control (16). The working class does not remain passive against that domination. *A continuous process of class struggle* takes place, where the working class also wins most significant

---

[1] By ideology, I mean, with Gramsci, the ethical, juridical, political, esthetic, and philosophic ideas about social reality, as well as the set of customs, practices, and behaviors which consciously or unconsciously reflect that vision of reality.

victories and determines changes in the boundaries, means, and instruments of that dominance (17). How this class struggle affects that dominance in the world of production, of politics, and of science is also covered in Sections I, II, and III, respectively. In all three sections, I have chosen medicine and medical knowledge as the primary points of reference.

SECTION I
WORK, MARKET IDEOLOGY, AND
THE REPRODUCTION OF POWER RELATIONS

How is class dominance being reproduced? By different means. For example, the division of labor within the working class, by dividing the labor force into different categories, erodes a sense of class solidarity. As a leading trade unionist of the health sector in Great Britain recently said (18), "By dividing workers into a multiplicity of sections and grades, management tries to lead them to believe that they have no common interests and that their interests are opposite." Also reproducing those dominant/dominated relations are the conditions of work, highly hierarchical and authoritarian, which tend to create a habit of submission and subordination, further accentuated by a fear of unemployment or dismissal which tends to produce an obedient body of workers and citizens.

There are two other factors which explain the reproduction of these relations. One, very important ideologically, is that this type of work is presented not as a result of specific power relations in society, but rather as a *logical, rational, and natural* outcome of the unavoidable and unchangeable industrialization and technologization of the work process. Thus, the culprit of workers' pains is seen in the unchangeable industrialization and technology of work rather than in the social power relations which determine this specific type of oppressive industrialization and technology. Needless to say, the absence in the current historical period of models of alternative processes of production and work strengthens the ideology that ours is the only logical, rational, and natural way of organizing production. But dominant ideology tries to impress on the worker that those relations are not only *natural*, but also *fair*. This dominant/dominated relationship in the world of production appears as a fair exchange in the labor market in which those exploitative relations are veiled and mystified by making them appear as a matter of free, unfettered, and equal exchange between the laborer who sells his labor and the capitalist who pays a wage for it. Needless to say, bourgeois ideology may even be willing to admit and accept that much work today is oppressive and does not offer the possibility for self-fulfillment to the worker. But this same ideology will quickly add that the worker is compensated with a fair wage and that fair wage will allow the worker to obtain the key to the door to his self-fulfillment in the house of consumption. The worker, denied the possibility for creativity and self-fulfillment in the world of production, is said to be given that possibility in the world of consumption. Moreover, while he has no control over the work process, he is being told that he has control over the product of that process where, not as a worker but as a consumer, he can, through the free expression of his wants in the market, allocate the resources in that society. Thus the sovereignty denied to the worker in the world of production appears as the sovereignty of the consumer in the world of consumption. In this scenario, the criteria and discussion of fairness center not on the control of the process of work but, rather, on the price to pay the worker for his work so that he may reach a sense of fulfillment, control, and pursuit of happiness in the world of consumption.

Suffice it to say, it is of paramount importance for the reproduction of the capitalist system that all struggles at the point of production be shifted to the area of consumption, *with the focus of the struggle being the cost of labor—personal and social wages—rather than the control of the process of production.* The acceptance of this shift in the struggle from the world of production to the world of consumption by the trade unions, and their consequent focus on the price of labor, has been a primary reason for the reproduction of capitalist relations. As Gramsci indicated (19, p. 30): "trade unionism by organizing workers not as producers but as wage earners had accepted and submitted to the rationale of the capitalist system where workers are merely sellers of their labor power." The shift from workers to wage earners is a key mechanism of reproduction of capitalist relations and responds to the intrinsic need of capitalism to separate the world of consumption from the world of production, focusing all areas of conflict on the former and not on the latter. Capital, in its position within the class struggle, clearly perceives the correctness of Marx's position when he wrote in the *Grundisse* (20) that, ". . . the important point to be emphasized here is that whether production and consumption are considered as activities of one or separate individuals, they appear as aspects of one process in which production forms the starting point and therefore the predominant factor. . . ." A predominant factor whose control capital cannot allow to be questioned.

A consequence of that bourgeois ideological dominance and acceptance of the *unalterability* of the process of work (and shift of the struggle from the world of production to the area of consumption) has been the acceptance by the unions of damage created at the workplace as being unavoidable, and thus the *champ de bataille* has been on the compensation for that damage. Consequently, occupational medicine, a branch of forensic medicine in its beginnings, had as its initial task to define for management the nature and size of the damage which needed to be compensated. Occupational doctors, still called company doctors in many countries today, had as a primary function to defend management interests and obfuscate or veil the actual damage created at the workplace. The struggle was, and still continues to be, between labor, which demanded a higher compensation, and capital (helped by occupational doctors), which wanted to minimize that compensation, denying for as long as possible that there was any relationship between work, disease, and death. Let me add here that not only occupational physicians directly employed by management, but many in academe, medical schools, and schools of public health, supported directly and indirectly by grants or funds from industry or industry-financed foundations, contributed to veil and mystify that relationship between work and disease (21).

A further consequence of the separation between the worlds of production and of consumption was that the damage created at the workplace, when and if recognized, was perceived to be unrelated to the damage produced outside the work context. Thus, a dichotomy was established between the branches of medicine responsible for the definition and administration of disease at the workplace (occupational medicine) and at the non-workplace, in the world of consumption (medical care). That dichotomy, production/consumption, is still present today and is being reproduced in the structure of health services with different administrations responsible for those two separated branches of medicine.

In summary, that shift of the struggle around the workplace from (a) control of work to compensation for damage; and from (b) the world of production to the world of consumption has led to the establishment of occupational medicine as a separate branch of medicine historically controlled by management in charge of defining damage and compensation. Needless to say, the priorities within the social system were higher for the medicine of consumption than for the medicine of production, particularly considering that a primary function for the latter—the one of policing the labor force—was achieved under capitalism by other more effective means than occupational medicine.

All these struggles on compensation were, for the most part, carried out under the supervision of the state institutions where capital was far more influential than labor, which leads me to discuss the second area where those dominant/dominated relations are being reproduced: in the realm of the political institutions.

SECTION II
WORK, POLITICAL IDEOLOGY, AND
THE REPRODUCTION OF POWER RELATIONS

In the same way that it is of paramount importance for the reproduction of the dominant/dominated relations at work to shift all struggles around the control over the process of production to the world of consumption, it is equally important to shift those same struggles from the world of work to the world of representative politics. Indeed, just as the worker/subservient relationship is concealed at the economic level of our society under the ideology of consumer sovereignty, the worker/subservient situation is concealed at the political level, with the dominated worker being presented as citizen-sovereign. According to bourgeois ideology, people decide through the market what they consume and through the political process what they want. A clear representative of this position is Eli Ginzberg, professor in the Business School at Columbia University, who begins his book entitled *The Limits of Health Reform: The Search for Realism* with the following sentence (22, p. 3): "In our society, it is still the citizens who, through their voice in the market place and in the legislature, ultimately determine how their resources will be allocated." According to this ideology, workers become citizens and, as such, have the same rights as the controllers of their work. Assembly line workers are supposed to have the same political and juridical weight, according to legislative discourse, as the Henry Fords of America. Both categories—bosses and workers—are abstracted into a new category: the citizens who determine, with equal weight, the major political decisions. In the political-juridical realm, they are both equal. But is it really true that both have the same power to choose, decide, and develop different political alternatives? Many studies have been prepared showing that the Henry Fords of America, or of any other

Western capitalist country, have far more power—an overwhelming power to shape the nature of what is discussed, voted upon, and presented in the political debate—than assembly line or other types of workers (23).

In order to consider them with equal political power, Ginzberg and others with him have had to consider them as individual citizens, an abstract category which levels off everyone independent of his position in the world of production where goods and services are being produced. But men and women under capitalism are not equal. That assumed equality in the realm of politics is continually shown as inequality in the realm of production. Under capitalism, the relations of production allocate men and women into different social classes, defined by their differential access to and possession of the means of production (24). Agents within those classes have, indeed, different political and thus juridical power. The class which owns, controls, and possesses the means of work has a dominant hegemony in the political-juridical apparatus of the state and in the ideological-cultural apparatus of society (25). It goes without saying that the intellectual representatives of that class deny this, dismissing it as a simplification, tolerable for "ideologs" but not for reasonable people. They present it as a matter of fact that the political-juridical institutions are an outcome of the will of the people who, via the electoral process in representative democracy, periodically elect those in whom authority is being bestowed. Consequently, bourgeois dominance in the apparatus of representation is denied by bourgeois ideology, in which bourgeois domination is veiled and mystified as representing the popular sovereignty and the *vox populi*. According to this ideology, the workers, regardless of how exploited in the economic arena they may be, are still supposed to be free and equal citizens who, by their will, have chosen, and continue to choose, a system which reproduces that system of exploitation. This is the most important ideological legitimation of the bourgeois rule, i.e. people want it and choose it.

It is worth stressing that in this scheme of things, democracy is not—as Lincoln said—government by the people, but one occasionally *approved* by the people. Democracy is thus defined differently from self-governance. In such a democracy, governments come and go at the approval of the people. In this respect, the government is assumed to represent *we, the people,* and what happens in our societies is what we, the citizens, want. As Etzione recently indicated in *The Washington Post* (26), "We, in the United States, have decided that we value production more than risk or damage at the work place." And that *we* is supposed to mean, of course, the American people, who have expressed their political will through their political institutions. We, the citizens, have chosen to maximize production rather than safety at work. It speaks of the overwhelming dominance which the bourgeois position has in official and academic discourse that authors such as Ginzberg, Etzione, and many others can consider these expressions as merely factual and absent of ideological meaning. They would strongly deny, of course, that they are bourgeois ideologists who reproduce the scheme convenient and favorable to dominance of our lives by the bourgeoisie. It is easy to predict that the bourgeois theorists would dismiss as "rhetorical" the interpretation that it is not we, the American people, but the capitalist class, which primarily—although not exclusively—dominates the state functions; and that it is not we, but the controllers of work, who decide on the nature of production and consumption in society. They would, indeed, dismiss that as Marxist "rhetoric." But they do not realize, or want to realize, that theirs is also a rhetoric and one which reproduces a pattern of class power relations where the minority and not the majority makes the major decisions. In summary, each ideological position has its own discourse dismissed as "rhetoric" by its adversary. The untenability and incredibility of bourgeois rhetoric, which assumes that we, the American people, decide on major issues in society, is increasingly clear for all to see. The majority of American citizens who belong to the working class and lower-middle class know reality far better than the bourgeois theorists. In many polls, they have expressed their belief that the two major parties are controlled by corporate America and that the government institutions work principally for the benefit of Big Business—that folksy term used to refer to the capitalist class (27).

In summary, then, the dominant/dominated relations at the workplace are being reproduced by shifting struggles from the world of production to the world of representative politics where the bourgeoisie is the dominant force. It is of paramount importance for the bourgeois order that a clear separation be established between the *economic* class struggle confined within trade union battles (primarily concerned with the price of labor and compensation of work and damage) and the *political* struggles carried out primarily by the political parties in the realm of representative democracy. As many points in history—from the General Strike in Britain in 1926 to the May events in France in 1968—show quite clearly, the shift of the place and focus of struggles from the place of work to the arena of representative politics has had a most important effect in diluting threats to the bourgeois order. But why this dilution, this weakening of that threat when the arena of struggle shifts from the floor of the factory to the parliament? One reason is that representative democracy converts the process of participation *from active to passive,* delegating popular power to elected and/or selected representatives. These representatives, however well they may represent the interests of the working class and popular masses, have to conform to a set of rules and operate within a set of state institutions where *the bourgeoisie is, by definition, dominant*—a bourgeois dominance which gives its character to those institutions, including the institutions of representation and mediation (28). Thus, it has always been in the interests of the bourgeoisie to demobilize the mass struggles occurring in the places of production by shifting those struggles to the parliament or its equivalent.

The previous paragraphs should not be understood as shying away from or slowing down the struggles which need to be carried out within the state and organs of representative democracy. *The class struggle carried out within the apparatuses of the state can lead to substantial victories for the working class.* The National Health Service (NHS) in the United Kingdom, for example, was no doubt a remarkable achievement for the British working class. But it would be wrong to consider the NHS as a socialist apparatus within a bourgeois state (29). I have shown elsewhere how the NHS is under the hegemony of the bourgeoisie, a hegemony which appears in the ideology, composition, and distribution of medicine in the U.K. (30). Similarly, the occupational health legislation which has appeared in the United States from the late 1960s and early '70s has to be seen also as a great achievement for the U.S. labor movement. But the fact that these achievements have occurred within a state that is under bourgeois dominance explains the limitations and the nature of that progressive legislation. The consequences of bourgeois dominance are many. One is that programs established by legislative mandates tend—*in the absence of continuous pressure from the working class*—to be manipulated by the components and strata of the bourgeoisie which are affected by that legislation. Lobbies of those groups are "always there, close to the corridors of power" to limit and change the progressive impact and nature of those programs. But, more importantly, those programs have to operate within parameters which are defined by the overall power relations in that society and which cannot be touched upon by those programs. For example, great stress is made by all governments that occupational health programs cannot interfere with the overall pattern of capital accumulation. Capital formation and the subsequent class power relations which it sustains cannot be affected by that type of legislation. And when they are, enormous pressures are brought to bear on governments to assure that that situation be reversed.

Last, but certainly not least, another consequence of bourgeois dominance in the apparatuses of the state, including those progressive programs, is that the implementation of those programs is carried out within the ideological framework convenient to the reproduction of the bourgeois order. For example, the prevalent approach of state regulatory agencies in occupational medicine is to protect the worker against an environmental agent such as a toxic substance which can cause harm. Consequently, a struggle takes place around the allowable exposure of the worker to that toxic substance (31). That struggle is *a very important and necessary one.* But it is still carried out within that ideological dichotomy of worker versus environment, which assumes an independence and autonomy where the worker is on one side of the working scene and the environment is on the other. The dichotomy of patient or potential patient versus environment characterizes, as I will discuss later on, the conception of risk and disease in bourgeois science. To the same degree that bacteria were perceived to be the external cause of disease, toxic substances are now perceived to be the cause of occupational disease. In either case, however, such a dichotomy is a faulty one. The social power relations which determine the environment of exposures also determine the nature of the work process and of the agents of that process, i.e. the workers. The social power relations which determine the working environment also determine how the worker fits within that environment, relates to that environment, and perceives himself in relation to fellow workers and to the controllers and managers of that environment. In other words, by focusing only on a specific item of that environment (the toxic substance) and by not touching on the power relations which shape both the environment and the worker, the bourgeois order is reproduced.

SECTION III
BOURGEOIS DOMINANCE, IDEOLOGY, AND KNOWLEDGE IN MEDICINE

In previous sections, I have discussed how bourgeois dominance appears in the world of production and in the political-juridical level of society, and how that dominance has many implications in medicine as well. In this section, I will focus on how that class dominance appears also in the production of knowledge in medicine. Many studies have been written showing how bourgeois dominance of our research institutions, including medical research institutions, has determined a set of priorities that, while presented as apolitical, are in fact clear political statements reflecting the class dominance of those institutions. Elsewhere, I have discussed how that overwhelming class dominance of our research institutions explains, for example, why most cancer research in Western capitalist countries has focused on biological and individual behavior, but not on other factors, such as carcinogens that exist in people's workplaces, which could be threatening to the sections of the bourgeoisie that have a major influence in the funding institutions for cancer research (32).

It would be erroneous, however, to believe that those cancer research priorities are merely a result of the influence of powerful interest groups in the top corridors of power in funding agencies. There is more to it than that. These groups belong to a class—the bourgeoisie—which has an ideology or vision of reality with an internal logic and consistency which, in turn, leads to the support of some positions, conclusions, and priorities and to the exclusion of others. This bourgeois ideology is the dominant one under capitalism. That it is dominant, however, does not mean that that bourgeois ideology is the only ideology. In this regard, it has to be stressed that each social class has its own vision of reality and ideology. In other words, there is not, under capitalism, just a single ideology which is upheld by all classes, races, and sexes. I stress this, because on both sides of the ideological spectrum, there are ideological currents (33) which postulate that there is in any society *just one ideology*—the dominant or ruling ideology—which has resulted from that society's choice, wills and wants (as the bourgeois theorists believe), or from an overwhelming dominance, tantamount to control, which the bourgeoisie has in that society. Agreeing with Marx (34, pp. 117-118) I believe that classes have different ideologies which also appear in different forms of culture:

> Upon the different forms of property, upon the social conditions of existence, rises an entire superstructure of distinct and peculiarly formed sentiments, illusions, modes of thought and views of life. The entire class creates and forms them through tradition and upbringing.

But one of them, the ideology of the dominant class, is the dominant ideology. As Marx and Engels indicated (35, p. 64):

> ... *the ideas of the ruling class* are in every epoch the ruling ideas, i.e., the class which is the ruling *material* force of society, is at the same time its ruling intellectual force. (Emphasis added)

But this "ruling" does not imply that the working class ideology is either non-existent or absorbed in the bourgeois one. Nor does it imply that a clearcut division exists between the two ideologies with a well-delineated boundary between them. Class struggle is continuously taking place, with victories and defeats which influence both ideologies. For example, I have already indicated in previous pages how bourgeois values appear in the working class. An example is when the working class accepts the belief that the nature of work is determined by industrialization. And vice versa, the rhetorical (although not actual) acceptance by the bourgeoisie of democracy as a part of dominant ideology was forced by the working class on the bourgeoisie, when the latter social class needed an alliance with the former in its struggle against the aristocracy, then hindering the rise to power of the bourgeoisie (36). In other words, democracy was not a set of values and practices spontaneously created by the bourgeoisie but, rather, an ideology forced on the bourgeois ideology by the working class. The bourgeoisie has always fought by all means the expansion of democracy, including the expansion of universal suffrage, freedom of association, freedom of the press, and many other freedoms which the working class has had to win with great sacrifice and not without heroic struggle.

In summary, there is, under capitalism, a dominant ideology which appears in all institutions, including the institutions of science and medicine.

Class Dominance in Scientific Medicine

How does the bourgeois vision of reality appear in science and medicine? In many ways. Let us outline some of them.

Dichotomy Science versus Ideology. An extremely important view within bourgeois ideology is that there is a clearcut dichotomy between science and ideology. Actually, science was the creation of the nascent bourgeoisie and was contraposed to religion (seen as the ideological expression of aristocratic dominance), which it was considered to transcend and supersede. Science was supposed to be a new global vision of reality which would rationalize and legitimize the new bourgeois social system. Galileo, who was one of the founders of the scientific revolution—and who, incidentally, was working as an advisor to coal owners on how to increase the rate of exploitation of coal miners (37)—established the basis for the creation of new knowledge based on what was called objective observation and not on theology. And that dichotomy—objectivity versus subjectivity, science versus ideology—has persisted throughout the history of science. Science was thus perceived as a body of neutral and value-free knowledge built in a painstaking and linear process in which each new scientific discovery was constructed upon a previous one. Science and technology became part of the forces of production and, as such, their development was considered to be intrinsically positive. According to bourgeois ideology, science and technology (and the process of industrialization which they determine) were forces of progress, determining, almost in a fatalistic way, the nature and shape of society. The most recent versions of those positions are the ones taken by Daniel Bell (38) and others, who indicate that power has shifted from the owners of the means of production to the managers of the process of that production and, more recently, to the producers—the scientists—of what is perceived as the most important ingredient of production: science and technology.

It is worth stressing here that the bourgeois interpretation of the value-free character of science has also appeared within the labor movement, particularly since Stalin (39). As Sweezy and Bettelheim (40), as well as Lecourt (41), have eloquently indicated, the forces of production, including science and technology, under Stalinism were perceived as neutral. Their development was perceived to be a primary condition for the achievement of a change in the relations of production at a later stage. That change in relations of production was perceived as needed, because they were retarding and hindering the full development of the forces of production.[2] In this dichotomy—forces versus relations of production—the forces of production were primarily understood as the instruments of production, and their development was considered to be the primary motor of history. The point that has to be stressed here, and Lecourt ignores it, is that that instrumentalist understanding of forces of production already appeared in Lenin. It was Lenin who believed that the Western forces of production (including Taylorism) should be imported and put to proper and better use by the Soviet Revolution. Lenin was an enthusiast of Taylorism. As Claudin-Urondo (42) has indicated, Lenin conceived science and technology as neutral entities, rather like tools, the function of which can be changed depending on the use being made of them. It should be pointed out that immediately after the October Revolution, a massive democratization in scientific institutions, such as in the medical ones, took place with changes in the pattern of class control of medical schools and other scientific institutions and with changes in the class origin of the medical profession and other scientists. These changes had quite an impact on redefining the nature of those institutions, and in redefining the process of creating scientific knowledge. That democratization had a very significant impact in redefining the nature of both scientific institutions and science itself. The priorities within medicine, for example, changed quite substantially, and initial changes in the understanding of medical knowledge started taking place. This process of democratization, however, was strongly reversed later on, in particular under the Stalin regime. Class control of scientific institutions and class origin of the scientists were reversed most dramatically under Stalin, giving strong political weight to the experts (scientists and technocrats) who became the controllers and administrators of scientific knowledge, closely supervised by the party apparatus. In this scheme of things, the development of the USSR meant primarily the fantastic growth of the forces of production (including science and technology) and the better redistribution of the product of that process. But it did not change the process of production and work, nor those forces of production. The nature of science and technology (and, as I have shown elsewhere, medicine) did not change under Stalinism (43).

Forces of production are not neutral, however. They carry with them the social relations of production which determine them. In other words, a factory or a hospital is not a neutral institution. They are bearers of power relations which determine how work in those institutions is done, by whom, and with what type of instruments. How the work process takes place in those and other institutions in society is determined by the power relations existent in that society. It is not the process and forces

---

[2] Social relations of production are the relations which exist in a given process of production between the owners of the means of production and the producers, a relation which depends on the type of ownership, possession, capacity for allocating and designing those means of production, and the use of the products of that process of production. Forces of production are the forces, instruments, labor, and knowledge which are organized to produce goods and services in a society. How the forces of production are organized, designed, and interrelated is determined by the social relations of production.

of production which determine the social division of labor (as the theorists of industrialism postulate), but, rather, it is the social division of labor, its concomitant power relations, and the ideological relations which those power relations carry which determine the forces of production, including science and technology. The power relations in society appear also *within* scientific knowledge, and the bourgeois ideological dominance appears and is being reproduced in the production of knowledge itself. The dominant ideology reproduces itself in scientific knowledge. And this reproduction takes place not only by selecting the subjects of inquiry, but also by choosing the method of inquiry, and the relations which the researcher or inquirer has within the overall process of production. Needless to say, this position—that bourgeois ideology reproduces itself in science and thus science is value-laden and not value-free —is continuously denied by scientists and other bourgeois theoreticans. Science appears as the epitome of objectivity. And all series of ideologies rush to be called sciences to gain legitimacy and credibility in bourgeois society. Not only natural sciences, but a long list of ideological positions appear with the sanction of sciences, e.g. business sciences, management sciences, social sciences, political sciences, economic sciences. Sciences become the newly accepted vision of reality which would enable the citizenry to cope with the world in a better fashion. All types of ideologies are thus made compulsory subjects in our scholarly institutions, from schools to academe, provided they are presented as sciences (i.e. value-free and neutral). In this way, while the parents of a ten-year-old child would strongly object to having him subjected to compulsory classes on a certain religion or certain ideology, they would not object, or would not be given the right to object, if that subject were, or is, presented as a science, e.g. economic science. Science becomes that magic word which allows the transformation of value-laden knowledge into a value-free one. Thus, the dichotomy of science/ideology constitutes a most powerful ideology for the reproduction of bourgeois relations.

The Division between Experts and Laymen. Once this dichotomy of science/ ideology is established, then we have to ask, What is science? And the bourgeois response is that science is an objective body of value-free, classless, and universal knowledge, based on testable observations of reality. As such, the production and reproduction of scientific knowledge take place in scientific institutions by individuals who—in the overall social division of labor—have been assigned the task of producing and reproducing that knowledge, i.e. the scientists. *Science then becomes what scientists—a small group of individuals in society—do. And scientific medicine is what medical scientists and practitioners do.* Needless to say, all systematic knowledge which is produced outside those institutions, and by individuals other than scientists, is not considered science. According to this criteria, the documents produced by research groups in occupational medicine that concluded in the 1930s, '40s, '50s, and even '60s in the United States that there was not a relationship between black lung and coal mining were supposed to be "scientific documents and conclusions" and thus trustworthy. On the other hand, the knowledge accumulated by generations of coal miners—knowledge which appeared in their culture as folk songs, popular writings, etc.—that work in the mines was destroying coal miners' lungs was dismissed as cultural, folksy, ideological, and, in summary, untrustworthy. Thus, knowledge is legitimized only and exclusively when it comes from scientists. This dichotomy of science/ideology then appears operationally as the dichotomy of expert/non-expert in which the control of the definition of science and expertise is delegated by the dominant bourgeoisie to another class, the petit bourgeoisie or professionals who carry on that task, namely, the production of knowledge under the hegemony of bourgeois ideology.

This last point of delegation raises the question of the autonomy of science. Can science become autonomous from the dominant ideology? My answer is yes and no (44). Yes, in the limited sense that once established, it has an internal logic of its own, i.e. the logic of that discipline or branch of science. No, in the major sense that scientific knowledge is continuously growing under the dominance of bourgeois ideology. In other words, scientific knowledge and scientific institutions are under bourgeois dominance, and that reality shapes the nature of that knowledge. For example, and as I will explain in the next section, bourgeois dominance in medicine established a vision and an understanding of disease in which that disease was seen as the lack of equilibrium within the different parts—organs and humors—of the body. This specific understanding of disease generated a medical knowledge which developed autonomously. But the division of labor within medicine—specialization—developed according to the bourgeois understanding of disease. Consequently, this internal logic of scientific medicine led to the creation of specialties which follow organic bases: cardiologists, nephrologists, and so forth. Thus, medical knowledge developed according to its internal logic given by that bourgeois conception of disease. In other words, *bourgeois dominance always determines in the ultimate instance what occurs in the realm of scientific knowledge* (45).

How Bourgeois Ideology Appears in Medical Knowledge

In the previous section, I indicated how the bourgeoisie's definition of science—knowledge produced by an elite, the scientists—appears and is reproduced in our society. In this section, I will discuss how that bourgeois ideological dominance over science appears in the production of knowledge. But, first, let us clarify what we mean by production of knowledge. It is the process whereby a perception of reality is transformed into a specific product, i.e. knowledge, a transformation which in science takes place by intellectuals whose primary instruments of work are the theories and methods of science. Scientific theories in each science consist of a group of concepts which belong to that specific branch of science (e.g. the law of gravity in physics). Scientific method is the way in which those concepts are used. Both theory and method allow that intellectual—the scientist—to transform this perception into knowledge (46). Needless to say, this knowledge is being reproduced not in abstract but in specific institutions, subjected to class hegemony, and by scientists whose very specific visions of reality are molded by the ideology of the dominant class (the bourgeoisie), their own social class (the petit bourgeoisie), their race, their sex, their discipline, their political position, among other factors. The scientist does not leave all those ideologies outside the walls of the scientific institutions. He carries those visions of reality in the production of knowledge as well. That production is submerged into and is part and parcel of those ideologies, of which the most important one is the ideology of the dominant class or bourgeoisie.

How does this bourgeois dominant ideology appear in medicine? By the submersion of that medical knowledge into the positivist and mechanistic ideology which typifies science created under the hegemony of the bourgeoisie, and which I would call bourgeois science. Actually, positivism and mechanicism appeared as the main ideologies of the bourgeoisie in the 19th and 20th centuries in Europe with the works of Hume, Comte, and, later on, Durkheim. According to positivism, science must focus on specifics to build up the general, looking at social phenomena as if those phenomena were natural, ruled by natural and thus harmonious rules. As Durkheim (47) indicated, positivism reduces social phenomena to natural phenomena. And within that interpretation, causality was supposed to be explained by association of immediately observable phenomena.

Positivism appears in medicine in its definition of disease as a biological phenomenon caused by one or several factors which are always associated and observed in the existence of that disease. For example, in one of the most widely used textbooks on epidemiology in the Western world, MacMahon (48) describes epidemiology—the science of studying the distribution of health and disease—as an extension of demography, and he defines that distribution according to age, sex, race, geography, and so on, giving major importance to those individual characteristics which are either biological or physical. Moreover, in explaining causality, MacMahon quotes Hume and indicates that that causality can only be seen but not explained, since we can only focus on the degree of association between several subsequent events.

A legitimate question at this point is to ask how that positivist conception of medicine came about. To answer that question, we have to go to the origins of scientific medicine as we understand it today. And these origins appeared primarily in the 19th and 20th centuries during the same time that science emerged as a recognized and legitimized area of endeavor. Those were times of large social upheavals and unrest in Europe. Capitalism was being established, changing from a mercantile system to an industrial one. Those changes had an overwhelming importance in defining the nature of medicine, as well as that of health and disease. One version advanced by the working class and by the revolutionary elements of the bourgeoisie, such as Virchow, saw disease as a result of the oppressive nature of existent power relations of society, and thus saw the intervention in smashing (the revolutionary) or modifying (the reformist) those power relations. Epitomized by the dictum that medicine is a social science and politics is medicine on a large scale (Virchow), its best representative was Engels, whose work on the conditions of the working class in England was a dramatic document showing the political nature of the definition and distribution of disease. His solution was written, with Marx, in the *Communist Manifesto,* with his call for revolutionary change, where the first steps included the actual democratization of political, economic, and ideological spheres in society. This version of medicine, however, did not prevail. The bourgeoisie, once it won its hegemony, supported another version of medicine that would not threaten the power relations in which it was dominant. The bourgeois social order was considered from then on as the natural order, where its class rules would be veiled and presented as rules of nature. Accordingly, disease was not an outcome of specific power relations, but rather a biological individual phenomenon where the cause of disease was the immediately observable factor, i.e. the bacteria. In this redefinition, clinical medicine became the branch of scientific medicine to study the biological-individual phenomena and social medicine became that other branch of medicine which would study the distribution of disease as the aggregate of individual phenomena. Both branches shared the vision of disease as an alteration, a pathological change in the human body (perceived as a machine), caused by an outside agent (unicausality) or several agents (multicausality). This mechanistic vision of health and disease is still the prevalent and dominant interpretation of medicine. Witness a recent definition of health and disease in Dorland's *Medical Dictionary* (49) in which health is defined as "a normal condition of body and mind, i.e. with all the parts functioning normally," and disease is defined as "a definite morbid process having a characteristic train of symptoms—it may affect the whole body or any of its parts, and its etiology, pathology, and prognosis may be known or unknown." From this mechanistic understanding of health and disease, it follows that the division of labor (specialization) in medical knowledge and practice has evolved around component parts of that body machine, i.e. cardiology, neurology, and so forth.

A related point is that the mechanistic interpretation of medicine was built upon knowledge which had been generated previously (blood circulation by Harvey in 1628, the microscope by Van Leeuwencheck in 1683, and others). But it would be erroneous to consider scientific medicine as a mere linear evolution starting with those previous discoveries. *These discoveries did not lead to or create scientific medicine.* Rather, it was the victory of the industrial bourgeoisie which established that positivist conception of science and of medicine. The fact that those previous discoveries were used and presented as the originators of scientific medicine was due to the change in the correlation of forces and subsequent victory of the bourgeoisie as the dominant class under industrial capitalism. In this respect, scientific medicine was not the linear growth of previous knowledge. Rather, and to use a Kuhnian term (50), a shift of paradigm took place, establishing another paradigm carrying a new, positivist vision of disease which added to what had already been built. This point has to be repeated, because it is part of the bourgeois understanding of scientific knowledge that this knowledge evolves linearly with "new" discoveries based on previous ones, as if these discoveries were the bricks on which the scientific building was constructed (51). According to this understanding, science and technology grow and determine the nature of power relations in our societies; and the history of humanity becomes divided into stages determined by the discovery of new technologies, which shape the nature of that historical stage, e.g. industrial revolution, nuclear age, and so on. Science and technology thus appear as the "motor" of history. But, as Braverman (52), among others, has shown, the so-called technological breakthroughs were not the ones which established new social orders; rather, the reverse was the case, i.e. a new correlation of forces used those *already known* technological breakthroughs which were, later on, presented as the actual cause of that change in the social order. But those breakthroughs or scientific and technological discoveries were used and put forward by new correlations of forces.

The victory and subsequent hegemony of the bourgeoisie, for example, was the one which stimulated science, including scientific medicine. It was this political reality which determined the advancement of the positivist and mechanistic conception of medicine, health, and disease. In other words, the power relations which existed under the bourgeois order were the ones which determined the form and nature of medicine. It led to a scientific inquiry where the aim of that inquiry was the discovery of the cause or microorganism, and the instrument of that inquiry was the microscope. By focusing on the microcausality of disease, however, science ignored the analysis of the macrocausality, i.e. the power relations in that society. Scientific inquiry in medicine developed into a search for the cause: bacteria, parasite, virus, or, later on, the toxic substance. Consequently, the strategy of intervention was the eradication of what was supposed to be the cause of disease. Needless to say, that interpretation of disease and of medical intervention was supposed to be presented and perceived only and exclusively as scientific and certainly not political. The dichotomy of science vs. ideology was made quite clear and explicit. The alternative explanation, i.e. the assumed "cause" was a mere intervening factor and the actual cause of disease resided in the power relations of that society, was dismissed as political, anti-scientific, and, in some circles, perceived also as needing "eradication." In a report of the Rockefeller Foundation on Health in Latin America (53), it was stressed that there was a great need "to eradicate disease in vast areas of rural South America, otherwise the virus of the tropics will soon attack the metropolis, a virus that can be biological or, even worse, *political.*" A clear call for scientific eradication of undesirable ideological explanations! The limitations of this strategy of eradication based on the unicausal interpretation of disease led to the later strategy of control instead of eradication. But, most importantly, that unicausal explanation was, and is, increasingly abandoned for the multicausal explanation of disease. Disease was later supposed to be determined by several causes, some of which included socioeconomic variables. But these socioeconomic variables were added to other causes as if they were independent variables, independent of each other. Social class thus appears as one more variable which may be indirectly associated with the direct and most important explanatory variables. But this limitation of the concept of causality to the immediately observable association between disease (e.g. cancer) and other specific events, such as smoking and occupation, is intrinsically limited since it leaves the key question unexplained, i.e. how those different events are related. As a recent report on cancer research (54) published by the United States government indicates, "a major defect in most cancer research in the Western world [and, I would add, other worlds as well] is that most cancer research has been based on looking for a single or multiple cause, ignoring the interrelations among those assumed causes." What this report touches on is that the primary cause for our ignorance of the causality of cancer has been a limited understanding of causality, a limitation that comes from the positivist understanding of knowledge which I have indicated. By focusing on statistical association, positivists are touching on the appearance but not on the reality of the phenomena. In other words, what are presented as "causes" are not the actual causes (55). The epistemological problem thus created cannot be solved either by indicating that those assumed causes are intermediate causes, part of a network of causalities whose linkage among the knots (intermediate variables) can be measured by statistical associations. The actual way of studying disease in any society is by analyzing its historical presence within the political, economic, and ideological power relations in that specific social formation. And by this, I do not mean the analysis of the natural history of disease, but rather the political, economic, and ideological determinants of that disease, determinants resulting from the overall power relations which are primarily based on the social relations of production. These power relations are the ones which determine the nature and definition of disease, medical knowledge, and medical practice. The understanding of the evolution and causality of black lung in the United States, for example, cannot come from an analysis of the natural history of black lung. It has to come from an understanding of the class power relations in the United States and how the class struggle shaped both the scientific definition, recognition, and knowledge of black lung in the United States and the actual production and distribution of that disease.

What I have said so far should not lead, however, to the opposite conclusion that the inquiry should be limited to the discovery of associations between specific power relations and disease. In other words, it is not enough to establish an association between specific forms of capital accumulation or, say, economic cycles and certain diseases. It is not enough to say that capitalism, for example, determines a certain disease profile. It is necessary to research how those power relations appear, how they are being reproduced, and how they determine the nature of death and disease in society. The different categories of analysis, such as world of production, consumption, and legitimation, need to be understood in detail and related to the specific mediating mechanisms that those sets of relations have with the apparent "causes" of disease. In other words, what is needed is not the incorporation of the social as mere additions to "environmental" variables which act on the individual; rather, what is needed is an understanding of how diseases mediate social relations, i.e. how the social power relations determine both the social and physical environment and the individual's experiences within that environment, including disease. Actually, there is an urgent need to break with that new dichotomy of individual/environment, which is as false as the old dichotomy of mind/body.

Consequently, the terms of the discourse have to be changed. Instead of using the dichotomy individual/environment, we should analyze how social power relations determine disease. Taking black lung as an example, we have to understand how the social power relations defined and determined the working and living conditions of the coal miners; how the workers struggled against them; and how, in that context, medical knowledge and medical practice came into being to obfuscate or clarify the nature of the damage inflicted on the coal miners. Needless to say, in the process of this struggle individuals and classes have different knowledge, perceptions, and ideologies regarding their own experiences, which leads me to the last point I want to stress: the existence of bourgeois science and working class science.

Bourgeois Science or Working Class Science—Utopia or Reality?

Knowledge is accumulated, stored, produced, and reproduced in the daily practice of people's lives. And the nature of that knowledge varies considerably, depending on the social class practices. Each social class has its own practice which appears in its own ideology and culture, i.e. a vision of reality, and vice versa, that ideology and culture also appear as class practices. Thus, there is a bourgeois ideology, culture, and knowledge given and reflected in bourgeois practice. And there is a working class ideology, culture, and knowledge given and reflected in working class practice. There is a bourgeois knowledge and a working class knowledge. Both classes have different practices which generate different types of knowledge. The knowledge (legitimized under the name of science) produced by the bourgeoisie and reproduced in scientific institutions, which denied, for example, that there was any relationship between work and cancer, was bourgeois knowledge aimed at reproducing bourgeois power and practices. The knowledge (perceived in scientific discourse as "hot air," "folklore," or populist culture) produced by the working class and reproduced in its cultural forms, affirming that work was killing its members, was, and is, working class knowledge based on experience. From this, I conclude that there can be two types of sciences: a bourgeois science and a working class science, each one based on different sets of knowledge and practice. To deny the above dichotomy is to assume a classless nature of knowledge, and thus a knowledge absent of practice. These two different and even conflicting visions of reality—the bourgeois and the working class visions—are not separated by clearcut boundaries without one influencing the other. Through the process of class struggle, the working class develops and imposes its own vision of reality on bourgeois science: witness current interest in researching the relationship between work and cancer. This new development is due to a large degree to the working class and the general population's outcry on the damage being created at the workplace. But still, the hegemony which the bourgeoisie has in all scientific institutions explains the nature and bias of that response, a bias reflected both in the choice of areas to be researched and the means and ways of researching it. The scientist does his job in institutions *with* the bourgeoisie. In this respect, the scientist is, to use a Gramscian term, an organic intellectual of the bourgeoisie who explains the reality with and for the bourgeoisie. This relationship of scientist/bourgeoisie is overwhelmingly clear in the United States, where most research is sponsored either by private foundations or by the state where capital's representatives are extremely powerful and influential.

The alternative, the socialist alternative, would be to carry on scientific inquiry *with* the working class, analyzing reality based on the extremely powerful knowledge given by the daily practice of the working class, and *under* the direction of the working class. In this area I see a great area of struggle: to democratize the institutions and to change the patterns of accountability of intellectual workers, and to work together with manual workers until eventually that dichotomy of intellectual/manual will be questioned and diluted. No doubt, this change of accountability requires a tough struggle: the one of democratizing our institutions. In this respect, it was a great victory for the Italian working class when it won the right to control occupational health services at the factory level and also when it won the right to undertake research at the factory with the researchers chosen by the workers. This is a clear example of how the struggles for democracy and for knowledge are one and the same.

Let me finish by saying that I am aware that many eyebrows will be raised when reading this section of my article. The nightmare of the Stalinist distinction between bourgeois science and proletarian science will undoubtedly be remembered. And the case of Lysenko will be immediately raised as a warning against those dichotomies. My answer to that legitimate concern is that the Stalinist version of proletarian science was not the science developed by the working class (which was not in power), but rather the version given by the Stalinist leadership of the party which identified proletarian science with dialectical materialism as defined and controlled by them. The fact that that agency of control was mislabeled proletarian science did not make that science proletarian, nor does it make the whole concept of class-bound knowledge meaningless. That is the mistake of Lecourt (56). It throws the baby out with the bathwater. There is proletarian knowledge and mass knowledge which will fully appear and will flourish unhindered when there will be mass democratization in the process of the creation of knowledge with the deprofessionalization of science, changing not only the class composition of scientists but, most importantly, the method and creation of knowledge, knowledge created not by the few—the scientists—but by the many—the working class and popular masses. As Gramsci once indicated, while all human beings are capable of being intellectuals, only a few are assigned that task. Similarly, while all human beings are capable of creating knowledge, only a few are given that task. Mass democratization would imply a redefinition and redirection of that process of the creation of knowledge. *This process would not mean, of course, the absence of a division of labor.* But it would mean a change in the power relations in the creation of knowledge, with a dramatic expansion of the capability of creation of knowledge, with the working class and popular masses being the agents and not the objects of that knowledge.

In other words, science is a *social relation* and, as such, the key operational issue is not only *for* what class that knowledge is being produced (the uses of science) but, most importantly, *by* what class, and its related question, *with* what class (the class character of science) that knowledge is being produced. The failure to understand the importance of these points explains the overabundance of references in which authors continue to search for the perfect socialist scientific method that would enable them to find the socialist truth. That search is not only a theoretical but a practical task as well. *And it requires a political and professional commitment to the working class.* In other words, it requires the scientist to break with the role to which he is assigned under bourgeois order and to ally himself with the working class, not to lead that class but to assist it in its potential for human liberation and creation of knowledge. Let me try to be very specific and advance an example of the proposed relationship with which I have experience, namely, two different ways and approaches to finding reality at the workplace.

One would be the bourgeois or positivist approach to finding the nature of a specific health problem (e.g. toxic exposures) in a factory and a way of solving it. The "expert" (epidemiologist or any other social scientist) usually called in by management would first establish a *hypothesis de travaille* based on his previous knowledge of that problem. Needless to say, it is part of the scientific ideology that he should be "objective" and unemotional about the issue under study. His only aim is to find the truth. As such, he would have a "healthy skepticism" about any subjective statements or situations, relying more comfortably on facts, and very much in particular on quantifiable facts. Second, he should try to obtain as much information as possible from each individual worker in order to ascertain the facts. Through questionnaires, interviews, medical records, and so on, he would try to obtain from each worker as much "objective" and quantifiable information as he could get and find relevant. He would also try to locate the collective dimensions of the problem by adding up the individual problems. Last but not least, he would try to test the hypothesis by statistical manipulation of quantifiable (objective) information.

He would finally submit a report for management's implementation. In that *modus operandi* of research, workers appear as passive subjects of research, remaining in the background and not in the forefront in the analysis and solution of the problem. This method of inquiry and data gathering is the most frequent tool used in social science research. Citizens, workers, blacks, women, etc. are studied individually, providing information through key instruments of inquiry, questionnaires or interviews. In all these approaches, three ideological positions—presented as scientific conditions—are present: (a) theory and fact are two separate entities, of which the former is supposed to be built upon the analysis of the latter; (b) the expert, the holder of proper methods of inquiry, is the active agent, while the studied object, the worker or citizen, is a passive one, i.e. the mere provider of information; and (c) collective information is the aggregate of individual information. The process and findings of this scientific inquiry are, of course, presented as objective and value-free (universal and classless) (57).

It is not surprising that in the late 1960s, when many anti-authoritarian movements appeared in the Western capitalist world, many of those analyzed passive objects—workers, blacks, women—rebelled against that science and against those scientists. At that time, alternative relations of production of knowledge were established. In many Italian and Spanish factories, for example, workers' committees and assemblies were established which rebelled against the type of science that was carried out in those factories. From then on, they did not allow any scientists to come inside the factory and ask them questions (58). Instead, they developed another approach in which the process of inquiry was carried out under their direction. Consequently, a new production of knowledge took place in which all information regarding the specific health problem was (and is) produced and discussed collectively with the correct understanding that a collective problematic is far more than the mere aggregate of individual problematics. Moreover, workers' assemblies have a collective memory and experience that puts their perception of reality in a collective and historical perspective. They know what is going on and what has been going on in that factory process and environment for a long time. And they have first-hand experience with what that problem has meant for their collective and individual health and well-being. Out of their collective discussion, they develop a hypothesis of what is happening in the factory regarding the specific health problem. In that process of generating and collecting data, subjective feelings, anxieties, and uneasiness are the propelling forces which guide all processes of gathering both objective and subjective data. Next the workers call in scientists of their own choosing to assist them in the collection and analysis of whatever data the workers feel need study. In this process, the workers keep a healthy skepticism about the meaning of science, expertise, and objective information. They scrutinize all objective data, and through the process of mutual validation, they accept the value of the data depending on how it fits within their own perception of reality. It is worth stressing here that many years of exposure to occupational medicine have taught workers the lesson that science is not value-free knowledge but very value-laden knowledge, reflecting the values of institutions where science is created and the values of scientists who create that science. Finally, once agreed collectively on the nature of the problem, the workers demand to participate collectively in the solution of that problem.

This collective production of knowledge based on collective practice is an alternate form of production of knowledge to the individual production of knowledge, characteristic of the bourgeois model. Needless to say, it puts the scientist in *a different social relation with the subject of study*. It puts him in an assistant role with his information and knowledge being just a part of a broader and more important knowledge which is created by the practice of the working class. Needless to say, the majority of scientists would oppose that diminution of their protagonism, since it would diminish their power. Many arguments are likely to be used against that change in power relations—ideological arguments presented as scientific arguments to defend specific class interests. The bourgeoisie and the majority of professionals will oppose that change by every means possible, including sabotage. To believe, as Julian Tudor Hart (59) does, that the majority of doctors are willing to join the working class in that change is to dangerously ignore history. From the October Revolution (60) to Allende's Unidad Popular (61), the medical profession has always fought by all means the process of change led by the working class. Still, that the majority of professionals would oppose change does not mean, of course, that a minority within those professions cannot play a very important role in taking sides with the forces for change. But in that process of changing class alliances, they will have to change not only their role (from leaders to assistants) but also their methods of work and the social and political context in which they use them. And it will be in that new realm of practice that new social relations and a new science will be created.

CONCLUSION
THE STRUGGLE FOR DEMOCRACY

I have shown in the three sections of this article how bourgeois ideological dominance reproduces dominant/dominated relations in the spheres of production, politics, and science, including medicine. Also, I have shown how the working class rebels against this bourgeois domination in a continuous process of class struggle, which leaves its mark on all those spheres. The class struggle takes many different forms, but aims at changing and/or breaking with those patterns of domination which oppress the working class and popular masses. It follows from what has been said that their liberation requires the breaking of that pattern of control where the few and not the many decide on the nature of our societies. And, by democratization I do not mean the mere existence of a plurality of parties and of civil rights. I mean far more than that. I mean a profound change in the pattern of control of the spheres of production, consumption, representation, ideological discourse, and scientific endeavor where the many and not just the few have control. Specifically, democracy cannot be seen as limited to the passive and indirect realm of representative politics. It has to be seen, as Marx and Engels said, as the massive, active, and direct involvement by the collectivity of workers and citizens in the governance of societal institutions where they work, reside, study, enjoy themselves, and are being taken care of. As Hal Draper (62) has indicated, the greatest contribution which Marx and Engels gave to the history of humanity was to reveal the clear symbiosis between socialism and democracy. As he put it, "Marx's socialism (communism) as a political program may be most quickly defined, from the Marxist standpoint, as the complete democratization of society, not merely of political forms." The struggle for democracy needs to combine struggles in the institutions of representative democracy, where power is delegated to full-time representatives—the "experts" in politics—with, most importantly, struggles to achieve forms of direct and mass democracy where power is retained by the users and workers in all societal institutions. For example, in order to change not only the priorities but also the nature of medical and scientific institutions, there is a need to win control of those institutions, not only indirectly through elected officials in the realm of representative democracy, but most importantly, through direct and assembly-type of democracy where workers, employees, users, and communities control those institutions. In other words, a socialist transformation will not occur without a massive and direct participation by the majority of the population in that process of transformation. As Marx once said, voting in a representative democracy gives an individual the right but not the power to change society. Eugene Debs put it in a more folksy manner: ". . . voting for socialism is not socialism any more than a menu is a meal." This right—the right to decide—has to be accompanied by the power which comes from actual direct participation and control by the majority of the population of their institutions.

To sum up, there is a need for the working class, through its different instruments and forms of struggle, to aim at a massive democratization of our societies, understanding democracy not only as an exercise in voting every so many years, but, most importantly, as a direct form of participation on a daily basis by the working class and popular masses in all economic, political, and social institutions (including the medical and scientific institutions). It is only in this way that the democratization of our institutions will imply a massive transformation of the majority of our working populations from being passive subjects to active agents in the redefinition of those societies, a transformation that takes place as part and parcel of their becoming the agents and not the objects of history.

Acknowledgments—I want to express my deepest appreciation to Sirkka Lee for assisting in the preparation of the manuscript. The comments made on earlier drafts by Elizabeth Fee, Kim Hopper, Howard Waitzkin, Eli Messinger, Eric Holtzman, and Len Rodberg are also appreciated.

REFERENCES

1. Trilateral Task Force on the Governability of Democracies. *The Governability of Democracies.* Trilateral Commission, New York, 1975.

2. By "capitalism," I mean a mode of production in which a class, the capitalist class, extracts as much labor power from each worker as possible, labor power that is needed to (a) put the means of production (owned, controlled, and possessed by the capitalist class) to work; and (b) produce value, including profit. Labor power is the human energy and competence that the worker provides to enable the means of production to work. It is usually referred to as work.

3. A most representative view of this position is found in Marcuse, H. *One Dimensional Man.* Beacon Press, Boston, 1975.

4. Ehrenreich, J. Introduction. In *The Cultural Crisis of Modern Medicine,* edited by J. Ehrenreich. Monthly Review Press, New York, 1979. After having been criticized for his deafening silence about the working class struggles around health and their consequences for the redefinition of medicine, the author added "coal miners' struggle" as a mere perfunctory note to that introduction of his volume, without actually referring to it. As with many other U.S. radicals, Ehrenreich ignores the dramatic and continuous struggles around health-related issues that are being carried out by the U.S. working class.

5. See Marshall, D. The miners and the UMW: Crisis in the reform process. *Socialist Review* 40/41: 65-115, 1978 for a detailed account of those struggles.

6. Quoted by Berlinguer, G. *Malaria Urbana.* Editorial Villalar, 1978, p. 428.

7. For an interesting account of the resurgence of class struggles around work, see Crough, C., and Pizzorno, A. (eds.). *The Resurgence of Class Conflict in Western Europe Since 1968,* Volumes I and II. Macmillan, New York, 1978. Also, see Basaglia, F., et al. *La Salud de Los Trabajadores.* Editorial Nueva Imagen, 1978.

8. Assennato, G., and Navarro, V. Workers' participation and control in Italy: The case of occupational medicine. *Int. J. Health Serv.* 10(2): 217-232, 1980.

9. Personal Observation, Autumn 1979.

10. Mentioned by Berlinguer, G. at XV International Congress on Sexuality, Rome, 1978.

11. Struggles against the nature of work under capitalism occur not only because of the actual damage imposed on the worker at the workplace, but also because of the harm created to the workers and their dependents in all spheres of their lives.

12. See Braverman, H. *Labor and Monopoly Capital: The Degradation of Work in the Twentieth Century.* Monthly Review Press, New York, 1974. Also, for an analysis of how the process of class struggle has shaped the form of bourgeois dominance in the process of work, see Friedman, A. L. *Industry and Labor: Class Struggle at Work and Monopoly Capitalism,* Macmillan, New York, 1977.

13. Bosquet, M. The prison factory. *New Left Review,* 73: 23, 1972. Also, see Linhart, R. *L'etabli.* Minuit, Paris, 1978.

14. See The working class goes to Hollywood. *Cineaste* 9(1), 1978. Also, Review of "Blue Collar." *Cineaste* 10(3), 1978.

15. Quoted from Doye, R. J. *Management Accounting,* 1970.

16. Class dominance is a process of continuous endeavor on the part of the capitalist class or bourgeoisie to maintain, regain, strengthen, and extend their interests in all economical, political, ideological, and cultural spheres of society over the ones of the dominated class or working class. In this article, dominance and hegemony are used interchangeably.

17. Class struggle is the conflict among classes that appears in all economic, political, ideological, and cultural spheres of society and takes place in the pursuit of class interests. Under capitalism, the main conflict is between the capitalist class and the working class.

18. Taylor, M. Creating a health workers' democracy. In *Trade Union Register 3,* edited by M. Brown and K. Coates. Spokesman Books, London, 1973.

19. Gramsci, A. *Quaderni del Carcere.* Einaudi, Turin. 1978. It is worth stressing that the unions are, of course, very important instruments of struggle by the working class. But the focus of those struggles on economic issues transforms them into limited and limiting instruments for revolutionary change, i.e. change from one to another mode of production.

20. Marx, K. *Grundisse.* Penguin Books, London, 1973.

21. See Kotelchuck, D. Asbestos research: Winning the battle but losing the war. *Health PAC Bulletin* 61: 1-32, 1974. Also, Epstein, S. *The Politics of Cancer.* Sierra Club Books, San Francisco, 1978, pp. 86-87.

22. Ginzberg, E. *The Limits of Health Reform: The Search for Realism.* Basic Books, New York, 1977.

23. See Greenberg, E. *The American Political System. A Radical Approach.* Winthrop Publishers, Cambridge, Mass., 1977.

24. By means of production, I mean not only the means that the workers use for their work, but also the infrastructure of production and distribution that enables the produced goods and services to be used and consumed.
25. For an expansion of this position, see Navarro, V. *Dictatorship and Democracy. Meanings and Implications for Class Struggle.* Mimeographed, 1979.
26. Etzione, A. Risk at the work place. *The Washington Post,* Dec. 28, 1978.
27. Hart Poll. *Common Sense,* Vol. 3, 1975. That lack of trust by American people in the U.S. political institutions represents a major crisis of legitimacy of bourgeois ideology in today's U.S.
28. Contrary to bourgeois ideology, which postulates that the state apparatus is neutral and can be used undistinctively by any class or group, I believe that the state's apparatus reflects the power relations of the whole of society and thus comes under the dominant influence of the capitalist class. That dominance explains its composition (the class position of the top echelons of the state personnel), its structure, and its function (i.e. to reproduce the capitalist relations). For a further expansion of this position, see State, power, and medicine: Part III. In Navarro, V. *Medicine Under Capitalism.* Neale Watson, New York, 1978.
29. Two examples of that perception are Hart, J. T. The point, however, is to change it. *Medicine in Society* 4(4), 1979, and Figlio, K. Sinister medicine. *Radical Science Journal* 9, 1979. Although different in their political position, both share that vision of the NHS as a socialist island in the capitalist state. Hart reduces socialism to a juridical-political category, i.e. the nationalization of the health sector. Figlio reduces socialism to the absence of market relations and to the mechanism of societal allocations done by the state for the "benefit of society." In that vision, socialism is defined by the relations of exchange, not by the relations of production. Socialism, however, is a social formation in which the working class and its allies are the dominant class. Thus, socialist control is working class control.
30. Navarro, V., *Class Struggle, the State, and Medicine.* Martin Robertson, Oxford, 1978.
31. Kirschten, D. Risk assessment. How much is a life worth? *National Journal* 7, 1979, p. 252. Also, for an excellent account of struggles in the U.S. to protect workers against the risky environment, see Berman, D. *Death on the Job.* Monthly Review Press, New York, 1978.
32. Navarro, V., The crisis of the Western system of medicine in contemporary capitalism. *Int. J. Health Serv.* 8(2): 205, 1978.
33. Representative of this position are Marcuse and most of the theorists of the Frankfurt School. A more recent example of this single society ideology is Kellner, D. Ideology, Marxism, and advanced capitalism. *Socialist Review* 42: 37, 1978. It is worth mentioning that the first major works of Althusser (*Pour Marx* and *Lire le Capital*) also carried that position of a single society ideology. Since 1968, however, Althusser has broken with that position. For an excellent and detailed critique of Althusser's position on this subject, see Vasquez, A. *Ciencia y Revolucion.* Alianza Editorial, Mexico, 1978.
34. Marx, K. *The Eighteenth Brumaire of Louis Bonaparte.* In Marx, K., and Engels, F. *Selected Works.* Lawrence and Wishart, London, 1968, pp. 117-118.
35. Marx, K. and Engels, F. *The German Ideology,* Lawrence and Wishart, London, 1974, p. 64.
36. Therborn, G. *What Does the Ruling Class Do When It Rules?* New Left Books, London, 1978.
37. Quoted in Interview con suclovico Geymont. El mito del progreso y de la neutralidad de la ciencia. In *El Viejo Topo,* No. 24, 1978, p. 13.
38. Bell, D., *The Post Industrial Society,* 1977.
39. See Stalin, J. *Dialectical and Historical Materialism.* A good critique of the work appears in Lecourt, D. *Proletarian Science: The Case of Lysenko.* New Left Books, London, 1976, pp. 110-11.
40. Sweezy, P. and Bettelheim, C. *On the Transition to Socialism.* Monthly Review Press, New York, 1971.
41. Lecourt, *op. cit.*
42. Claudin-Urondo, C. *Lenin and the Cultural Revolution.* Harvester Press, Sussex, 1977.
43. Navarro, V. *Social Security and Medicine in the USSR: A Marxist Critique.* Lexington Books, Lexington, Mass., 1977.
44. I am not using the categories of "yes" or "no" in an either/or type of relationship. Rather, I am using them in a dialectical way, i.e. that the autonomy of science takes place within a set of class relations that both influence and are influenced by science.
45. The meaning of "ultimate instance" is that although conflicts may appear between scientific developments and capitalist relations, those capitalist relations tend eventually to impose themselves on those developments.

46. Harnecker, M. *Los Conceptos Elementales del Materialismo Historico.* Siglo XXI, 1977, pp. 3-5.
47. Durkheim, E. *Las Reglas del Metodo Sociologico.* La Pleyade, Buenos Aires, 1974.
48. McMahon, B. *Principles and Methods of Epidemiology* (in Spanish, *La Prensa Medica Mexicana*), 1975, p. 2. For an excellent critique of ideology within epidemiology, see Breilh, J. *Critica de la Interpretacion Ecologica Funcionalista de la Epidemiologia,* Universidad Autonoma de Mexico, 1977 (mimeograph).
49. *Dorland's Medical Dictionary,* 1968.
50. Kuhn, T. *The Structure of Scientific Revolutions.* University of Chicago Press, Chicago, 1962.
51. For a critique of the concept of linearity in scientific knowledge, see Kuhn, *op. cit.* Also, for an alive but not always rigorous discussion on this subject, see Feyerabend, P. *Science in a Free Society.* New Left Books, London, 1978. Neither Kuhn nor Feyerabend touches on the socioeconomic and political determinants of the scientific breakthroughs, a key subject which leaves their positions wanting. A further fault of Feyerabend's work is the key determinant role that he considers scientists have in initiating or stopping changes. For example, in examining the situation of blacks, Chicanos, and American Indians, he writes that "much of the spiritual misery of the remnants of non-western culture in the U.S. is due to this uninformed intellectual facism of most of our leading philosophers, scientists, philosophers of science ..." (p. 207). The roots of the problems, however, are much deeper than Feyerabend seems to realize. He does not touch, for example, on the key issues of why those "fascist" ideas are the ruling or leading ideas.
52. Quoted in Braverman, *op. cit.*
53. Quoted in Breilh, *op. cit.*
54. Bridford, K., et al. *Estimates of the Fraction of Cancer in the United States Related to Occupational Factors.* Prepared by the National Cancer Institute, National Institute of Environmental Health Sciences, and National Institute for Occupational Safety and Health, 1978.
55. The fact that those assumed causes are only apparent but not the real ones does not make them irrelevant. They may allow for a description, but not for an explanation of reality. The vast array of empirical phenomena immediately observable in social life can only be explained if one analyzes the social reality behind those appearances.
56. Lecourt, *op. cit.*
57. For a critique of similar positivist approaches used in social sciences, see Scientific method in sociology. In Sherman, H. J., and Wood, J. L. *Sociology: Traditional and Radical Perspectives.* Harper and Row, New York, 1979, pp. 275-324.
58. For an analysis of the political and economic forces that determined the Italian experience and for a more detailed account of the process outlined here, see Assennato and Navarro, *op. cit.*
59. Hart, *op. cit.*
60. Navarro, V. *Social Security and Medicine in the USSR. op. cit.*
61. See Navarro, V. What does Chile mean? *Health and Society,* Spring 1974, p. 93.
62. Draper, H. Marx on democratic forms of government. *The Socialist Register,* 1974, p. 101.

CHAPTER 2

Black Lung: The Social Production of Disease

Barbara Ellen Smith

The recognition that certain forms of ill health are socially produced and therefore possibly preventable is one of the most important sources of progressive political vitality in the United States today. During the past decade, sporadic protest has erupted over hazardous situations in isolated workplaces and communities, from the controversy over toxic waste disposal in the Love Canal area to the protest against use of dioxin-contaminated herbicides in the Pacific Northwest. In some instances, more prolonged and widespread struggles have developed, such as the movement for black lung compensation and the current mobilization against nuclear power. These phenomena are admittedly quite diverse in their social bases, ideologies, and political goals. However, to varying degrees, all have involved the politicization of health hazards and illness, and thereby have drawn into the arena of political controversy one of the most elite professional domains in the United States—scientific medicine.

These controversies characteristically have originated in the bitter suspicions of lay people who fear that certain of their health problems are caused by industrial practices and products, but who have no scientifically credible proof to substantiate their concern. In some cases, scientists have scornfully dismissed as "housewife data" lay efforts to document these health problems (1). Indeed, health advocates' demands for compensatory or preventive action have often encountered their most formidable ideological opposition from the ranks of the medical establishment, who come armed with the seemingly unassailable authority of "science" and characteristically argue that no action is justified until further evidence is collected. Especially in contexts like that of the petrochemical industry, where workers and sometimes residential communities are exposed to manifold hazards about which little is known and whose effects may not be manifested for decades, health advocates can be forced into a no-win situation: they must prove their case with data that do not exist, using a model of disease causation that is ill suited to multiple and/or synergistic hazards, and which a growing chorus of critics argue is structurally incapable of explaining the major health problems of our place and time, such as heart disease and stress (2).

This article examines one health struggle, the black lung movement, during which the scientific authority of the medical establishment was itself questioned in the course of an intense political controversy over the definition of disease. The movement arose in southern West Virginia in 1968 and had as its initial goal the extension of workers' compensation coverage to victims of "black lung," a generic term for the ensemble of respiratory diseases that miners contract in the workplace. To elucidate the medical politics of this struggle, this article looks at three aspects of the history of black lung. The first section explores the major changes in medical perceptions of black lung and presents evidence suggesting that these shifting perceptions have been occasioned by social and economic factors ordinarily considered extrinsic to science. This section also points out the ideological and political functions of the medical definitions of this disease. The second part focuses on the history of black lung itself and argues that the respiratory disease burden is intimately related to the political economy of the workplace, the site of disease production. The final section describes the recent battle over black lung compensation, focusing on the strikingly different definitions of disease that miners and the medical establishment elaborated.

MEDICAL CONSTRUCTIONS OF BLACK LUNG

The history of science is popularly conceived as a continuum of concepts and paradigms evolving through time toward an ever more comprehensive and accurate understanding of a "given" external reality. However, there is a growing tradition of literature that challenges this positivist approach by classifying the scientific knowledge of any society as part of its historically specific belief systems, and viewing scientific concepts as both a consequence of and an influence upon the overall structure of social relations. Efforts to pursue this approach with regard to medical science have been especially fruitful and abundant. Scholarship has focused primarily on the ways in which medical practice has tended to reflect and uphold socially structured inequality (especially that based on class, sex, and race). Some analysts have also begun to investigate the exceedingly complex correspondence between the structures, forces, and dynamics that medical knowledge invests in the human body and the dynamics of social relations in the "body politic." (3)

The case of black lung provides an exceptionally clear example of the ways in which factors external to science have shaped and changed medical knowledge. In the United States, medical perceptions of black lung fall into three periods, bounded by major shifts in the political economy of the coal industry. Observations of miners' unusual respiratory disease burden and speculation as to its workplace origins characterized the first medical construction of black lung. This viewpoint originated in the anthracite coalfields of Pennsylvania during a period when medical knowledge and practice, health care delivery arrangements, and industrial relations between miners and operators were all in a state of flux. A completely different concept of black lung emerged in a later period from the expanding bituminous coalfields, where tight corporate control over the health care system, a stark class structure, and other factors were relevant to the medical outlook. A third concept of black lung developed gradually after World War II in the context of a highly unionized, increasingly capital-intensive industry with a union-controlled health plan for miners and their families.

The first written documents concerning miners' unusual respiratory trouble originated from the anthracite region of eastern Pennsylvania; here were located the first large-scale coal mining operations in the United States, dominated by the affiliates of nine railroads. During the 1860s and 1870s, a few physicians acquainted with this region began to publish articles remarking on miners' respiratory difficulties and speculating that they were related to the inhalation of dusts and gases in the workplace. These articles are remarkable for their detailed accounts of unhealthy working conditions and their inclusion of statements by miners themselves on their workplace health (4).

This period prior to the hegemony of scientific medicine was characterized by a relative eclecticism and fluidity in medical knowledge, practice, and health care delivery arrangements. Some medical historians argue that the uncertain financial, professional, and social status of physicians lent more equality and negotiability to the doctor-patient relationship than is customary today (5). In the anthracite coalfields, miners were beginning to finance their health and welfare needs through mutual benefit associations that gave financial assistance in cases of sickness, disability and death (6). This brief period of relative fluidity in the health care system was soon eclipsed, however, by the simultaneous eradication of the benefit associations and the growth of the company doctor system. The most significant episode in this process was the strike of 1874-1875, which led to the famous Molly Maguire murder trials and resulted in the disintegration of the major anthracite trade union, the Miners' and Laborers' Benevolent Association. The powerful Philadelphia and Reading Railroad, whose affiliate Coal and Iron Company was the largest anthracite coal producer, subsequently attempted to replace the union's health and welfare functions with a Beneficial Fund financed by miners and controlled by the company. During the last two decades of the nineteenth century, as mining corporations gradually extended their control over health care delivery through the company doctor system, physicians in the anthracite fields grew silent on the subject of miners' occupational lung disease. The anthracite industry subsequently entered a period of decline from which it never recovered; the center of U.S. coal production shifted to the bituminous fields, where physicians elaborated a completely different concept of black lung.

The bituminous industry of southern Appalachia achieved national economic importance around the turn of the century and by the end of World War I was rapidly becoming the heart of U.S. coal production. In the coal camps of this rural and mountainous region, physicians did not simply ignore the existence of black lung, as many have suggested; rather, they viewed miners' diseased state as normal and non-disabling, and therefore unworthy of scientific investigation. The sources of this perception may be found partly in the political economy of the coal industry, which left a peculiarly repressive stamp on the structure of health care delivery in Appalachia (7).

In the southern bituminous industry, coal operators initially assumed a direct role in establishing, maintaining, and controlling many social and political institutions, such as the public schools, churches, and the police. Their activities derived in part from practical necessity: companies often had to import much of their labor force into this sparsely populated area, and in order to keep these workers had to provide housing, food, and a minimum of public services. However, the operators' role was neither benign nor merely practical. The profits to be made from housing, food, and to a lesser extent medical care were often quite significant to companies attempting to survive in the highly competitive, unstable business environment of bituminous coal. Moreover, totalitarian control of coal communities, including issuance of a separate currency (scrip), domination of the police, and even control of the physical access to the towns, enabled these companies to forestall what they perceived as one of the most pernicious threats to their economic status—unionization.

Health care did not escape the logic of this competitive environment and direct domination of the work force. The company doctor was the only source of medical care in almost all rural Appalachian coal camps. Under this system, the coal company controlled the employment of a doctor, but miners were required as a condition of employment to pay for his services. The company doctors' accountability to the coal operators is one of the most obvious and fundamental reasons for the medical concepts of miners' occupational health developed during this period. Work-related accidents and later diseases spelled economic liability for the coal operators under the workers' compensation system. Any agitation for preventive action would have represented an even greater nuisance. There was instead a uniform tendency to ascribe accidents and diseases to the fault of the miner—his carelessness and personal habits, such as alcoholism. Thus, one physician in 1919, after reciting a litany of occupational safety and health hazards, including dust, gob piles, electricity, poisonous gases, and contaminated water supplies, managed to conclude: "Housing conditions, and hurtful forms of recreation, especially alcoholism, undoubtedly cause the major amount of sickness. The mine itself is not an unhealthful place to work." (8)

The medical ideology surrounding black lung was more complex than this outright denial of occupational causation. Physicians dubbed the widespread breathlessness, expectoration of sputum, and prolonged coughing fits "miners' asthma." These symptoms of lung disease were *constituted as a norm*; as such, they were to be expected and by definition were nondisabling. For example, in 1935, one physician in Pennsylvania wrote (9):

> As far as most of the men in this region are concerned, so called "miners' asthma" is considered an *ordinary* condition that needs cause no worry and therefore the profession has not troubled itself about its finer pathological and associated clinical manifestations (emphasis added).

A miner who complained of disability due to respiratory trouble was diagnosed as a case of "malingering," "compensationitis," or "fear of the mines." The social control aspects of this ideology are obvious: if disease was natural, inevitable, and nondisabling, then prevention was unnecessary. Moreover, exhibiting disability from a respiratory disease was a medically stigmatized sign of psychological weakness or duplicity (10).

Although the company doctor system provides one explanation for this medical concept, it may also be related to class interactions in the coalfields and to some of the basic precepts of scientific medicine. It may be speculated that the company doctor's social as well as medical perspective on the coal miner and his family was influenced by the relative status of each within the coal camp environment (11). The monoeconomy of the Appalachian coalfields produced a rather simple and vivid class structure, in which physicians, lawyers, and a few other professionals formed an island in a working-class sea. On the one hand, the superiority of the doctors' status relative to the working class was everywhere apparent—in their standard of living, language, etc. On the other hand, these physicians were in a distinctly inferior position by the standards of the medical profession as a whole, and moreover were denied numerous amenities available in more cosmopolitan surroundings. Their degraded social and physical environment was embodied in and no doubt in many cases attributed to coal miners themselves—their ramshackle houses, coarse language, "lack of culture," and so on. What was "normal" for miners, including even a chronic respiratory condition, was by no means normal for the company doctor (12).

The outlook of scientific medicine, which around the turn of the century was gaining hegemony over other forms of medical theory and practice, is also relevant to the company doctors' conceptualization of black lung. With the rise of scientific medicine, production of medical knowledge gradually became the province of research scientists, divorced from the human patient by their location in the laboratory. Building on the precepts of cell theory and the discovery of bacteria, their efforts focused on the isolation of specific aberrations in cell function, and their correlation with discrete disease agents. The "germ theory" of disease causation, which essentially holds that each disease is caused by a specific bacterium or agent, became the basis of scientific medicine. This theory confounded the microscopic *agent* of disease with the *cause* of disease; it thus implicitly denied a role to social and economic factors in disease causation and displaced the social medicine of an earlier period.

At the level of medical practice, diagnosis became a process of identifying separate disease entities, with confirmation of the diagnosis sought in the laboratory; the patient's own testimony as to his/her condition was relegated to a decidedly secondary status. Indeed, scientific medicine involved what Jewson (5) termed the "disappearance of the sick-man" from the medical world view. The patient increasingly appeared almost incidentally as the medium for disease, eclipsed by the focus on identifying discrete pathologies. In the absence of a verifiable clinical entity, the patient was by definition (health is the absence of disease) pronounced healthy. His/her protestations of feeling ill became a matter for the psychiatrist (13).

These features of the scientific medical outlook dovetailed with previously mentioned factors to produce the company doctors' conceptualization of black lung. To the extent that any company doctor seriously attempted to diagnose a miner's respiratory condition, the effort was informed by the search for previously established clinical entities, especially silicosis and tuberculosis. Up until very recently, silica was considered the only dust seriously harmful to the respiratory system. Moreover, silicosis possesses characteristics that scientific medicine is most conducive to recognizing as a legitimate clinical entity: it is associated with one specific agent; it produces gross pathological change in lung tissue, apparent upon autopsy; and it reveals itself relatively clearly in a characteristic pattern on an X-ray. Most coal miners were not exposed to silica in significant quantity, and their X-rays did not exhibit the classic silicotic pattern. To the extent that their X-rays revealed the pathological changes now associated with coal workers' pneumoconiosis, these too were considered normal—for coal miners (14). Moreover, as a group, miners seemed to experience a low mortality rate from tuberculosis, considered the prime public health problem of this period. Hence developed the perversely ironic "coal dust is good for you" theory: "It is in the highest degree possible that coal-dust possesses the property of hindering the development of tuberculosis, and of arresting its progress." (15)

The company doctor system did not go unchallenged by coal miners; unrest over its compulsory character occasionally led to strikes and generated the demand for a health care plan organized on the opposite basis—union control and industry financing. Following a protracted strike and federalization of the mines in 1946, miners finally won a contract establishing such a system, the Welfare and Retirement Fund. Financed by a royalty assessed on each ton of mined coal, the Fund provided pensions, hospitalization, and medical care for miners and their families. Although officially directed by a tripartite board composed of representatives from industry, the union, and the public, in reality the Fund was controlled by the United Mine Workers. At the time of its creation, progressives in the health care field almost unanimously viewed the Fund as an innovative leap forward in health care delivery. Contradictions embedded in coal's postwar industrial relations subsequently compromised this vision and constricted the Fund's activities. Nevertheless, in its first decade and heyday, the Fund transformed the structure and quality of health care in the Appalachian coalfields (16).

The establishment of the Fund made possible the beginning of a third period in the medical conceptualization of miners' respiratory disease. Progressive physicians, many organized in prepaid group practice financed through the Fund, undertook clinical research on the respiratory problems of their coal miner patients. The Fund also employed in its central office a physician whose primary responsibility was to educate the medical profession about coal miners' dust disease. These physicians were largely responsible for the trickle of literature on coal workers' pneumoconiosis that began to appear in U.S. medical journals during the early 1950s; of the articles they did not write, most depended on data from Fund-affiliated hospitals and clinics. All argued essentially that "authoritative opinion to the contrary notwithstanding," coal miners suffer from a "disabling, progressive, killing disease which is related to exposure to coal dust." (17)

Despite these efforts, medical recognition of coal workers' pneumoconiosis did not evolve in an orderly, linear fashion, advanced by the inquiring gaze of these scientists. They remained a minority within the medical establishment, and coal miners in most states continued to be denied workers' compensation for occupational lung disease. The recognition that black lung was rampant among U.S. coal miners did not evolve of its own accord within the boundaries of medical science. It was forced on the medical community by the decidedly political intervention of miners themselves.

BLACK LUNG AND THE TRANSFORMATION OF THE WORKPLACE

Since the changing medical concepts of black lung reveal more about the development of the coal industry and health care delivery systems than the nature and extent of respiratory disease among coal miners, observers may well wonder what the history of black lung actually entails. It is extremely difficult to reconstruct satisfactorily. Epidemiological data on miners' lung disease are simply nonexistent, except for the very recent period. The early commentaries cited previously suggest that pervasive respiratory problems accompanied the growth of the anthracite and bituminous coal industries, a conclusion corroborated by nonmedical sources (18); however, acceptance of "miners' asthma" and a dearth of medical literature swiftly followed. Between 1918 and 1940, a few scattered studies, primarily by the U.S. Public Health Service, uncovered "extraordinary" excess mortality from influenza and pneumonia among anthracite and bituminous coal miners; their susceptibility was likely due to the work-related destruction of their respiratory systems. However, all U.S. Public Health Service research on miners' occupational respiratory disease focused on silicosis; the resulting data were mixed, but the invariable conclusion was that bituminous miners were not exposed to silica in significant quantity and were not seriously disabled by work-related lung disease (19).

Although the lack of statistics precludes documentation of the extent of black lung, it is possible to trace the changing causes of disease by analyzing the site of disease production—the workplace. By "workplace" is meant not only the physical characteristics of the site of coal production but also the social relations that shape and are part of the workplace. The interaction between miners and operators under historically given circumstances has shaped the timing and character of technological innovation, the nature of the work process, the pace of work, and other factors relevant to the production of occupational disease. The history of black lung is thus internally related to the history of the workplace, as a physical site and a social relationship.

This history may be divided into two major periods, distinguished by their different technologies, work organizations, industrial relations, and sources of respiratory disease: handloading and mechanized mining. During the initial handloading era, which persisted until the 1930s, of utmost importance to the production of coal and disease was the highly competitive and labor-intensive character of the industry. Fragmented into thousands of competing companies, bituminous coal suffered from chronic bouts of overproduction, excess capacity, low profit margins, and fluctuating prices. Because labor represented approximately 70 percent of the cost of production, a prime tactic in the competitive struggle was to cut the cost of labor, principally by lowering the piece rate. In addition, the craft nature of the labor process rendered companies relatively powerless to control productivity and output, except by manipulating the miners' wages (20).

These economic dynamics had important implications for the workplace as a site of disease production. The instability of the industry frequently resulted in irregular work and a lowering of the piece rate, both of which forced miners to work faster and/or longer hours in an attempt to maintain their standard of living. The impact on health and safety conditions was almost invariably negative, as miners necessarily reduced nonproductive, safety-oriented tasks, such as roof timbering, to a minimum (21). Working longer hours in mines where "towards quitting time [the air] becomes so foul that the miners' lamps will no longer burn" (22) no doubt increased the respiratory disease risk. Moreover, a financially mandated speedup encouraged miners to re-enter their work areas as soon as possible after blasting the coal loose from the face, an operation that generated clouds of dust and powder smoke (23).

Respiratory hazards often were especially grave in non-gassy mines, where ventilation tended to be poorest. The prospect of losing their entire capital investment in one explosion encouraged mine owners to install better ventilation systems in mines where methane gas was liberated; the non-gassy mines, however, tended to "kill the men by inches." (4, p. 244) Writing around the turn of the century, one mine inspector described in detail the ventilation problem and its implications for miners' health (22, pp. 449-450):

> ... adequate ventilation is not applied in such [non-gassy] mines, because they can be wrought without going to the expense of providing costly and elaborate furnaces or fans, air-courses, stoppings, and brattice. From four to six cents a ton are thus saved in mining the coal that should be applied in ventilating, but saved at the expense of the workmen's health. ... Constant labor in a badly-aired mine breaks down the constitution and clouds the intellect. The lungs become clogged up from inhaling coal dust, and from breathing noxious air; the body and limbs become stiff and sore, the mind loses the power of vigorous thought. After six years' labor in a badly ventilated mine—that is, a mine where a man with a good constitution may from habit be able to work every day for several years—the lungs begin to change to a bluish color. After twelve years they are black, and after twenty years they are densely black, not a vestige of natural color remaining, and are little better than carbon itself. The miner dies at thirty-five, of coal-miners' consumption.

During the 1930s, the introduction of mechanical loading equipment dramatically altered the workplace, while the organizing successes of the United Mine Workers transformed relations between miners and operators. Although mechanical cutting devices were introduced into underground coal mines as early as 1876, their adoption was gradual and associated with only a partial reorganization of the craft work process. The classic changes produced by mechanization and Taylorization, such as elevated productivity, loss of job control, de-skilling, and an increased division of labor, appeared slowly in bituminous coal during the first three decades of the twentieth century. However, the widespread introduction of loading machines in the 1930s broke the craft organization of work once and for all. More technological innovation swiftly followed, with the introduction of continuous mining technology after World War II. This technology did not increase the already specialized division of labor as much as it replaced several tasks (and miners) with one central production worker—the continuous miner operator.

Virtually all sources agree that the mechanization of underground mining greatly increased dust levels and magnified the existing problems with respiratory disease (24). Miners were quick to rename the Joy loaders "man killers" and to protest the unemployment, physical hardships placed on older miners, and health and safety problems that attended their introduction. For example, at the 1934 UMWA convention, miners debated at length a resolution demanding the removal of these machines from the mines; the few delegates who spoke against it were nearly shouted down by the tumultuous convention. One miner argued (25, p. 192):

> I heard one of the brothers say that they don't hire miners over forty years of age in their locality. I want to tell you brothers that there is no miner that can work in the mines under those conveyors [loading machines] and reach the age of forty. Those conveyors are man killers and I believe this convention should do its utmost to find some way whereby those conveyors will be abolished. ... The young men after they work in the mine six or eight hours daily become sick, either getting asthma or

some other sickness due to the dust of the conveyors and they can no longer perform their duty.

Another miner, during debate over continuous mining machinery at a UMWA convention 22 years later, echoed those comments (26):

> ... [T]hey are putting coal moles [continuous miners] in our mines, and I hope they don't put them in anybody else's mines. We had one man die from the effects of that procedure. We had to give them a 15-minute shift. We have had any number who have had to get off because of health. It seems that someone forgot the miners who have [to operate] the moles. . . . He stands up there and inhales the fumes and the oil and the steam that is created by the heat from the mole. He doesn't get sufficient oxygen. . . .

It would be mistaken to conclude that because mechanization was associated with increased dust levels, machines themselves were the cause of this problem. Here again, the economic and political circumstances of technological innovation were critical in determining its impact on the workplace. The large coal operators introduced continuous mining technology in the midst of a desperate competitive struggle with oil and natural gas, which by the 1950s had usurped coal's traditional markets in home heating and the railroads. By making coal a capital-intensive industry and vastly increasing labor productivity, the large operators hoped to force the small, labor-intensive producers into bankruptcy and win a respectable share of the growing utility market. Of crucial importance to the pace, nature, and success of this mechanization strategy was the role of the union. Headed by the authoritarian but charismatic John L. Lewis, the United Mine Workers not only accepted but aggressively promoted mechanization, believing that it would lead to institutional security, high wages, and economic prosperity (27). Although there was widespread rank-and-file discontent with mechanization, the very process replaced labor with machinery, rendering miners redundant and their protest ineffective. Despite scattered strikes and other expressions of unrest, miners were unable to modify the policy of their union or exert significant control over the impacts of mechanization on their workplace and communities.

The result was not simply increased respirable dust in the workplace, but social and economic disaster in the coalfields. In the space of 20 years, between 1950 and 1969, the work force shrank by 70 percent. For the unemployed, the monoeconomy of the Appalachian coalfields left no alternative but migration. Coal-dependent communities became ghost towns, as some counties lost half their population in the space of 10 years. Those who managed to keep their jobs in large mines confronted increased dust, noise, high-voltage electricity, and other hazards. Supervision intensified, as the operators attempted to recoup their investments in machinery by pushing productivity higher and higher (28).

The black lung controversy that erupted in 1968 was very much a product of and a challenge to this history. The movement represented an effort by miners and their families to reclaim the political and economic potency denied them for almost 20 years. Black lung disease in a sense became a metaphor for the exploitative social relations that had always characterized the coalfields, but worsened during two decades of high unemployment, social dislocation, and rank-and-file weakness vis-à-vis the coal industry. The goal of black lung compensation represented, in part, a demand for retribution from the industry for the devastating human effects of its economic transformation.

THE BATTLE IS JOINED

By 1968, when the black lung movement arose, the union's overt cooperation with the large operators had outworn its usefulness to the industry and outlived its tolerability for the rank and file. The major producers had thoroughly mechanized their mines, reduced intraindustry competition from small companies, and held their own against external competition from alternative fuels. Capital was flowing into the industry not only through the enormously increased productivity of its workers, which tripled between 1950 and 1969, but also in the form of investment by the oil industry. Electric utilities seemed to offer unlimited market potential. Threatening the rosy forecasts, however, were an increasingly rambunctious work force and a projected manpower shortage. An enormous turnover was beginning in the work force, as the miners who managed to keep their jobs during postwar mechanization were now retiring en masse, replaced by young workers with no necessary allegiance to the UMWA leadership. The economic prosperity rankled workers already beginning to question the sluggish collective bargaining advances of their union leaders and made strikes a more potent weapon (29).

The first unmistakable evidence that rank-and-file rebellion was afoot erupted in the winter of 1968-1969 with the birth of the black lung movement. Originating in southern West Virginia, the movement was based in the older generation of workers who were leaving the mines. They faced retirement with a sparse pension of $100 per month (if they could meet the Fund's increasingly arbitrary and strict eligibility requirements), without the traditional cushion of the extended family and without compensation for the respiratory disease from which so many suffered (30). Discontent focused on the demand that the West Virginia legislature pass a bill recognizing black lung as a compensable disease under the state's workers' compensation statutes. Opposing the movement were the combined forces of the coal industry and the medical establishment. A member of the latter insisted, "There is no epidemic of devastating, killing and disabling man-made plague among coal workers." (31) Another argued, "The control of coal dust is not the answer to the disabling respiratory diseases of our coal miners." (32)

Exasperated by strident opposition and legislative inaction, miners began to quit work in February 1969 in a strike that eventually brought out 40,000 workers and shut off coal production throughout the state. Their solidarity and economic muscle forced a black lung compensation bill through the legislature; although less liberal than what miners had hoped for, they declared a victory and returned to work after the governor signed the bill into law.

This was the most dramatic and widely reported phase of the black lung movement, but it marked only the beginning. Coupled with the death of 78 miners in the violent Farmington mine explosion in November 1968, the black lung movement generated a national political debate over health and safety conditions in U.S. coal mines. In December 1969, the Congress passed a Coal Mine Health and Safety Act, which detailed to an unprecedented degree mandatory work practices throughout the industry and offered compensation to miners disabled by black lung and the widows of miners who died from the disease. Large coal companies vigorously opposed certain, but not all of the act's provisions. Most notably, they fought the extremely strict respirable dust standard of 3.0 mg/m^3, scheduled to drop to 2.0 mg/m^3 after three years; this was designed to prevent black lung. The compensation program, by contrast, was to their liking: not only did it seem to promise that the turmoil over black lung would dissolve, the program also relieved them of liability for compensation by financing benefits with general tax revenues from the U.S. Treasury.

Ironically, passage of the act ensured that the issue of black lung compensation would not die but remain the focus of a continuing movement. In 1970, the Social Security Administration began administering the claims process for compensation benefits; within the program's first week of operation, 18,000 claims poured into agency offices (33). By the fall of the same year, letters of denial began to flow back into the coalfields. The bitterness and confusion that ensued derived partly from a pattern that repeated itself throughout thousands of these rural communities: several disabled miners and widows received black lung benefits, but their brothers or uncles or neighbors down the road were denied, even though by all appearances they were equally or even more disabled by lung disease. In other words, the criteria by which the Social Security Administration judged claimants' eligibility appeared completely arbitrary and violated local perceptions of who was disabled by black lung. Thus miners and their families pitted themselves against Social Security and the medical establishment in a bitter struggle over who would control the definition of disease and disability.

The Social Security Administration initially based its eligibility criteria on the orthodox medical conception of black lung, a view that reflects the rigidity and narrowness of the germ theory. According to this perspective, black lung is limited exclusively to one clinical entity—coal workers' pneumoconiosis (CWP); this is the only lung disease considered occupational in origin and therefore compensable. The agent (and cause) of CWP is, by definition (pneumoconiosis means "dust-containing lung"), the inhalation of respirable coal mine dust, which produces certain pathological changes in one organ (the lungs) and which are revealed in a characteristic pattern on an X-ray. The disease process is linear and quantitative; the stage of CWP is determined by the number and size of opacities on the lung field, as revealed through an X-ray. The first stages of disease, categorized as "simple" pneumoconiosis, are considered compatible with health, whereas advanced or "complicated" pneumoconiosis is severely disabling and sometimes fatal (34).

This conception of black lung has highly significant political and ideological functions. Most important, it minimizes and depoliticizes the problem. If the *cause* of CWP is respirable dust, then prevention is a technical matter of controlling this inanimate object, rather than a political question involving the relations of power in the workplace. Moreover, most surveys find a 3 percent prevalence of complicated CWP; if this is the only stage of disease considered disabling, then a relatively small number of coal miners are functionally impaired by occupational lung disease and deserve compensation. Respiratory disability in miners with simple CWP is attributed to nonoccupational factors, above all the victims themselves and their cigarette smoking. Obviously, this entire train of thought functions to shift medical and political emphasis away from the workplace as a source of disease and onto the worker (35).

The entire diagnostic and claims procedure also functioned to individualize what miners and other activists considered a collective problem. On a practical level, the dominant medical concept of black lung meant that claimants with evidence of complicated CWP, even if they experienced little disability, automatically received compensation; some with lesser stages who met a complex combination of other criteria also received benefits. But thousands of miners and the widows of miners, who by all appearances were equally or more disabled by respiratory disease, were denied compensation.

In the course of their movement to achieve more liberal eligibility criteria, miners and other activists implicitly elaborated a completely different understanding of black lung and its causes. Their view was not articulated by a single spokesperson or written down in a single position paper; it was woven into the culture and ideology of the movement, and in almost all respects ran counter to the dominant medical view of black lung. Indeed, the very act of insisting collectively on the reality of their own disease experience was in itself a challenge to scientific medicine, insofar as the latter tends to individualize health problems and denigrate the patients' perceptions of their own condition.

It should be stressed that the movement's ideology did not involve a wholesale rejection of science and was not based on fundamentalist religion or other anti-scientific sensibilities. Indeed, some activists made skillful use of the scientific arguments of a few physicians who, because of their research findings, lent support to the black lung cause (36). Overall, the movement's ideology was based in the collective experience of its participants. Their skepticism toward the medical establishment had historical roots in the company doctor system, which for many activists was a bitter and living memory. Their view of black lung itself was based in their own holistic experience of disease—its physical as well as psychological, social, and economic aspects. And their understanding of the causes of black lung derived from their experiences with the coal industry, as workers, as widows of men killed by the mines, and as residents of coal towns where "there are no neutrals" (37)—even scientists.

For movement participants, the medical definition of black lung as a single clinical entity principally affecting one organ of the body had little meaning, because black lung meant a transformation in their whole way of life. As one 56-year-old miner, disabled by black lung since the age of 48, described (38):

> Black lung is a cruel disease, a humiliating disease. It's when you can't do what you like to do; that's humiliating. I had to lay down my hammer and saw, and those were the things I got the most pleasure out of. The next thing I liked to do was work in my garden; now my garden's the biggest weed patch in Logan County. There were times in 1971 when I was still working that it was difficult for me to get to the bedroom when I was feeling bad. Now, of course, that's humiliating.

Many miners' analysis of the agents and causes of black lung also contrasted with the orthodox medical view. They argued that many features of the workplace had damaged their lungs, such as working in water over their ankles or breathing the fumes from cable fires. Moreover, they asserted that although respirable dust was the agent of CWP, the cause of the whole disease experience ultimately was economic:

> Where do we get the black lung from? The coal companies! They've had plenty of time to lessen the dust so nobody would get it. It's not an elaborate thing to keep it down: spray water. They just don't put enough of it on there. They don't want to maintain enough in materials and water to do that. . . . (39)

> Should we all die a terrible death to keep those companies going? (40)

Thus, miners developed a belief that they were *collectively entitled* to compensation, not at all because of individualized medical diagnoses of CWP but because of the common health-destroying experience that defined them as a group: work in the mines. Implicit in this view was the idea that black lung is a destructive process that begins when a miner starts work, not something that acquires legitimacy only when a radiologist can find it on an X-ray.

A disabled coal miner reported (41):

> I worked in the cleaning plant, an outside job. I had four conveyors to bring to the storage bin. I had, I'd say, 16 holes in this galvanized pipe, two rows, that's 32 holes in all, little tiny holes, to keep down the dust. I stood many a time across from that conveyor and somebody'd be on the other side, and all you could see was their cap lamp. And that's in the cleaning plant; that's outside! That's not even at the face.
>
> In the Black Lung Association, we're asking due compensation for a man who had to work in the environment he worked in. Not that a man can't choose where he works. But he's due more than just a day's wages. He and his family ought to be compensated for the environment he worked in.

These beliefs found expression in a multitude of political demands concerning the black lung compensation program, eventually and most clearly in the demand for automatic compensation after a specified number of years' work in the mines. Federal legislation to effect this change went down to defeat in 1976. However, medical and legal eligibility requirements for compensation were so liberalized by amendments passed in 1972 and 1978 that most miners and the widows of miners who worked a substantial period of time in the mines are now receiving black lung benefits (42).

The black lung movement has been rightly criticized for its lack of a preventive focus. Despite the clear and widely held perception that the coal companies were to blame for black lung, activists never directed their struggle at the heart of the problem, prevention in the workplace. This was partly due to the initial, erroneous view that the cost of state compensation (financed by industry) would force the companies to improve health conditions in the mines. A lasting and effective prevention campaign would have required a tighter alliance between working miners, disabled miners, and widows; a much firmer conviction that black lung is not inevitable; and, at least eventually, a political vision of how miners might improve their occupational health by asserting greater control over the workplace.

However, the black lung movement suggests that even within the confines of an after-the-fact struggle for compensation, important and intensely political issues may be at stake. This article has explored the history of black lung on many levels—as a medical construct, a product of the workplace, a disease experience, and a political battle. The evidence presented suggests that miners' experientially based view of black lung and challenge to the medical establishment have historical justification. Medical science's understanding of black lung has not derived from observation unencumbered by a social and economic context, but has been profoundly shaped by that context; as a result, it has performed crucial political and ideological functions. In one era, it served to "normalize" and thereby mask the existence of disease altogether; in the more recent period, it has tended to minimize and individualize the problem.

By contrast, black lung activists succeeded in challenging the scientific medical establishment by insisting on the validity of their own definition of disease. They viewed black lung as an experience affecting the whole person in all aspects of life. Rather than focusing on a causal relationship between one discrete agent and one disease, they looked at the workplace as a total environment where the miner confronts an array of respiratory hazards. Finally, activists defined black lung as a collective problem whose ultimate cause was economic. In its entirety, the history of black lung suggests that a similar task of redefinition awaits other health advocates if they wish to challenge effectively the social production of disease.

Acknowledgments—This article was written under a research fellowship at the International Institute for Comparative Social Research in Berlin, West Germany. I wish to thank the Institute and its staff for their financial support, friendship, and intellectual stimulation. Conversations and correspondence with Norm Diamond, Gerd Göckenjan, and Meredeth Turshen were also an invaluable part of the process that led to this article.

REFERENCES

1. NOVA. A plague on our children. WGBH Educational Foundation, Boston, 1979, film transcript, p. 35.
2. For a clear presentation of the overall argument, see Doyal, L. (with Pennell, I.). *The Political Economy of Health*. Pluto Press, London, 1979. See also Turshen, M. The political ecology of disease. *Review of Radical Political Economics* 9(1): 45-60, 1977. See also Eyer, J. Hypertension as a disease of modern society. *Int. J. Health Serv.* 5(4): 539-558, 1975.
3. Many analysts have pointed out this relationship on a theoretical level, but only a few have attempted to apply it in concrete investigation. See the discussion concerning the relationship between capitalist work relations and technology and the scientific model of brain function (as factory manager, telephone exchange, and, today, computer) in Rose, A. *The Conscious Brain*. Alfred A. Knopf, New York, 1974. For a more general discussion, see Figlio, K. The historiography of scientific medicine: An invitation to the human sciences. *Comparative Studies in Society and History* 19: 262-286, 1977. See also Foucault, M. *The Birth of the Clinic*. Vintage Books, New York, 1975.
4. The most comprehensive discussion I found was Sheafer, H. C. Hygiene of coal-mines. In *A Treatise on Hygiene and Public Health*, edited by A. H. Buck, vol. 2, pp. 229-250. William Wood and Company, New York, 1879. Sheafer wrote: "Any one who has seen a load of coal shot from a cart, or has watched the thick clouds of dust which sometimes envelop the huge coal-breakers of the anthracite region so completely as almost to hide them from sight, can form an idea of the injurious effect upon the health of constant working in such an atmosphere. The wonder is not that men die of clogged-up lungs, but that they manage to exist so long in an atmosphere which seems to contain at least fifty per cent of solid matter" (p. 245). See also Carpenter, J. T. Report of the Schuylkill County Medical Society. *Transactions of the Medical Society of Pennsylvania*, fifth series, part 2, pp. 488-491, 1869.
5. Figlio (3). Jewson, N. D. The disappearance of the sick-man from medical cosmology, 1770-1870. *Sociology* 10(2): 225-244, 1976.
6. On early financing of medical care in the coalfields, see Ginger, R. Company-sponsored welfare plans in the anthracite industry before 1900. *Bulletin of the Business Historical Society* 27(2): 112-120, 1953. See also Falk, L. A. Coal miners' prepaid medical care in the United States—and some British relationships, 1792-1964. *Med. Care* 4(1): 37-42, 1966.
7. A comprehensive survey of health care under the company doctor system was extracted from the U.S. government by the United Mine Workers of America during temporary federalization of the mines in 1946. The result was the so-called Boone report. U.S. Department of the Interior, Coal Mines Administration. *A Medical Survey of the Bituminous-Coal Industry*. Government Printing Office, Washington, D.C., 1947.
8. Hayhurst, E. R. The health hazards and mortality statistics of soft coal mining in Illinois and Ohio. *J. Ind. Hygiene* 1(7): 360, 1919.
9. Rebhorn, E. H. Anthraco silicosis. *Med. Soc. Reporter* 29(5): 15, Scranton, Pennsylvania, 1935.

10. Those who persisted in their complaints of breathlessness were eventually referred to psychiatrists, according to the testimony of miners and their families during interviews with the author. The argument that miners' symptoms of lung disease were psychological in origin may be found in Ross, W. D., et al. Emotional aspects of respiratory disorders among coal miners. *J.A.M.A.* 156(5): 484-487, 1954.

11. My thoughts on this relationship were stimulated and clarified by Figlio, K. Chlorosis and chronic disease in 19th century Britain: The social constitution of somatic illness in a capitalist society. *Int. J. Health Serv.* 8(4): 589-617, 1978.

12. This view persists today. Abundant examples may be found, especially in journalistic and sociological literature on Appalachia. Miners are alternately romanticized and reviled; in either case, they are "a breed apart."

13. See Brown, E. R. *Rockefeller Medicine Men.* University of California Press, Berkeley, 1979. On the germ theory and its implications for the doctor-patient relationship, see Jewson (5), Figlio (3), and Berliner, H. S., and Salmon, J. W. The holistic health movement and scientific medicine: The naked and the dead. *Socialist Review* 9(1): 31-52, 1979.

14. "One radiologist in southern West Virginia says until five years ago he regularly encountered chest X-rays from physicians that showed massive lung lesions labeled 'normal miner's chest.' " Aronson, B. Black lung: Tragedy of Appalachia. *New South* 26(4): 54, 1971.

15. Meiklejohn, A. History of lung disease of coal miners in Great Britain: Part II, 1875-1920. *Br. J. Ind. Med.* 9(2): 94, 1952. This view apparently originated in Britain and was picked up by physicians in the United States.

16. See Seltzer, C. Health care by the ton. *Health PAC Bulletin* 79: 1-8, 25-33, 1977.

17. Martin, J. E., Jr. Coal miners' pneumoconiosis. *Am. J. Public Health* 44(5): 581, 1954. See also Hunter, M. B., and Levine, M. D. Clinical study of pneumoconiosis of coal workers in Ohio river valley. *J.A.M.A.* 163(1): 1-4, 1957. See also the numerous articles by Lorin Kerr in this period, especially Coal workers' pneumoconiosis. *Ind. Med. Surg.* 25(8): 355-362, 1956.

18. Nonmedical literature from all over the world suggests that coal miners have long experienced black lung. Friedrich Engels discusses miners' "black spittle" disease in *The Condition of the Working Class in England.* Alden Press, Oxford, 1971. Emile Zola's character Bonnemort in the novel *Germinal* is clearly a victim of black lung. And John Spargo, a progressive era reformer intent on the prohibition of child labor, discusses the respiratory problems of the anthracite breaker boys in *The Bitter Cry of the Children.* Macmillan Company, New York, 1906, p. 164.

19. U.S. Public Health Service. The health of workers in dusty trades, Part III. Public Health Bulletin Number 208, Government Printing Office, Washington, D.C., 1933; U.S. Public Health Service. Anthraco-silicosis among hard coal miners. Public Health Bulletin Number 221, Government Printing Office, Washington, D.C., 1936; U.S. Public Health Service and Utah State Board of Health. The working environment and the health of workers in bituminous coal mines, non-ferrous metal mines, and non-ferrous metal smelters in Utah. 1940.

20. A lucid discussion of the labor process in this period may be found in Dix, K. *Work Relations in the Coal Industry: The Hand-Loading Era, 1880-1930.* Institute for Labor Studies, West Virginia University, Morgantown, West Virginia, 1977. On the economics of the industry, see Suffern, A. E. *The Coal Miners' Struggle for Industrial Status.* Macmillan Company, New York, 1926. See also Hamilton, W. H., and Wright, H. R. *The Case of Bituminous Coal.* Macmillan Company, New York, 1925.

21. One study actually found an inverse statistical relationship between employment levels and the rate of fatal accidents. See the discussion in Dix (20), pp. 101-104.

22. Roy, A. *History of Coal Miners of the U.S.* J. L. Trauger Printing Company, Columbus, Ohio, 1907, p. 119.

23. In some cases, state law or local practice dictated that coal be shot down at the end of the day, allowing the atmosphere to clear overnight. However, this was not uniform practice throughout the industry.

24. Physicians, miners, and government officials seem to agree on this point; representatives from industry in some cases demur. There is also disagreement about the magnitude of any increase in respiratory disease. See *Papers and Proceedings of the National Conference on Medicine and the Federal Coal Mine Health and Safety Act of 1969.* Washington, D.C., 1970. Debate on these questions also runs through the many volumes of testimony on the 1969 act. See U.S. Senate, Committee on Labor and Public Welfare, Subcommittee on Labor. *Coal Mine Health and Safety.* Hearings, 91st Congress, 1st Session. Government Printing Office, Washington, D.C., 1969.

25. United Mine Workers of America. *Proceedings of the 33rd Consecutive Constitutional Convention.* United Mine Workers of America, Indianapolis, Indiana, 1934, vol. 1.

26. United Mine Workers of America. *Proceedings of the 42nd Consecutive Constitutional Convention.* United Mine Workers of America, Washington, D.C., 1956, see pp. 306-331.

27. Lewis clearly articulated this position in his book, *The Miners' Fight for American Standards.* Bell Publishing Company, Indianapolis, Indiana, 1925.

28. This paragraph compresses an enormous social and economic transformation into a few sentences. For a detailed description of the changed industrial relations in this period, see Seltzer, C. The United Mine Workers of America and the coal operators: The political economy of coal in Appalachia, 1950-1973. Ph.D. dissertation, Columbia University, 1977.

29. See David, J. P. Earnings, health, safety, and welfare of bituminous coal miners since the encouragement of mechanization by the United Mine Workers of America. Ph.D. dissertation, West Virginia University, 1972. David demonstrates how miners fell behind workers in certain other unionized industries during this period.

30. In 1969, the U.S. Surgeon General estimated that 100,000 coal miners were afflicted with CWP. A study of 9,076 miners, conducted between 1969 and 1972, found a 31.4 percent prevalence of the disease among bituminous miners; among those who had worked 30 to 39 years in the mines, prevalence rose to over 50 percent. See Morgan, W.K.C., et al. The prevalence of coal workers' pneumoconiosis in U.S. coal miners. *Arch. Environ. Health* 27: 222, 1973. Current prevalence in the work force runs around 15 percent. These data are all on CWP. Black lung, i.e. the whole disease experience that miners consider occupational in origin, is not considered a legitimate concept by scientific medicine, and its prevalence is unknown. In scientific medical terms, black lung includes CWP, bronchitis, emphysema, and possibly other unrecognized disease processes. The prevalence of this ensemble of diseases is of course higher than that of CWP alone.

31. Dr. Rowland Burns, as quoted in the Charleston (West Virginia) *Daily Mail*, January 15, 1969.

32. Dr. William Anderson, as quoted in the Charleston (West Virginia) *Gazette*, April 16, 1969.

33. U.S. House, Committee on Education and Labor. *Black Lung Benefits Program.* First Annual Report. Government Printing Office, Washington, D.C., 1971.

34. The views of W.K.C. Morgan and his associates represent the dominant position of the medical establishment on CWP. See Morgan, W.K.C. Respiratory disease in coal miners. *Am. Rev. Resp. Dis.* 113: 531-559, 1976.

35. For example: "The presence of severe shortness of breath in a coal miner with simple CWP is virtually always related to a nonoccupationally related disease, such as chronic bronchitis or emphysema, rather than to coal mining. . . . Smoking is by far the most important factor in producing respiratory symptoms and a decrease in ventilatory function." Morgan (34), pp. 540-541.

36. Several physicians took the side of miners in the black lung controversy, arguing that the degree of respiratory disability does not correlate with X-ray stages of CWP and that disability in miners with simple CWP is often occupationally related. Some explained this phenomenon by hypothesizing that the disease process is pulmonary vascular in nature, i.e. it affects the small vessels of the lungs, impairing their ability to exchange gases with the bloodstream. See Hyatt, R. E., Kistin, A. D., and Mahan, T. K. Respiratory disease in southern West Virginia coal miners. *Am. Rev. Resp. Dis.* 89(3): 387-401, 1964. See also Rasmussen, D. L., et al. Respiratory impairment in southern West Virginia coal miners. *Am. Rev. Resp. Dis.* 98(10): 658-667, 1968.

37. This is a line from a famous song by Florence Reese, "Which Side Are You On?", inspired by the mine wars in Harlan County, Kentucky, during the 1930s.

38. Author's interview with disabled coal miner, Logan County, West Virginia, September 6, 1978.

39. Author's interview with disabled coal miner, Raleigh County, West Virginia, September 19, 1978.

40. Author's interview with working coal miner, Raleigh County, West Virginia, August 24, 1978.

41. Author's interview with disabled coal miner, Raleigh County, West Virginia, September 19, 1978.

42. By 1978, approved claims exceeded 420,000, and amendments enacted in that year are pushing the total even higher. This does not mean, however, that eligibility requirements will not be tightened in the future. Indeed, the current trend is to do so. See General Accounting Office. *Legislation Allows Black Lung Benefits To Be Awarded without Adequate Evidence of Disability.* Report to the Congress. Government Printing Office, Washington, D.C., 1980.

CHAPTER 3

The Health Effects of Low-Dose Radiation on Atomic Workers

A Case Study of Employer-Directed Research

Theodor D. Sterling

The distribution of health services and benefits is very much influenced by political and socioeconomic conditions. Navarro (1) has shown that access to many health care resources, especially those determining the types of health problems to which major efforts and facilities are allocated, has a distribution that reflects the location of wealth and political power rather than of need.

One facet of political impact on the use of medical resources is the relationship of production methods to the health and safety of employees. A number of economic and political (along with medical) factors combine to affect the degree of hazards in the workplace to which employees are exposed.

First, there is a strong correlation between production costs and safety in the workplace. For instance, Threshold Limit Values (TLVs) are determined as much by the cost of the implementing technology as they are by the effects of chronic exposure. Large industries have been known to relocate, or threaten to do so, when costs of reducing harmful exposures to workers were felt to be excessive (2-4).

An earlier version of this paper—A Moral Problem for Science: The Hanford Study of Atomic Workers—was delivered at the Conference on Health Implications of New Energy Technology, April 4, 1979, at the Rocky Mountain Center for Occupational Health, Park City, Utah.

Second, management has political power. Representatives of management not only serve in central decision-making posts, but management groups are active consultants and advisors to various government agencies. At the same time, the exercise of government authority (through regulating agencies) over industrial practices is curbed and shaped by the threat of possible adverse outcomes, e.g. unemployment, which are politically feared (5). The influence management may have, in and out of government, on restraining job-related safety measures was vividly demonstrated during the early days of the Occupational Safety and Health Administration (OSHA) and the National Institute of Occupational Safety and Health (NIOSH). Opposition by some industries to these two agencies affected their levels of funding, and there was strong evidence that OSHA failed to promulgate or implement "unpopular" standards in response to industry protests (2).[1]

Third, decisions at all levels of policy and practice are formed by health professionals (physicians, industrial hygienists, industrial toxicologists, etc.) who, for the most part, are employed by industry and culturally, economically, and socially belong to the management strata of society. Thus, many health professionals not only work for management but also *think* like management (1).

It is therefore reasonable to infer that research related to the health of the workplace is often influenced by considerations other than health, by considerations of the possible effect of the results of such research on industrial processes, especially on their costs. Indeed, in the early days of capitalism, when employers controlled all resources in society, very little (if any) research related to health and safety in the workplace.[2]

However, once the existence of hazards in the workplace has been demonstrated, this fact takes on a political reality and pressure of its own. There are relatively independent loci of influence in society that insist on a more equitable evaluation of health factors. The health of workers is, in itself, a strong motivation for action by those government forces responsible for the health of the overall population. More to the point, issues pertaining to the health of workers lend themselves to political manipulations by contesting forces (e.g. industry, regulatory agencies, unions) within the existing power structure. For objective reasons, there also is a great deal of community interest in the hazards of the workplace. In many ways, the industrial worker serves as a guinea pig for the rest of society. He is the first to experience the hazards of many substances to which the total community subsequently will be exposed and experiences these hazards under much more intense conditions than will others.

---

[1] One of the most blatant examples of the interaction of regulating agencies with business interests was uncovered among the papers of the Committee to Re-elect President Nixon. A memorandum from OSHA's chief administrator to the election committee suggested that the committee use, as one of its arguments for soliciting campaign contributions, the promise that OSHA would not promulgate "controversial standards" (e.g. for cotton dust) and so point out the desirability of "four more years of properly managed OSHA." (6)

[2] Until late in the 19th century, the employer's attitude was that workmen contracted for their labor and, as independent contractors, incidentals such as their health were their own problem. Much of this type of thinking is preserved in the orientation of many health professionals who view disease as a self-inflicted consequence of personal habits such as smoking, drinking, and faulty nutrition, rather than as a result of exposure to harmful substances in the community or to hazardous work (1, 7).

Thus, the fact that coke oven workers have a high incidence of lung cancer indicates that exposures to volatile fumes from carbonization will be instrumental in causing that disease in the population at large, albeit at a lesser incidence rate than among workers on and around coke ovens.

A dilemma may thus be created for industrial managers. On the one hand, demonstrations of health hazards in the workplace lead to increased production costs and government interference. On the other hand, there are forces in society that press toward regulation of industrial procedures once it becomes known that certain industrial practices are hazardous. One way in which management may deal with this conflict is by controlling the investigations that are carried out on the health of employees. That such controls are occasionally exercised has been suspected by some health workers, but substantive evidence for that suspicion has been difficult to come by. For that reason, the recently uncovered conflicts of interest relating to an investigation into the effects of low-dose radiation on workers at the Hanford Atomic Plant in Washington State provide valuable lessons for health professionals interested in the equitable distribution of health services. I am referring, of course, to the investigation initiated in 1965 by Dr. Thomas Mancuso of the School of Public Health at the University of Pittsburgh. That study followed workers at the Hanford plant and determined the causes of death in relation to levels of exposure in the Hanford Atomic Works (8, 9).

The 15-year history of that investigation demonstrates the workings of a number of powerful political factors. The purpose of the study was primarily political and economic. It was thought that the study could not possibly uncover adverse health effects, if such effects should in fact exist. The expectation was instead that the study would furnish proof to employees that their exposure levels were not harmful to their health. When it turned out that the Mancuso study was in danger of showing an increase of cancers among Hanford employees, control over the study was transferred from the independent, university-based investigator to the employer. Since then, publicly released analysis of the Hanford data reported by statisticians in the employ of management has been so construed that no health effects appear among Hanford workers as a function of low-dose radiation, even though others have shown that cancer rates have indeed increased among Hanford employees.

HIGHLIGHTS OF A PUBLIC HEALTH INVESTIGATION

Early understandings of the effects of radiation were based on the mortality patterns of Hiroshima and Nagasaki survivors and on the incidence of cancer among populations treated with X-ray therapy. Based on early observations, over a time span now thought to be inadequate, 5 r (rads) or less per year generally was assumed to be a "safe" exposure level.[3] Sparing accidents, a worker at the Hanford plant could expect an exposure level of less than 5 r in a one-year period.

Two features of the follow-up study of Hanford workers proposed by Mancuso were at variance with "good" research design. In the first place, Mancuso proposed

[3] An average chest X-ray has an approximate whole-body exposure of .025 r.

to test the health effects of exposure levels which were generally believed to be safe. In the second place, the number of employees working at Hanford was relatively small. Given the belief that a yearly exposure of 5 r was safe, the number of workers available for follow-up was thought to be too few to detect any possible small effects due to radiation, in the event there was such an effect after all. In general, studies which have too few individuals to detect an experimental condition are termed "inadequate." (See, for instance, reference 10.)

Nevertheless, the study was funded through the Atomic Energy Commission (AEC). The purpose of funding the study apparently was not to detect any adverse effects of the exposure to which Hanford workers were subjected. It was firmly believed by all scientific advisors and by management that the study design was not adequate to lead to such findings. Rather, the study was implemented and supported for frankly admitted *political* reasons. By not detecting an increase in cancer among Hanford workers, the study would serve to reassure employees that their safety was of concern to management and that management was monitoring the health effects of radiation levels to which they were chronically exposed. Thus, the study was an apparent ruse to demonstrate to the workers that the levels of radiation in the workplace would not result in disease.

These two major aspects of the study (its inadequate design and its political purpose) were frankly discussed in a number of memorandums which were subsequently obtained from the files of the AEC and Department of Energy (DOE) through the Freedom of Information Act. For example, on November 13, 1967, a major study consultant from Harvard School of Public Health, Dr. B. MacMahon (who also served as the chairman of the Ad Hoc Advisory Committee to the Federal Radiation Council of the National Academy of Science), wrote to Dr. L. A. Sagan, then contract officer for the AEC (11):

> In my opinion this study does not have, never did have, and never (in any practical sense) will have, any possibility of contributing to knowledge of radiation effects in man.... I recognize that much of the motivation for starting this study arose from the "political" need for assurance that AEC employees are not suffering harmful effect.

Another consultant, Dr. W. M. J. Schull, a geneticist from the University of Michigan, wrote Sagan on November 8, 1967 (12):

> It seems to be highly probable that if one went through the mechanics of calculating the kinds of radiation effects which a study of the present magnitude might detect, one would be led to conclude that the undertaking is a hopeless one. However, as earlier recognized, it may have other merit in that it may provide a firmer basis for settlement of claims against the Atomic Energy Commission.

Similarly, a number of memorandums within the scientific management structure of AEC disclosed that both scientists and management were generally aware of the purposes of funding the Mancuso study. On November 20, 1967, Sagan summarized the findings of the Advisory Committee for Biology and Medicine to Dr. J. R. Totter, who was director of AEC's Division of Biology and Medicine (13):

> It was the unanimous opinion of the group that, aside from a certain "political" usefulness, it is very unlikely that new information on radiation effects will accrue from this study.

Similar memorandums were written throughout the years during which the study was supported. For instance, as late as February 11, 1971, Dr. R. D. Moseley, who was then chairman of the Advisory Committee for Biology and Medicine for the AEC, wrote to Glen T. Seaborg, its director, that the study would not produce valid information on low-dose radiation effects (14). Perhaps the situation was described most frankly by Dr. S. Marks, who succeeded Sagan as project officer for the Mancuso study. In a memo to Totter dated February 28, 1972, Marks wrote (15):

> This study probably will not confirm or refute any important hypothesis but should permit a statement to the effect that a careful study of workers in the industry has disclosed no harmful effects of radiation (if the results are negative as they are likely to be). That statement, supported by appropriate documentation, would seem to justify the existence of the study. A corollary statement could presumably be made about other similar exposed populations.

Note the conflicting contention of the first sentence in this paragraph. On one hand it is acknowledged that "this study probably will not confirm or refute any important hypothesis," but on the other hand it is noted that this same study "should permit a statement to the effect that a careful study of workers in the industry had disclosed no harmful effects of radiation." It would be difficult to state with more honesty the true purpose of AEC's support of the Mancuso study.

In the end, two of the presuppositions underlying the funding of the Mancuso study turned out to be incorrect: (a) that there were definitely no radiation effects due to chronic exposure to low levels (5 r or less per year) of radiation; and (b) that the study's sample size was inadequate to detect such an effect if it should exist. However, the possible increase in cancers among Hanford workers was not detected by Dr. Mancuso. His study protocol aimed to correlate causes of death to monitored radiation levels over a prolonged period of time. That data had not yet been completely collected or analyzed when, quite accidentally, Dr. Sam Milham, from the State of Washington Department of Social and Health Services, stumbled in 1974 on an increased cancer incidence among Hanford workers. Dr. Milham had surveyed proportional morbidity by occupation of citizens in Washington (16). Among the occupations that showed a heightened incidence of cancer were atomic workers, almost all of whom worked at the Hanford plant. As Milham had conducted his study for purposes other than to test the effects of low-dose radiation,[4] he brought his findings, in person, to the attention of scientists and AEC representatives at the Hanford plant.

While the Hanford plant is under the management of a number of collaborating companies, Battelle Northwest Laboratories (now Pacific Northwest Laboratories) is actually the major employer responsible for both measuring the effects of radiation on workers and for their health. Since 1964, AEC (and later DOE) has contracted with Battelle for operation and management of the Hanford Laboratories, including extensive research and development programs as well as continuation of the Hanford plant radiation dosymmetry program (17). AEC representatives turned to management at Battelle with the request to undertake a *covert* study to verify Dr. Milham's claims.

---

[4] Dr. Milham has made many contributions to the study of health effects of wood processing on workers in the wood industry. His discovery of heightened cancer rates among Hanford atomic workers thus was not within his major area of interest.

Contrary to usual custom, no bids were put out for such a study. In fact, no written request was made. Battelle management apparently responded to the concerns expressed during discussions with AEC management. A check of Milham's findings was conducted by Dr. Alpen. Alpen's findings confirming Milham's were imparted in a number of memorandums from a Mr. A. G. Fremling and a Mr. R. P. Fasulo to central AEC management in July 1975. Fasulo noted (18):

> The message of Dr. Alpen's draft is clear that Battelle data suggest that Hanford has a higher proportion of cancer deaths for those under 65 than the United States as a whole or than the State of Washington as a whole.

And again (19):

> But even more disturbing from our standpoint is that in Battelle's analysis of incidence of cancer within the Hanford employees who had been exposed to varying amounts of radiation, the analysis tends to show a much higher incidence of certain types of cancers among those who have had 6 r and above throughout their lifetime.

And again (20):

> From this, Battelle, in the report, concludes that they have established that there is a relationship between cancer as a cause of death and a total external dose of radiation received, even though the exposures have been without [sic] their permissible amount. The relationship is particularly pronounced for lung cancer. In essence, where we are is that we hoped to get a good answer to the Milham report, and, instead, it looks that we have support for it.

At that point, moves were instituted to remove Mancuso from the study, or rather to remove the study from Mancuso. Administrative reasons cited for that action were later examined by the Subcommittee on Health and Environment of the Committee on Interstate and Foreign Commerce (21). In summary, the reasons given for removing Dr. Mancuso were that: (a) he was about to retire; (b) he had failed to publish his findings; and (c) his scientific peers had recommended limiting, terminating, or selecting another investigator in his place.

However, Congressional hearings brought out quite an opposite set of facts. Dr. Mancuso was not about to retire. An internal memorandum of the Department of Energy actually praised Mancuso for not "prematurely" publishing earlier positive findings of increased cancer rates among Hanford employees. Moreover, a peer review committee had actually recommended continuation rather than termination of Mancuso's contract (17). It is probably more correct to assume that the contract was removed from Dr. Mancuso because of his record of publications of health hazards in the chemical, chromate and rubber industries on the effects of beta-naphthylamine, benzidine, and asbestos. There is no doubt, given Mancuso's distinguished record of occupational health work, that his name would lend considerable credibility to a study that showed no effects of low-dose radiation to atomic workers. It is also clear from Mancuso's record that if he would have discovered what Milham found earlier and Battelle had verified, he would vigorously have published his findings and been just as convincing about them.

The transfer of the investigation apparently was done to give the employer control over the collection of further data and the dissemination of results. The study was first transferred to the so-called Oak Ridge University group, and then to Battelle

Northwest. In the meantime, Dr. Marks, who was previously project officer for the Mancuso study, moved from his position at the Department of Energy to Battelle, where he is now, along with Dr. Gilbert, the scientist responsible for the conduct of the study.

In a number of publications (22, 23), Drs. Gilbert and Marks have written that no detectable effects due to radiation exposure can be found among Hanford workers. Two aspects of these reports are of interest. First, no use is made of previous work by Milham (although a reference to his work is included by Marks) or of the data on which the internal memorandums of Alpen had been based, both of which verify a higher-than-average proportional mortality ratio for Hanford workers when compared to other occupations and groups in the State of Washington. Second, their analysis differs from that by Kneale, Mancuso, and Stewart (9) in several important aspects, most noticeably in not relating cancer among radiosensitive tissues to internal measures of radiation penetration, especially radiation bioassays of urine. Thus, not only is the continuation of the Hanford investigation in the hands of the employer, but the analysis of data appears to be designed to at least play down the possible effects due to radiation.[5,6]

DISCUSSION

The public record of the Mancuso affair offers a rare opportunity to observe the political process through which occupational health studies may be managed. Of course, it is not known how many other important investigations were thus managed, diverted from their original goal, suppressed, or used for political purposes. However, the ease with which AEC, DOE, and Battelle managers exercised their control over the Mancuso investigation would suggest that they were honoring a practice not distinguished by being unusual.

What made the Mancuso affair different from other similar incidents and may have led to the disclosure of management manipulations was Dr. Mancuso's strong support among labor unions. It was the protest of the unions with whom Mancuso has worked on other occasions—most notably, of the International Association of Machinists and Aerospace Workers and the Oil, Chemical and Atomic Workers International Union—which, in conjunction with the Nader group of public-service-oriented attorneys, forced public hearings on the affair itself.[7]

---

[5] It is not my purpose here to analyze the existing wealth of data on low-dose radiation effects. Nevertheless, the lesson may be to examine with some suspicion adversary positions taken by scientists and statisticians who are employed by DOE at Battelle. Justification for this suspicion appears, for example, in the failure of either Marks or Gilbert to refer to Alpen's work. Yet Alpen worked for Battelle Northwest, as do Marks and Gilbert! Surely the fact that a Battelle scientist had originally checked and verified Milham's findings is of relevance.

[6] A review by Hutchison et al. (26), appearing in September 1979, was published too late to be included here. However, this review fails to resolve conflicting claims about the same data.

[7] The pressure from unions and the Nader group may have actually forced reconsideration of Dr. Mancuso's status as principal investigator. Apparently in response to pressure exerted on him by labor, former Secretary of Health Joseph A. Califano directed Dr. William Foege, Director of the Center for Disease Control, and Dr. Anthony Robbins, Director of the National Institute of Occupational Safety and Health, to contact Mancuso and request that he submit a proposal to continue and complete the study which he had begun with the Department of Energy (24).

One lesson that emerges from this incident is that labor may need to take a stronger hand than in the past in all aspects of the management of health resources, including and starting with health-directed investigations. The Mancuso affair demonstrates that society cannot rely upon an ethic of health professionals to equitably investigate and disseminate results of studies on possible work hazards.[8] It may be useful, therefore, to write specifications for proper health investigations directly into negotiated contracts. Or it may be required that labor unions develop their own research resources and negotiate the right to investigate working conditions, again as part of overall work condition settlements.

There is also a lesson here relating to the accountability of health officials. It is clear that scientists are not held accountable for their actions. There are no mechanisms by which scientists who participate in promoting investigations which they know, or suspect, will not result in findings useful to the health of employees but which will primarily serve political purposes can be held accountable. Similarly, there is no way to force scientists to publish findings that would be contrary to the interests of management. The work of scientists under conditions of conflicts of interest is in no way restricted. In fact, most studies on workers' health are conducted by management-supported medical staffs.

Yet, the honest and equitable action of scientists needs to be assured. Rational and public-oriented health policy emerges more and more as a resultant vector generated by opposing forces. It is only when labor or environmentally oriented citizens dispute the claims of industry that facts relating to the health of the total community seem to surface and influence decisions about public health policies. One precondition of rational public health policy may be the establishment of an adversary process, ensuring that environmental and labor interests are properly represented in the health-policy-setting process. But the proper representation of adversary arguments relies upon an assumption of the basic honesty and integrity of the scientists and health professionals who help form them. In turn, it is difficult to see how the merit of scientific contributions can be evaluated if there is no accountability for scientists whose work is dishonest, incompetent, or both. Perhaps the time has come to legislate fines, and even jail sentences, for public actions by scientists and health professionals which are detrimental to the health of the public. After all, in law lies the final resort for enforcing responsible behavior of citizens and, if public health scientists cannot formulate a code of ethics of their own, then their conduct may have to be regulated through legal means.

The lessons from Hanford may not be restricted to health professionals. What of the role of management? Certainly the design and execution of health investigations are not within the purview of managing an industry. It is useless, therefore, to rail against the role of management in protecting its operations against inefficient and costly encroachments to satisfy extraneous health criteria or, at least, in carefully

---

[8] Most scientists in the Western world, and probably in many countries with more autocratic governments, seem to adhere to a sort of oral tradition of freely disseminating results. One factor fostering openness in science may rest in the circumstance that scientific claims are not creditable unless they are public. But there are no "codified" ethics governing scientific behavior with respect to collection and dissemination of findings, even in the health sciences.

examining the need for these encroachments. As long as professional health workers can be found who will tell management what management wants to hear (which often is that extra expenditures are not required because of possible health reasons), it would be useless to wait for management to become overly zealous in guarding the health of its employees. Nevertheless, the action of management needs closer scrutiny. Here, perhaps, an educational rather than a legal approach might be considered.

It appears to me that one difficulty lies in the reaction of management to the discovery of health problems among its employees. Two models of response can be delineated. The first, the *cooperative* model, seeks to determine the sources of problems and the ways and means to eliminate them. The second, the *competitive* model, seeks to dispute the existence of health effects and attempts to manipulate information in such a way that these health effects are made to disappear—at least in the short run. Management followed the competitive rather than the cooperative model in the Mancuso affair. However, it is questionable whether there were any gains to management from following such a course. After all, the operation of the Hanford and similar plants is largely tax-supported, and increases in costs of operation do not necessarily detract from profits or judgments of operational efficiency. Thus, to acknowledge difficulties in operation and to devise procedures to decrease exposure of workers to penetrating radiation would not have conflicted with other management aims. It is quite possible that the reaction of management to the discovery of health hazards was a reflex preference of the competitive to the cooperative model. It would seem that an educational effort may be the only solution, short of holding management responsible for not conducting properly conceived scientific investigations.

REFERENCES

1. Navarro, V. The underdevelopment of health of working America: Causes, consequences and possible solutions. *Am. J. Public Health* 66: 538-547, 1976.
2. Ashford, N. *Crisis in the Work Place.* MIT Press, Cambridge, Mass., 1976.
3. Berman, D. M. *Death on the Job.* Monthly Review Press, New York, 1978.
4. Stellman, J. M., and Daum, S. M. *Work Is Dangerous to Your Health.* Pantheon Press, New York, 1973.
5. Lindblum, C. E. *Politics and Markets.* Basic Books, New York, 1977.
6. A.F.L.-C.I.O. G. C. Guenther letter. *Facts and Analysis,* July 22, 1974.
7. Sterling, T. Does smoking kill workers or working kill smokers? *Int. J. Health Serv.* 8: 437-452, 1978.
8. Mancuso, T. F. Radiation exposures of Hanford workers dying from cancer and other causes. *Health Physics* 33: 369-384, 1977.
9. Kneale, C. W., Mancuso, T. F., and Stewart, A. M. A Cohort Study of the Cancer Risks from Radiation to Workers at Hanford. Paper presented at the Annual Meeting of the American Association for the Advancement of Science, Houston, Texas, January 1979 (in press).
10. Sterling, T., and Pollack, S. *Introduction to Statistical Data Processing.* Prentice Hall, Englewood Cliffs, N.J., 1968.
11. MacMahon, B. Letter to L. A. Sagan, November 13, 1967.
12. Schull, W. M. J. Letter to L. A. Sagan, November 8, 1967.
13. Sagan, L. A. Memorandum to J. R. Totter, November 20, 1967.
14. Moseley, R. D. Letter to G. T. Seaborg, February 11, 1971.
15. Marks, S. Footnotes to Brief Report by Dr. Mancuso (memorandum), February 1972.
16. Milham, S. Occupational Mortality in Washington State, 1950-1971. National Institute for Occupational Safety and Health Publication No. 76-175-A, Washington, D.C., 1976.
17. Rogers, P. G. Letter to J. R. Schlesinger, May 4, 1978.
18. Fasulo, R. P. Draft note to files on Milham/Mancuso occupational radiation exposure studies, July 1, 1975.

19. Fasulo, R. P. Draft note to files on further developments in Mancuso/Milham studies, July 21, 1975.
20. Fremling, A. G. Draft replies, July 17, 1975.
21. *Effects of Radiation on Human Health. Effects of Ionizing Radiation.* Vol. 1. Hearings before the Subcommittee on Health and the Environment of the Committee on Interstate and Foreign Commerce, U.S. House of Representatives, 95th Congress, Second Session, Serial Number 95-179, January 24-26 and February 8, 9, and 28, 1978. U.S. Government Printing Office, Washington, D.C., 1978.
22. Marks, S., Gilbert, E., and Breitenstein, D. Cancer Mortality in Hanford Workers. Vienna, International Atomic Energy Agency, SM-224-509, 1978.
23. Gilbert, E. S. Mortality of Hanford Radiation Workers. Paper presented at the Environmental Health Conference on Health Implications of New Energy Technology, Rocky Mountain Center for Occupational Health, Park City, Utah, April 4, 1979.
24. Califano, J. A. Letter to M. Bancroft (Public Citizens Litigation Group), February 1, 1979.
25. Hutchison, G. B., MacMahon, B., Jablon, S., and Land, C. E. Review of report of radiation exposure of Hanford workers. *Health Physics* 37: 207-220, 1979.

PART 2

The Nature of
Work and Health

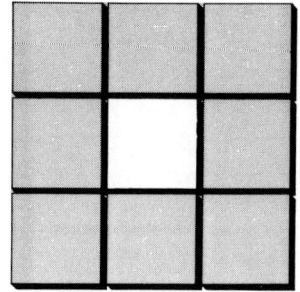

CHAPTER 4

Work and General Psychological and Physical Well-Being

David Coburn

The theme of a recent Canadian conference was "Life-style—Freedom of Choice," referring to life-style in relationship to health or well-being. The stimulus for much of the recent concern with life-style has arisen from the Lalonde Report, *A New Perspective on the Health of Canadians* (1). This is in one respect unfortunate because the Lalonde Report, while obviously an advance over previous unicausal examinations of health and illness, has not yet received critical evaluation. In particular, it would be premature and misleading to accept the Lalonde classification of life-style (versus environment) as that over which the individual exercises control or can make choices because the degree to which individuals really have "choices" is a matter of dispute. Freedom of choice in the health field is an area for study rather than one on which to base a classificatory schema. Inasmuch as the degree of choice is in question, assigning events to "environment" or to "life-style" components of the health field concept is a hazardous and arbitrary undertaking.

Furthermore, while the Lalonde Report may contain a "new perspective," it

A draft of this paper was presented at the Canadian Public Health Association annual meeting held at Vancouver, British Columbia in June 1977. The study on which this paper is based was supported in part by a U.S. Department of Health, Education, and Welfare Grant (No. CH00235) to the Health Services Research Center, Kaiser Foundation Hospitals, Portland, in part by the Social Science Research Center, University of Victoria, and in part by the Canada Council (S71-0407).

certainly is the embodiment of some old (Liberal Government) values. For example, the policy implications of the report have a largely individualistic bias in which such events as alcohol addiction, smoking, drug abuse, over-eating, malnutrition, and lack of exercise are all attributed to "self-imposed" risks, and in which the health education and health promotion of individuals appears as a strong component (1, pp. 16-17).

The health field concept also produces a fragmented rather than a holistic picture of health problems—each must be accommodated under one, or a combination, of the headings of human biology, environment, life-style, and health care organization. The interrelationships among these categories and the interaction between individuals and their environments as determinants of health status and exposure to health risks are downgraded in importance.

Having said this, it is my contention that a person's job is an only partially voluntary aspect of life-style, or, more accurately, life-space, is closely tied to wider phenomena in the social structure such as the class system, and has important implications for workers' well-being. This paper tackles the last of these assertions, namely, the work-health linkage.

Although in recent years there has been a renewed interest by politicians and others in the study of occupational health in Canada, these concerns have focused primarily on noxious physical, chemical, or biological stimuli at work, on physical health, and on manual workers in industry. However, there is increasingly wide recognition among researchers that this focus is an excessively narrow one which, on the macro-level, neglects not only the political economy of work and health, but also (a) the psycho-social or sociotechnical aspects of the work environment as they influence health; (b) the influence of work on mental or psychological states as well as on physical health; and (c) occupational as opposed to industrial health, i.e. the fact that many types of jobs or professions (including the practice of medicine) entail health risks—manual workers in industry are not the only persons whose work influences their health (this broadening of emphasis is not to deny the prime importance of the protection of industrial workers from work hazards).

The main assumptions underlying this broader approach, one which has seen in recent years a worldwide revival, are: that man and his environment are in a symbiotic, interactive relationship; that everything a person does or experiences has psychological and physiological implications; that other people and organizations are an important part of an individual's environment; and that much of our present environment is man-made and to some extent modifiable. The notion of adaptation as used by Dubos (2) conveys most of the essence of this new approach (or revival of an old approach). Selye puts the interaction of man in environment as follows: "Adaptation to our surroundings is one of the most important physiologic reactions in life: one might even go so far as to say that the capacity of adjustment to external stimuli is the most characteristic feature of live matter" (3).

One of the prime questions at issue, of course, is precisely the notion of adjustment, i.e. should we (or can we) adjust the environment or the individual? This question brings up the problem of the degree of man's malleability and the extent to which man has certain inherent characteristics, the violation of which contravenes his basic nature, producing either distortion of "normal" development or deleterious moral or health consequences. While far beyond our current discussion, these problems will ultimately have to be faced in assessing various approaches to health and their underlying assumptions.

It is not necessary to document in detail the fact that in Canadian society, and in industrialized societies in general, the work role is a highly important one. Not only is work an area of life which might have general health implications, but also the time spent at work can itself be judged as desirable or undesirable. Assuming a 40-hour work week and 8 hours a day sleep, for example, 36 percent of a normal week's waking time is spent on-the-job and much of the remaining time revolves around preparing for work, getting to and from work, and human maintenance activities. Even apart from the influence of work on self-esteem or self-identity, it is through work that most Canadians seek to express their human potential, their contribution to society, and it is through work that they are tied in to the larger society. Work-life provides the setting in which individuals utilize general societal resources in exercising authority and manipulating physical, cultural, and human materials. Thus, time on-the-job is time free for production, time for people to be productive and creative. In assessing the influence of work on well-being, then, we must examine life on-the-job as well as work's more general effects.

The bored, frustrated automobile assembly-line worker, the pressured ulcer-ridden executive—these stereotypes depict man at opposite ends of the work complexity continuum. They indicate the radically different types of work environment that coexist in our society and emphasize their possible impact on the worker. Perhaps the most recent in a long line of speculations regarding the influence of work on health is that of Navarro (4), who follows Marx's concept of alienation in contending that: "A continuous process of alienation and frustration is created by the capitalist system that reflects itself in despair and much disease and unease." This is partly because work "serves not primarily as a source of creativity or self-expression, but rather as a means of obtaining one's satisfaction elsewhere . . ." and because of the "lack of control felt by the citizenry over their own work . . ." (4, p. 447). This concern with the effects of overly simple work is balanced by interest in the possibly stressful demands of highly complex jobs. Thus, at one end of the continuum we have possible alienation and frustration, at the other end we have stress.

Work might affect well-being on-the-job and/or off-the-job. It is also conceivable that work can effect health without the worker being aware of these effects, i.e. a man may have positive attitudes toward, and be satisfied with, a job which by other measures is having a deleterious influence on his well-being. Therefore, both work factors or characteristics of the job and work attitudes and feelings about work are examined here in their relationship to general well-being.

This is not the place to review extensively previous research on psychosocial aspects of work and health. For example, a list of publications from the Institute for Social Research at Ann Arbor, Michigan, alone, is 23 pages long. In brief, however, one of the prominent models of the work-health relationship is a Person times Environment (P × E) one in which the impact of work on health is hypothesized to be greater for those whose work (on a variety of dimensions, complexity, responsibility, etc.) is incongruent with their personal preferences, capacities, or needs (5-8). In general, research tends to confirm the hypothesis that routine, repetitive work leads to psychological symptomatology or to lower levels of mental health. Kornhauser (9) and Gardell (10) both note that the degree to which the worker finds the job satisfying (Kornhauser) or interesting-monotonous (Gardell) mediates between objective job complexity and levels of mental health, i.e. it is perceptions of or reactions to work rather than objective job characteristics that are the prominent predictors of mental health. Assuming that feelings of satisfaction or interest-monotony reflect Person times Environment interaction, these latter findings also support the P X E model. The present paper examines both the joint and separate effects of work factors and work attitudes on feelings of worker well-being.

METHODS

Data were obtained from a questionnaire survey of male workers in Victoria, British Columbia in 1970. Usable questionnaires were returned by 1143 of 2180 men, for a response rate of about 52 percent. In the current analysis, however, several groups were omitted (self-employed men, men working 25 hours a week or less, and men on their current jobs less than one year), leaving a total of 780 men for analysis. This smaller number includes men in a variety of white- and blue-collar jobs from professionals and high-level government administrators to unskilled manual workers. It is the case, however, that the occupational structure in Victoria includes a lesser proportion of men in the most alienating jobs, i.e. industrial assembly-line work, than is typical of some other Canadian cities.

This study is part of a larger one which included, in addition to the above sample, interview and clinical record data on a sample of about 900 men, part of a random sample of families enrolled in the Kaiser Foundation Health Plan in Portland, Oregon. This paper focuses mainly on the results from the Victoria men, although supporting data from the Portland sample will be mentioned in passing. With the exclusions mentioned above, the final Portland sample size is 670.

Measures

We are faced with the task of measuring work factors, work attitudes, and general psychological and physical well-being. Variables included under these three main headings are indicated in Table 1.

There is as yet no generally agreed-upon way of dividing up a person's job into relatively few dimensions. In fact, even when we tried to do so empirically, factor analysis did not reveal a simpler and interpretable underlying set of factors which would adequately represent those listed in Table 1. The work factors included are those such as job control and variety which tap various aspects of job content or job tasks (intrinsic job factors) as well as those such as pay, job security, or the bureaucratic nature of the work organization, which reflect more the context within which job tasks are performed (extrinsic job factors). It should be emphasized that all of the job factors were taken from worker self-reports. Some of these are fairly straightforward items (how many hours a week do you work?), while others, such as the degree of control the worker experiences, involve some interpretation by the

Table 1

Listing of work and health variables included in the analysis

	Work Factors	Work Attitudes	Psychological and Physical Well-Being
1.	Career contingencies Job security Opportunity for promotion Years in present job	Job alienation[a] Job satisfaction[a] Job stress[a]	Psychological well-being Happiness Psychological symptoms[a] Physical well-being Self-assessed health Role incapacity[a]
2.	Work organization Degree of bureaucracy[a] Percentage of union members in workplace Union membership of respondent		
3.	Working conditions Nonsocial Indoor-outdoor Shift work Fringe benefits[a] Social Has fellow workers Meets the public		
4.	Job content Number of people supervised Physical demands Job control[a] Supervision by others[a] Variety[a] Chances of error Deadlines		
5.	Work overlap with family life[a]		
6.	Class-related Pay Job prestige		

[a] Indices formed of two or more items; otherwise, all single-item measures (see Appendix).

respondent. We are thus dealing mainly with worker perceptions rather than objectively measured factors of the job.

Turning to job attitudes, three main concepts have been used to assess the immediate impact of a person's job, namely, satisfaction or job morale, alienation, and stress. Measures of these concepts were formed consisting of two or three individual questionnaire items (see the Appendix). Although the other two measures are largely self-explanatory, it must be pointed out that the alienation index is a subjective measure referring to the degree to which the worker finds the job monotonous/interesting and nonchallenging/challenging (as opposed to various other objective or subjective conceptions of alienation).

How does one measure health, or, as the World Health Organization puts it, well-being? Not only do varying ways of measuring physical health *not* highly intercorrelate, but the conceptualization and measurement of mental health or psychological well-being are even more complex and disputed. While the indices used here do not have a well-developed history of validity and reliability, they do encompass the range of concerns usually included in definitions of health while also meeting certain logical criteria.

An index of psychological well-being was constructed by combining (equally weighted) an item tapping self-assessed happiness (11) with a ten-item index measuring the number of psychological symptoms experienced ("psychological" items from the Langner index of psychophysiological symptomatology) (12, 13). That is, it is assumed that a person is high in psychological well-being if he is both happy and shows few psychological symptoms, and vice-versa.

Physical well-being was measured by combining (equally weighted) an item tapping self-assessed health with an index measuring the number of days in the past year of worker incapacitation because of health problems (disability days). (In Portland, an index measuring the number of symptoms experienced was used instead of disability days.) Those high on the physical well-being index were men describing themselves as healthy and as experiencing a low number of disability days in the past year, and vice-versa.

The correlations between the psychological and physical well-being scales are moderate to low (Victoria $r = .26$; Portland $r = .37$), indicating only partial overlap between the two. One might, of course, expect that the relationships between the two aspects of well-being might be casual (in either direction), i.e., men in poor physical health might experience lower psychological well-being or vice-versa.

An overall well-being index combined (equally weighted) the above two indices.

Analysis

The basic model with which we can begin the discussion is shown in Figure 1. It is assumed that certain facets of work tend to produce certain work attitudes, which in turn influence workers' general psychological and physical well-being. This model must be elaborated in facing some of the problems of causal inference regarding the work-nonwork relationships. Given the cross-sectional nature of the data, it is impossible to make firm causal conclusions. We can, however, attempt to infer

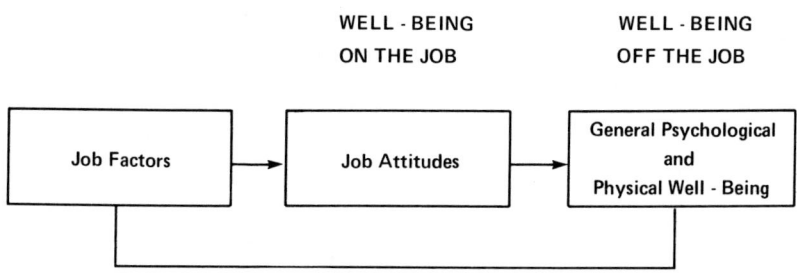

Figure 1. Effects of work on health.

causation by eliminating the chief competing hypotheses regarding the work-health link, leaving the "work produces well-being" hypothesis as the most plausible.

It might be claimed that any correlations found between work and general well-being are due to selection factors, to possible spurious relationships, to measurement artifacts, or to factors in the work environment not explicitly included in the analysis, e.g. physically noxious stimuli. The chief alternative explanations to the "work effects health" hypothesis are as follows:

1. Less psychologically or physically healthy men are selected into particular types of jobs (e.g. those low in income, prestige, variety, control, etc.).
2. Various nonwork concurrent life conditions or personal characteristics are producing spurious relationships between work type and health.
3. Since one of the dependent variables includes items tapping health or illness behavior rather than health status (disability days in the Victoria sample) it is a measure of the former rather than the latter.
4. The work-health correlations are caused by co-varying physical, chemical, or biological noxious stimuli rather than by the various job conditions we have measured.
5. Lowered general well-being produces a more pessimistic view of the job rather than vice-versa.

A series of indices was constructed to test alternative hypotheses 1 to 3. These included pre-job or background variables such as age, education, social origins (father's socioeconomic status (SES)), self-assessed childhood health, size of family of origin, Canadian versus foreign birth, and an index tapping factors predisposing the individual to experience stress (negative background index) (hypotheses 1 and 2). Concurrent life characteristics included marital status, number of financial dependents, length of time in the Victoria area, propensity to see a physician, religion and religiosity (hypotheses 2 and 3).

The model with which we began, then, must be expanded to include the first three possible alternative explanations (Figure 2).

Our first task is to identify the key determinants of the job attitudes (satisfaction, alienation, stress). Next, we examine the influence of the work factors and work attitudes on general well-being. We then use step-wise multiple regression in estimating

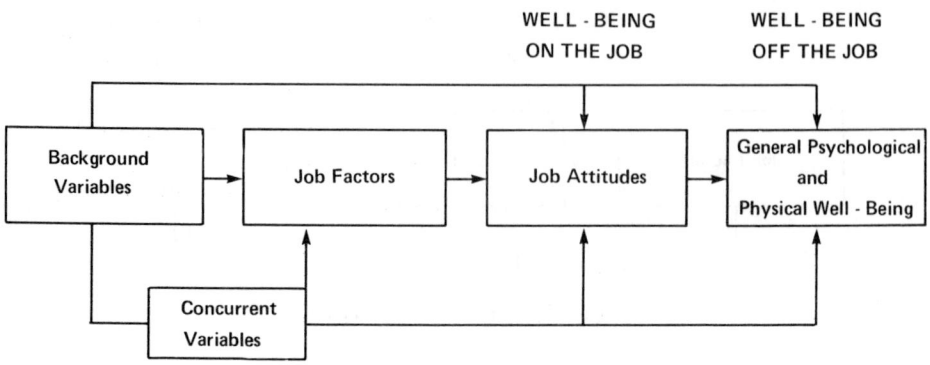

Figure 2. An expanded model of the effects of work on health.

the additional percentage variance explained by the job factors and the job attitudes over and above that accounted for by the thirteen control variables. This procedure is a very conservative one, since it allows the control variables to account for as much of the variance in the well-being variables as they can, and then asks how much of the leftover variance is accounted for by the work factors and attitudes. Finally, a test is made of the likelihood of the final two alternative hypotheses, i.e. the influence of other noxious stimuli and the possibility of a causal direction the reverse of that hypothesized.

It is assumed that most of the important relationships between work and health will be revealed using a linear model. Tests of this assumption using Multiple Classification Analysis (14), a technique which makes no assumptions of linearity, showed few substantial improvements in predictive ability, hence regression techniques are used throughout.

FINDINGS

Before examining the influence of the various job factors on the three job attitudes, the interrelationships among the job attitudes themselves are of interest. Table 2 indicates that men who find their work interesting and challenging tend also to be satisfied with their jobs. Yet interesting work brings with it a good deal of stress. On the other hand, feelings of stress are unrelated to job satisfaction. The stress levels of men satisfied with their jobs are about the same as those of the less-satisfied men.

The relationships shown are remarkably similar for both the workers from Victoria and those from Portland. The alienation-satisfaction correlation is also close to that shown between boredom and satisfaction, $r = .63$, among a sample of workers in the United States (7).

How widespread are feelings of discontent or job strain in this population of working men? Eighteen percent are undecided or dissatisfied with their jobs (Portland, 16 percent), 14 percent say they dislike their jobs or like them only a little, while 47 percent state they would choose a different type of job if they could start all over again. Thirteen percent feel their jobs are mostly dull and monotonous or worse, while

Table 2

Interrelationships of alienation, job satisfaction, and stress (Pearson r's)

	Satisfaction	Stress
Alienation (monotonous-interesting)	-.60 (-.58)[a]	-.32 (-.33)
Satisfaction (satisfied-dissatisfied)	—	.07 (.02)
Stress (high-low)	—	—

[a] Correlations in the Portland sample.

32 percent state their jobs subject them to a great deal of stress (Portland, 33 percent). Combining responses, we find the following percentages:

Monotonous *or* dislike, 18 percent
Monotonous *or* dissatisfaction, 24 percent
Monotonous *or* different type of work, 56 percent
Monotonous *or* different type of work *or* high stress, 72 percent

Taking into account differences in response categories, these findings are similar to those shown in both Canadian and U.S. national samples (15, 16). The data also indicate that the extent of job discontent is highly dependent on question wording and on the stringency of the criteria of discontent used.

Which job dimensions best predict satisfaction, alienation, and stress, our measures of well-being on the job? Controlling for all other job factors, four facets of the job stand out as having the greatest independent influence on job satisfaction and on feelings of alienation, namely: prestige, control, variety, and opportunity for promotion. But a wider variety of different job factors effect feelings of stress, the two strongest referring to the number of deadlines experienced and the degree to which the job is perceived as interfering with one's family life (Table 3).

Table 3

Influence of work factors on work attitudes (standardized partial regression coefficients)

Alienation		Satisfaction		Stress	
Variety	-.39[a]	Prestige	.23	Deadlines	.21
Control	-.20	Control	.21	Work overlaps with family life	.17
Promotion	-.10	Variety	.20	Hours worked	.13
Prestige	-.08	Promotion	.13	Meets public	.12
				Chances of error	.11
R = .75		R = .56		R = .53	

Percent variance explained:
(adjusted)[b] = 54%   30%   26%

[a] All unstandardized betas at least two times the standard error.
[b] Adjusted for the number of variables included in the regression equation.

Certain types of job factors produce higher morale and different types produce stress. Whether or not low stress is a desirable or undesirable phenomenon is another question. While we might agree that interesting and satisfying work is desirable, could we also agree that a low-stress job is attractive? Writers concerned with worker self-actualization would probably insist that a person needs a certain amount of stimulation and challenge in order to function effectively and in order to grow as a person. The mastery of potentially stressful situations in fact contributes to individual growth and competence. It is that stress which a person cannot handle with the external and internal resources at his command that contributes to an unhealthy work situation. This leads us in turn to postulate, as others have, that felt stress is partly attributable to a lack of adequate resources or coping mechanism either within the person or in his environment and partly to the absolute levels of (objective) stressors. Furthermore, just as some psychosocial factors have been implicated as causes of stress, others, such as support provided by a positive family life or by an understanding work supervisor, have been said to mediate or muffle the effects of a stressful job (17). In order to assess fully the effects of work stressors, however, we need to know not only whether or not the worker experiences tensions but also whether or not work stressors have consequences independent of worker feelings of stress.

So far, we have been talking about those work factors which make an important independent contribution to the explanation of job satisfaction, alienation, and stress. Perhaps just as significant are aspects of the job which do not appear on this list. The most prominent omission is pay. In fact, neither pay nor, to a lesser extent, job security, are substantially associated with higher overall job satisfaction once we take into account the other job factors. These findings confirm other studies in indicating that in general populations money makes a relatively slight independent contribution to feelings of satisfaction.

What do the correlations given in Table 3 mean in percentage terms? Of the men fairly high or high on all four best predictors of satisfaction (prestige, control, variety, opportunity for promotion, $N = 69$), 64 percent are high in satisfaction compared to 5 percent for men low on the four job factors ($N = 41$). Similarly, less than 1 percent of those high in variety and control are high in subjective alienation, compared to 67 percent of the low variety and control workers. Finally, of those men who indicate that their work overlaps with their family lives and that their jobs have a lot of deadlines, 65 percent are high in stress compared to only 7 percent of the men low on the above two variables. These findings also indicate that results that appear moderate in "variance explained" terms can show striking effects when percentage differences are used.

Even though the set of work factors included in the analysis of the Portland sample was somewhat different from that analyzed in Victoria, the results are fairly congruent. Variety, opportunity for promotion, and prestige are strong predictors of job morale in Portland as in Victoria, along with decision making (Portland) and job control (Victoria). The Portland data again point to the lesser import of pay as an independent influence on morale. The perceived stressors did differ somewhat, with the four most important among the American men being decision making, hours worked per week, number of men supervised, and the degree to which the work was physically tiring.

Quite clearly then, in both samples, the determinants of satisfaction (and alienation) are different than those influencing felt stress. These two quite different syndromes or reactions to life on the job may also have differing consequences for the worker off the job.

INTERACTION MODEL

It is evident that a good deal of the variance in satisfaction and stress is left unexplained, and it has been claimed that a better predictor of job attitudes and other reactions to work is provided by examining both aspects of the work environment and aspects of the person conjointly. Regarding satisfaction, for example, the P X E model would take into account the fact that men low in need for control might be highly satisfied in a low job control situation while men high in need for control, in the same job, would be dissatisfied.

Ideally, as French and Kahn have pointed out (18), a testing of this thesis requires commensurate measures of the job and the person, e.g. degree of control versus the need for control. The current data do not permit this type of measurement. We can, however, by making certain assumptions, provide a tentative test of this hypothesis.

The background characteristics of the individual, his social origins (father's SES), and his level of education were assumed to reflect aspects of the person. Father's SES was taken to be a partial measure (or determinant) of expectations regarding the job environment, particularly regarding extrinsic job rewards. That is, the higher the father's SES, the higher the assumed needs or expectations for a high paying, high status, secure, etc., job. Education is somewhat more problematic in the sense that it more obviously reflects both aspects of preparation for work (worker abilities or capacities, inherited or learned) and needs and expectations. Which is to say, we cannot separate out various aspects or characteristics of the person. Higher educational attainment is simply assumed to indicate higher needs and expectations (regarding extrinsic job rewards) as well as greater worker preparation or abilities (referring more to intrinsic job factors).

In testing the P X E thesis, the major job factors were formed into three indices measuring job responsibilities (chances of error, deadlines, number of people supervised), job content (variety, control), and job rewards (pay, prestige, security). The zero-order correlations of these composite measures with the job attitudes in all instances were higher than those for corresponding measures tapping the incongruence or mismatching of education (or father's SES) with responsibilities, content, or rewards. Inspection of the cross-tabulations of groups incongruent regarding education and various job factors (all eight separate factors mentioned above) also showed no clear trends for the incongruent groups to show particularly high or low satisfaction or stress (the exceptions: low education/high pay men are highest in satisfaction; low education/high number of men supervised are highest in stress).

These findings, on the surface at least, tend to contradict the findings of previous researchers (7, 8). It should be pointed out, however, first, that the incongruency indices used here were relatively crude, and, second, that the present data do not exclude incongruence effects, they simply indicate that the main effects of the job factors themselves are much stronger than the incongruence effects. An additional explanation might be that as in a previous study, we found few workers to be in *highly* incongruent jobs (8).

WELL-BEING OFF THE JOB

Does a man's job, in its sociotechnical aspects, influence his general well-being? Is it true, as some have claimed, that what a man does on the job not only affects his work attitudes but also casts a pervasive shadow over his whole life and on his health? If so, what aspects of work are particularly important correlates of well-being?

Table 4 shows the relationships between the work factors (enumerated earlier) and the work attitudes and well-being, and the combined influence of the work factors and work attitudes on general psychological and physical well-being both before and after allowing the thirteen background and concurrent life condition variables to explain as much of the variance as they can. What Table 4 indicates is that, in absolute terms, work-life has a low but substantively important relationship with general well-being (we would expect findings of this magnitude by chance much less frequently than one time in a thousand). However, work-life, compared to most social science findings in the field of health and illness, is relatively quite a strong contributor to the experience of well-being.

And again we find percentage differences to be sizeable. For example, constructing an index of the four job factors best predicting overall well-being (prestige, security, work overlap, opportunity for promotion) plus the three job attitudes (alienation, satisfaction, stress), the 58 men high on the index (i.e. low on job prestige, high on alienation, etc.) show 66 percent low in overall well-being compared to only 11 percent low in well-being among the 55 men at the other end of the continuum.

The job variables are much more highly related to psychological than to physical well-being (primarily because of the strong relationship of the job attitudes to the general measures of psychological status). And, the job factors and attitudes retain a major portion of their co-variation with well-being even after the stringent control measures are introduced. With all variables in the analysis, work accounts for 62 percent of the *explained* variance regarding psychological well-being and 45 percent of the *explained* variance regarding physical well-being.

Which of the work factors are of particular importance? Table 5 indicates the most important work factors and the most important work attitudes (taking these two sets of work variables independently before and after introducing the control variables). In the case of psychological well-being, the two most important items are: (a) the degree to which the job overlaps with family life, or, in sociologists' terms, inter-role conflict; and (b) the prestige attached to the job, a self-esteem-related variable. Lower physical health is particularly related to working a lesser number of hours per week and to lower job security. In the case of hours worked, however, the causal direction is problematic, i.e. it seems more likely that poorer health leads to working a lesser number of hours per week than vice-versa. Omitting hours per week from the analysis, however, only slightly decreases the work/physical well-being relationship and does not substantially alter the order of the remaining variables.

Regarding job attitudes, a point of note is the low relationship of job satisfaction to psychological well-being and its negligible relationship to physical well-being once

Table 4

General well-being by job factors and job attitudes controlled on
13 background variables (percent variance explained (adjusted))

Job Variables	Psychological Well-Being		Physical Well-Being		Overall Well-Being	
	Zero-Order	Controlled	Zero-Order	Controlled	Zero-Order	Controlled
Job factors	9.9	7.3	6.1	3.4	10.8	5.0
Job attitudes	13.0	11.0	3.2	2.7	11.2	9.6
Factors plus attitudes	15.3	12.0	7.9	5.6	15.7	12.2
	R = .391		R = .281		R = .396	
Variance explained by all background and job variables		19.3		12.5		21.2

the other job attitudes are controlled. While lesser satisfaction has few implications for physical health, work perceived as monotonous and lacking in challenge does tend to be associated with lower health, although it is difficult here to separate health status from health behavior, i.e. the use of illness as a form of "escape" into the sick role. There is, of course, a good deal of overlap between alienation and satisfaction. Alienation as measured could even be considered a component of satisfaction rather than as an independent construct. And, omitting alienation from the analysis does increase the contribution of satisfaction; with alienation excluded in all instances satisfaction has a greater effect on well-being than does stress.

If we assume that the three job attitudes do reflect person times job matching, then person-job congruence is obviously an important correlate of psychological well-being and somewhat less of a concomitant of physical well-being. Part of the influence of the job factors on health is mediated through their effect on the job attitudes. However, some of the effect of the job factors on general well-being is direct rather than indirect. In particular, work overlap with family, job prestige, and security have important independent influences on psychological well-being, while hours worked and security have substantial independent influences on physical well-being.

Looking at the overall results (Table 6), it is interesting to note that the background characteristics, particularly childhood health and age, account for more of the variance regarding physical health than they do for psychological well-being, while concurrent life characteristics account for more of the variance regarding psychological than for physical well-being (although even here childhood health is the single most important variable). A person's psychological state is apparently more responsive to current events than is physical health while both mental and physical states are influenced by events during childhood.

We can now turn to the final two alternative hypotheses. Alternative hypothesis 4 postulated that the work-health correlations might be due more to the physical or

Table 5

Work factors and work attitudes related to general well-being (standardized partial regression coefficients)[a]

Psychological Well-Being			Physical Well-Being			Overall Well-Being		
Work factors			Work factors			Work factors		
Work overlaps	-.20[b]	(-.17)[c]	Hours	-.12[b]	(-.12)[c]	Prestige	.14[b]	(.13)[c]
Prestige	.15	(.14)	Security	.11	(.11)	Security	.14	(.14)
Security	.11	(.11)	Pay	.09	[d]	Work overlaps with family life	-.16	(-.13)
Variety	.09	(.09)	Promotion	.09	[d]	Promotion	.10	[d]
Control	.09	[d]	Length	.08	(.08)			
Promotion	[d]	(.08)						
Work attitudes			Work attitudes			Work attitudes		
Alienation	-.16	(-.12)	Alienation	-.18	(-.10)	Alienation	-.22	(-.13)
Satisfaction	.20	(.11)	Satisfaction	.02	(-.03)	Satisfaction	.14	(.05)
Stress	-.24	(-.21)	Stress	-.13	(-.18)	Stress	-.23	(-.25)

[a]All unstandardized betas at least twice the standard error except job satisfaction with physical well-being.
[b]Not controlled.
[c]Controlled on 13 pre-job and concurrent life characteristics (in parentheses).
[d]Instances in which the unstandardized betas are less than twice the standard error are omitted.

chemical work environment than to the psychosocial and sociotechnical work variables examined. That this is not a good explanation is indicated by data from analyses for white-collar and blue-collar men separately, the former presumably free from exposure to noxious stimuli. Work has a very similar impact (in size) for both white- and blue-collar men, approximately as large as for the sample as a whole.

Finally, does lower (psychological) well-being lead to more pessimistic views of work (alternative hypothesis 5) rather than work leading to lowered well-being? Two available crude objective measures of jobs, drawn from the *Dictionary of Occupational Titles* (D.O.T.) (19), classify jobs as repetitious and/or as lacking in autonomy. Those men whose perceptions of the degree of variety and autonomy (perceived job factors) differed widely from the *D.O.T.* assessment ($N = 140$) were eliminated from the sample and the analyses were rerun for the remaining 640 men. This sample presumably consists of men with an accurate perception of their jobs (i.e. those whose job perceptions are not strongly affected by general psychological well-being), yet again, work influences well-being much as before. The findings, therefore, do not seem to be caused by lower psychological well-being influencing perceptions of the job more than the reverse.

The magnitude of the influence of work on health, controlling for the background and concurrent life characteristics variables, is slightly less in the Portland sample than among the Victoria men (Table 6).

Finally, a word on one of the individual measures of psychological well-being, happiness. Multiple regression analyses reveal that, of all the background, concurrent, and work variables, the following have the greatest independent effect on general feelings of happiness: job prestige (standardized beta = .15); job satisfaction (beta = .14); work overlap with family life (beta = -.11); religiosity (beta = .11); and childhood health (beta = .10). Happiness, then, is a product of higher job prestige and satisfaction, having a job which does not interfere with one's family life, and interesting and less stressful work. Religious people tend to be happier than the nonreligious, and those having a healthier childhood are happier than those having

Table 6

Work variables and well-being controlling for background and concurrent life characteristics (additional percent variance explained with sets of variables introduced in order)

	Psychological Well-Being		Physical Well-Being		Overall Well-Being	
Background characteristics	4.8	(5.4)[a]	6.3	(9.3)	7.0	(9.2)
Concurrent characteristics	2.5	(3.4)	0.6	(0.0)	2.0	(1.8)
Job factors	7.3	(4.5)	3.4	(3.6)	7.0	(4.5)
Job attitudes	4.7	(3.6)	2.2	(2.2)	5.2	(4.5)
	R = .488		R = .416		R = .505	

[a] Portland results are given in parentheses.

Table 7

General happiness by job prestige (percentage "very happy")

	Job Prestige[a]					
Marital Happiness	Excellent		Good		Average or Poor	
Extremely happy	57.4	(54)	44.6	(148)	25.4	(67)
Pretty happy or not especially happy	37.2	(47)	12.6	(245)	4.1	(123)

[a] "Would you say people you know think of you as having: an excellent job . . . a poor job?" This item proved a better predictor of well-being than measures of *occupational* prestige.

Table 8

General happiness by job satisfaction (percentage "very happy")

	Job Satisfaction					
Marital Happiness	High		Medium		Low	
Happy	52.1	(96)	50.7	(67)	27.8	(108)
Pretty happy or not especially happy	28.3	(113)	10.7	(131)	4.0	(174)

the opposite experience (although these two relationships are not particularly strong). Excluding the job attitudes (satisfaction, alienation, stress) from the analysis leaves the remaining variables in the same order of importance. Incidentally, pay and job security have no independent effect on happiness, once other factors are taken into consideration. And, again controlling for other factors, to be married or to have higher educational attainments are associated with only miniscule increments in happiness. Even comparing the influence of the job variables on happiness with the effect of marital happiness (itself perhaps a partial product of work factors such as work overlap with family life) indicates the strong independent effect of the job (Tables 7 and 8).

SUMMARY AND IMPLICATIONS

A first step in establishing causal links between any elements of the environment, social or nonsocial, and well-being, is to demonstrate co-variation. The data presented support recent research in other countries indicating that various dimensions of work are indeed related to a worker's general psychological and physical well-being. The analysis, I believe, also warrants the further inference that the work conditions described do indeed produce variations in general well-being, particularly regarding psychological status.

We found that satisfaction/alienation and stress are two differing modes of response to the job. The intercorrelations of these two work attitudes are low and their chief determinants differ. The degrees of variety and control men experience are particularly strong predictors of satisfaction and alienation, while number of deadlines and overlap of work with family life are prime causes of work stress.

The work factors explain 7-10 percent of the variance in psychological well-being (maximum = uncontrolled, minimum = controlled on background and concurrent variables) and 3-6 percent of the variance in physical well-being. Job factors and job attitudes combined explain 12-15 percent of the variance in psychological well-being, 6-8 percent in physical well-being, and 12-16 percent in overall well-being.

The degree to which work overlaps with family life (negatively) and job prestige best predict higher psychological well-being, while hours worked per week (negatively) and job security best predict higher physical well-being. Work stress is a (relatively) strong predictor of all three health indices as is, to a lesser extent, work alienation. Job satisfaction shows a relatively strong correlation only with psychological well-being, but, as noted, eliminating job alienation from the analysis greatly increases the influence of satisfaction on general well-being. If the job attitudes are assumed to reflect Person times Environment interaction, then such interaction does add substantially to the prediction of general well-being, although consistent P X E interaction effects were not found regarding well-being on the job.

Tests of various alternative hypotheses support a causal "work leads to well-being" model. Data from the Portland sample are also largely consistent with the findings from Victoria.

The main caveats to these findings concern the self-report nature of much of the data. All the data on work, health, and background information came from the worker himself and were collected in a single questionnaire. It may be that a generalized tendency to optimism or pessimism influenced reports of both work and health, although we did find that workers whose perceptions of work (regarding control and variety) were fairly congruent with objectively measured job dimensions (control and variety) showed work-health relationships similar to those of the group as a whole.

It might be claimed also that the percent variance explained is, in absolute terms, low and therefore that some of the findings presented here should be accordingly discounted. And, it is true that the weakest individual findings related to physical health and specifically to the relationships between the work variables and disability days (Victoria) or number of physical symptoms experienced (Portland). There are four main points to be made against the contention of no substantive significance. First, compared to most findings relating social structural factors to health or well-being (e.g. the literature on recent life events and illness), those described here are sizeable. Second, compared to the numerous nonjob background and concurrent life variables included in the study, the job factors and attitudes are the most potent predictors of well-being. Third, the percentage differences between groups of men high versus low on the job variables are quite large. Fourth, the findings are generally supported in two different samples of working men, one from Victoria (Canada), the other from Portland (U.S.).

The findings presented are congruent in at least some respects with recent studies in the area. Furthermore, these studies tend to buttress the claims to a causal rather than simply a correlational relationship. A study in the United States of 2000 white- and blue-collar workers (7) produced an analytical model fairly close to that presented here, i.e. work factors leading to work attitudes leading to health status. It was also shown that high-stress jobs lead to high levels of strain "even within occupations where people have roughly the same nonwork environments." And, workers on machine-paced assembly lines (objectively classed) were lower in psychological and physical well-being than men in similar work but whose pace was set by the work group rather than by the assembly line.

A Swedish study of blue-collar workers (20) reinforces these causal inferences in showing that physiological measures, i.e. the production of adrenaline and noradrenaline, are intimately associated with job characteristics. The most consistent correlations were found "between psychophysiological variables and job characteristics referring to different aspects of monotony and machine control." The worst jobs were those which combined a heavy work load with routine repetitive work. Subjective states of well-being tended to co-vary with adrenaline excretion.

A particularly interesting series of studies was carried out on a sample of about 1800 male rubber workers in North Carolina (21). A self-administered questionnaire tapped job conditions, felt stress, illness experience, and exposure to physical and chemical agents in the plant, i.e. location within the plant. It was found that psychosocial work stress directly influenced certain illness symptoms (regarding angina, ulcers, neurotic symptoms) regardless of exposure to chemical agents. However, among those men exposed to noxious chemical stimuli, men high in psychosocial stress were much more likely to exhibit dermatological and respiratory symptoms than those low in work stress. A later study (17) showed that particular types of social support mitigated the potentially deleterious effect of work stress on health. The most important of the social supports were wives and supervisors (as opposed to coworkers, friends, and relatives).

The model to which these studies point, then, is a traditional public health model, i.e. a host × stimuli × context one in which illness can best be predicted and explained by examining the critical areas in which a susceptible host is exposed to noxious stimuli in an environment lacking (social) supports. The degree of host susceptibility, the toxicity of the stimuli, and the mediating or enhancing effect of the environment can all refer to (and be effected by) psychosocial as well as to physical or biochemical variables.

The series of studies by the Institute for Social Research at the University of Michigan (7) has led to the development and delineation of a variety of ways of conceptualizing and analyzing work stresses, from role conflict and role ambiguity to qualitative and quantitative work underload and overload. Indeed, work in Europe in these areas is advanced enough that psychosocial work standards or goals have been written into legislation in the Scandinavian countries. It seems likely that sooner or later workers in North America will begin to press for legislation to cover aspects of their work previously neglected. We may also see possible cases of worker compensation involving psychosocial work stress or other aspects of the work environment mentioned here.

Most of all, however, the work-health relationship involves seeing the interaction of man in his environment in a new way, or at least taking seriously old paradigms involving stimuli, host, and environment or context. Unicausal theories of illness and disease based on the germ-illness paradigm are finally being replaced by a more complex but hopefully more accurate model of the determinants of well-being.

If the suggested causal patterns are correct, the way we view work and its place in society will have to be reexamined. We can no longer view work in isolation from other life activities or goals. Occupations and jobs will have to be assessed both as to their effects on worker well-being on the job and as to their influence on health and nonwork activities in general. We need a much more inclusive tally of the side-effects of work-life in examining any input-output calculus in the area of the production of goods and services. The health effects of work are another example, perhaps analogous to the pollution problem, of individuals and the general public paying the costs of a particular system of production, the public costs of private fortunes.

There is little doubt as to prevailing values regarding work, at least insofar as these are reflected in current production organizations. As Fox notes: "The modern criterion of job design . . . is oriented towards minimum cost and maximum output rather than towards self-realization and fulfillment" (22). These work values are a reflection of a social structure and a supporting value system which are increasingly recognized as containing inherent strains, not the least of which are the contradictions between private expropriation and control and public responsibility, between self-interest and the interests of other individuals, groups, or collectivities. There is the paradox of a means to the attainment of well-being, private enterprise, being elevated to the status of an end in itself. Intrinsic to the capitalist system is a predominant emphasis on capital accumulation as the engine of progress with a concomitant de-emphasis on the actual development of man.

If the roots of well-being are indeed embedded in current social structural arrangements such as in the place of work in society at large, then what we are examining is not only the alteration of individual habits or fashions a la Lalonde (change *within* the system) but change *of* the system. As the contradictions of current economic and social policies come to the fore, the legitimacy of the status quo is increasingly called into question.

Finally, the findings of work and health relationships need to be placed within a wider conceptual framework. We have analyzed data for men only, but what are the effects of work (outside or inside the home) on women? If, as some research indicates (23), housework is as boring, repetitive, or stressful as even the most alienating industrial work, what are the consequences for well-being? Furthermore, what are the conditioning factors which lead to work stressors producing poorer health in some men but not in others? Indeed, what facets of work might serve as buffers to the possible impact of nonwork stressors on health i.e. what about work is health enhancing or preserving? While this is not the place for an examination of some of the assumptions underlying research on work and health, it is well to ask if *any* event or activity, if viewed as constraining or demanding, itself has health consequences and whether or not work has the same influence on health for other groups in society as it apparently does for the working men considered in this study.

Acknowledgments—Thanks are owed to Dr. C. R. Pope for his collaboration and support and to W. Peace for assistance in preparation of this paper.

REFERENCES

1. Lalonde, M. *A New Perspective on the Health of Canadians.* Information Canada, Ottawa, 1974.
2. Dubos, R. *Man Adapting.* Yale University Press, New Haven, 1965.
3. Selye, H. The general adaptation syndrome and the diseases of adaptation. *Journal of Clinical Endocrinology* 6: 117-231, 1946.
4. Navarro, V. Social class, political power and the state and their implications in medicine. *Soc. Sci. Med.* 10: 437-457, 1976.
5. Jaques, E. Executive organization and individual adjustment. *J. Psychosom. Res.* 10: 77-82, 1966.
6. French, J. R. P., Jr. Person role fit. *Occupational Mental Health* 3: 15-20, 1973.
7. Caplan, R. D., Cobb, S., French, J. R. P., Jr., Van Harrison, R., and Pinneau, S. R., Jr. *Job Demands and Worker Health.* National Institute for Occupational Safety and Health No. 75-160. U.S. Government Printing Office, Washington, D.C., 1975.
8. Coburn, D. Job-worker incongruence: Consequences for health. *J. Health Soc. Behav.* 16: 198-311, 1975.
9. Kornhauser, A. *Mental Health of the Industrial Worker.* John Wiley and Sons, Inc., New York, 1965.
10. Gardell, B. Alienation and mental health in the modern industrial environment. In *Society, Stress and Disease,* edited by L. Levi, pp. 148-180. Oxford University Press, London, 1971.
11. Bradburn, N. M. *The Structure of Psychological Well-Being.* Aldine, Chicago, 1969.
12. Langner, T. S. A twenty-two item screening score of psychosomatic symptoms indicating impairment. *J. Health Soc. Behav.* 3: 269-276, 1962.
13. Crandell, D. L., and Dohrenwend, B. P. Some relations among psychiatric symptoms, organic illness and social class. *Am. J. Psychiatry* 123: 1527-1538, 1967.
14. Andrews, F., Morgan, J., and Sonquist, J. *Multiple Classification Analysis.* Institute for Social Research, University of Michigan, Ann Arbor, 1967.
15. Burnstein, N., Tienheara, N., Hewson, P., and Warrander, B. *Canadian Work Values.* Manpower and Immigration Information Canada, Ottawa, 1975.
16. Quinn, R. P., and Shepard, L. J. *The 1972-73 Quality of Employment Survey.* Survey Research Centre, Institute for Social Research. University of Michigan, Ann Arbor, 1974.
17. Wells, J. A., McMichael, A. J., House, J. S., and Kaplan, B. H. Effects of Social Support on the Relationship Between Occupational Stress and Health. Duke University, Durham, N.C., 1976 (mimeographed).
18. French, J. R. P., and Kahn, R. L. A programmatic approach to studying the industrial environment and mental health. *Journal of Social Issues* 18: 1-47, 1962.
19. *Dictionary of Occupational Titles,* Ed. 3, Vols. I and II. U.S. Department of Labor, Washington, D.C., 1963, and supplement, 1966.
20. Frankenhaeuser, M., and Gardell, B. Underload and overload in working life. *Journal of Human Stress* 2: 35-46, 1976.
21. House, J. S., Kaplan, B., McMichael, A. J., Spirtos, R., and Wells, J. A. Effects of Occupational Stress on the Health of Rubber Workers. Duke University, Durham, N.C., 1969 (mimeographed).
22. Fox, A. *A Sociology of Work in Industry.* Collier-Macmillan, Ltd., London, 1971.
23. Oakley, A. *The Sociology of Housework.* Pantheon Books, New York, 1974.

APPENDIX

Index Construction

Indices were formed through inclusion of items of similar face meaning and/or factor analysis and/or examination of interitem correlations. Items of differing numbers of response categories were recoded before summation.

Job Satisfaction

Taking into consideration all the things about your job, how satisfied or dissatisfied are you with it?

Overall, how much do you like your present job?

If you had the chance to start again, would you take the same type of work you do now or not?

Job Alienation

My job is interesting nearly all the time—to—my job is completely dull and monotonous. How much challenge do you find in your work?

Job Stress

How much stress or pressure would you say there is in your work?
How mentally tiring is your job?
Do you sometimes get the feeling that your job is more than you can handle? How often do you feel this way?

Psychological Symptoms

The ten "psychological" items from the Langner Index of Psychophysiological Symptomatology (references 12, 13 in the article).

Bureaucracy

Number of people at place of employment plus number of levels of supervision.

Fringe Benefits

Days off work for sickness without loss of pay plus days of paid vacation per year.

Job Control

A six-item index, e.g. How much can you vary the pace at which you work if you want to? How often are you asked for your own comments or suggestions about your work?

Supervision

To what extent is your work checked by supervisory personnel?
How closely are you supervised on your job?

Variety

How much variety is there in what you do at your work? How often do you encounter new situations or new types of problems in your work?

Work Overlap with Family

A five-item index, e.g. Do you sometimes work on weekends? Do you ever bring home work to do?

Negative Background Index

A seven-item index, e.g. How happy would you say your childhood was? How did your parents seem to get along while you were growing up?

Propensity To See a Physician

A ten-item index tapping readiness to see a physician for ten different symptoms.

Religiosity

Church attendance, frequency of praying, self-assessed religiosity.

CHAPTER 5

Job Alienation and Well-Being

David Coburn

Work has been a renewed focus of interest for intellectuals ever since the Industrial Revolution and its accompanying rapid technological innovation and social change. The introduction of machinery and the factory system of production brought a greatly increased division of labor. Work was fragmented into numerous compartmentalized and minute tasks. Responsibility and decision making were vested in managers and supervisors rather than in the workers themselves. The use of mechanical sources of power produced a situation in which workmen became mere machine tenders. The average industrial worker was left with routine, repetitive tasks.

The main attempt to place the altered nature of work within a broader historical analysis of societal evolution was Marx's development (or redevelopment) of the concept of work alienation. This concept joined changes in the work environment to the progression from a feudal to a capitalist epoch. According to Marx, under capitalism the worker becomes estranged not only from the product of his labor (which is expropriated by the capitalist) but also (because of the division of labor, factory technology) from the activity of production itself. Since Marx claims that free, spontaneous activity defines the species life of man, routine, repetitive, forced work leads to man's estrangement from other men and from his own true nature. At work, the worker "does not affirm himself but denies himself, does not feel

The study on which this paper is based was supported in part by a U.S. DHEW Grant (No. CH00235) to the Health Services Research Center, Kaiser Foundation Hospitals, Portland, in part by the Social Science Research Center, University of Victoria, and in part by the Canada Council S71-0407.

content but unhappy, does not develop freely his physical and mental energy but mortifies his body and ruins his mind." Furthermore, because work is forced, it becomes not the satisfaction of a need but "merely a means to satisfy needs external to it" (1, pp. 110-111). In the production process, the needs of the worker are irrelevant.

Alienation, in Marx's terms, thus encompasses a syndrome of characteristics, one aspect of which is work which is intrinsically uninteresting and monotonous in which the worker lacks control over his work tasks. Other components of the syndrome concern the societal level of analysis and the alienative effects of ownership and control by the capitalist and the effect on the worker of commodity fetishism. Alienation as used here, however, refers only to the job task component of alienation. And, ever since the Industrial Revolution and Marx's formulation of the work alienation concept, monotonous and repetitive work has been claimed to have undesirable consequences for the worker, ranging from lowered job satisfaction and unhappiness to higher felt powerlessness and lower mental and physical health. In this paper, we use the idea of work alienation and one of its variants in tracing out the possible relationships between a man's work and his psychological and physical well-being. Indeed, if a man's work does affect his nonwork life, then the area of physical and mental health should be an important dependent variable since health is a prerequisite to all of man's other activities.

The present study, then, is restricted in two ways. First, we are examining only one component of alienation. Second, we are using as dependent variables or possible consequences of alienation only one of many possible outcomes. Despite these restrictions, we will have occasion to relate the work setting to the societal context of which it is a part. Furthermore, we are not saying that the only criterion for evaluating work is the examination of its consequences. The very fact of engaging in routine work over which one has little control, and which does not encourage or permit the growth of one's full capacities and abilities, is in itself one criterion of assessment.

The relationships between the sociotechnical aspects (versus the physical, chemical, biological, etc., dimensions) of work and health have received much recent attention (2-5) although little effort has been employed in directly testing the work alienation-health thesis (but see reference 6). A good deal of the previous research specifically examining the health effects of monotonous, repetitive work was carried out before and immediately after the Second World War in both Britain and the United States. Examples are the work of Kornhauser (7), Doll and Jones (8), and Fraser (9). In general, both the earlier and more recent research (3, 10) tend to confirm the hypothesis that routine, repetitive work leads to psychological symptomatology or to lower levels of mental health. Kornhauser and Gardell both note that satisfaction (Kornhauser (7)) or feelings of interest-monotony (Gardell (6)) mediate between objective job complexity and levels of mental health, i.e. it is perceptions of or reactions to work rather than objective job characteristics which are the main proximate predictors of mental health. Many of the studies, are, however, confined to blue-collar samples and/or fail to adequately control for the numerous possible confounding variables. Still, the evidence does point to a link between work monotony and poorer psychological and physical health.

Although alienation has occasionally been used as an orienting concept, the most prevalent research model is a Person times Environment (P X E) one in which the impact of work on health is hypothesized to be greater for men whose work (on a variety of dimensions, complexity, responsibility, etc.) is incongruent with their personal preferences, capacities, or needs (3, 11). The research mentioned previously which underscores the importance of worker perceptions or evaluations of work as related to mental health also tends to support the P X E model in that perceptions of or feelings about work may be assumed to be the result of P X E interaction.

The theory underlying the work alienation-health link has never been made very explicit. Presumably alienative work, that is work which is fragmented and routine, in which the worker has little control over what he does or how he does it, violates men's (assumed) basic needs for active, spontaneous, creative labor. The worker becomes (consciously or unconsciously) dissatisfied/frustrated, which in turn produces lowered psychological and physical health (the latter presumably through mechanisms relating the psyche to the soma, e.g. the stress mechanisms outlined by Selye and others (12, 13)).

One of the main substantive cleavages in the literature on alienation arises between those who define work alienation as sets of objective conditions versus those who view alienation as a subjective state of the worker. Another is between those who ignore the surrounding social structure versus those including social structural influences as part of their conceptual approach. The first dichotomy can be handled, if not resolved, if one studies both alienative work and the alienated worker (see Etzioni (14)). Thus, a number of writers (14-17) view alienation as having both a structural base and psychic or behavioral consequences. The resulting hypothesis is that particular work constraints or work types lead to psychic consequences for the worker and distinctive behavioral patterns or states, whether at work and/or in nonwork life. We include the "or" because we must leave open the possibility that certain work dimensions may be associated with particular general psychological or physical health consequences without the worker being aware of these effects or indeed reflecting them in his attitudes toward his work, although, as we have noted, the evidence to date does indicate a process whereby work type → work perceptions or attitudes → general well-being.

In making a direct examination of the "work alienation affects health thesis," we first use a conventional approach in defining alienative work as work which is fragmented and repetitive, in which the worker has little control over his work tasks. Later we test the work-health hypothesis using a modified conception of alienation.

METHODS AND MEASURES

Methods

The present study uses data collected in 1970 from a sample of male workers in Victoria, British Columbia. A random sample of 2180 male workers in the Victoria metropolitan area labor force was drawn from the Victoria City Directory. Data were collected by means of a mailed self-administered questionnaire. The return rate of 52.5 percent provided a final total of 1143 workers. In the present analysis only those men employed by others, currently working 25 hours a week or more, and who have been employed in their present jobs for 1 year or more, are included, for a total number of 780 (875 when the self-employed are added).

Compared to census statistics and to the occupational distribution of employed males as given in the City Directory, our sample tends to include respondents somewhat older and of higher educational and occupational status than both non-respondents and adult males in the Victoria metropolitan area generally. The respondents do, however, include a wide variety of socioeconomic status groups, from unskilled laborers to high-level government administrators and professional men, even though the occupational distribution of Victoria does not include large numbers of the most alienative work types, e.g. industrial assembly-line jobs.

Measures

Work Alienation. Three main measures of alienation were employed. The first was an objective measure of the degree of repetition and lack of autonomy of occupations taken from the U.S. *Dictionary of Occupational Titles* (18). That is, respondents' jobs were coded as to the levels of variety and autonomy the *D.O.T.* assigns these particular jobs. The main problems with this index are, first, the difficulties in equating individual *jobs* (from questionnaires) with *occupations* as described in the *Dictionary*, and, secondly, because the *Dictionary* does not code all occupations on the variety/autonomy dimensions (in the present study, all noncoded occupations were assigned the medium category on repetition or control). The repetition and control indices (both trichotomies) were summed into an index of alienative work, i.e. workers high on this index are those in less repetitive, more autonomous jobs; those low, the opposite.

The second measure (perceived alienation) was developed by factor analyzing a number of self-reports about work, out of which three main factors emerged: (a) job variety (two items); (b) job control (six items); and (c) supervision (two items). Three indices were constructed by summing the replies to the various items (see the Appendix for a listing of the questionnaire items). The first two of these indices were combined into an overall index of perceived alienation. (It was found that this index correlated more highly with the health indices than did an index including the supervision items. Since we want to make the strongest possible case for alienation, the supervision index was omitted in the final analysis.)[1]

A final index (subjective alienation) combined two items, one asking the worker how interesting versus monotonous his job was, the other how challenging or unchallenging it was (although it is recognized that there is a fine line between perceptions (perceived alienation) and evaluations (subjective alienation)). The more subjective the assessment, presumably, the more the measure taps the interaction of characteristics of the person with dimensions of the job.

The objective alienation index correlates $G = .40$ with both perceived and subjective alienation. Perceived and subjective alienation correlate $G = .68$. Apart from the

[1]Nevertheless, inclusion of the supervision index does not substantially alter the findings reported here.

measurement problems just mentioned in regard to objective alienation, the cross-tabulations indicate that job conditions perceived as monotonous by one person may appear more interesting for another, but that at the extremes there is a good deal of consensus. Even some men who perceive their jobs as high in control and variety, however, do not find their jobs interesting. The discrepancy probably arises because perceived variety/control is not the sole determinant of interest; personal preferences come into play, i.e. a plumber might prefer to be a mechanic or vice-versa. The subjective alienation measure then probably incorporates the additional aspect of preference.

We used two types of dependent variables, first, well-being on-the-job, and, second, general psychological and physical well-being.

Well-Being On-the-Job. Well-being at the workplace was measured by two indices. The first was an index of job satisfaction composed of questions tapping overall job satisfaction, job liking, and whether or not the worker would take the same type of job if he could begin again (summed). The second was a measure of work stress, which is simply the response to a question asking the worker the degree to which he feels the job is stressful or not stressful.

General Psychological and Physical Well-Being. An index of psychological well-being was constructed by combining (equally weighted) an item tapping self-assessed happiness with a ten-item index measuring the number of psychological symptoms experienced ("psychological" items from the Langner index of psycho-physiological symptomatology (19, 20)). That is, it is assumed a person is high in psychological well-being if he is both happy and shows few psychological symptoms, and vice versa.

Physical well-being was measured by combining an item tapping self-assessed health with an index measuring the number of days in the past year incapacitated (disability days). Those high on the physical well-being index are men describing themselves as healthy and as experiencing a low number of disability days in the past year and vice versa.

The correlations between the psychological and physical well-being scales are moderate ($r = .26$), indicating some overlap between the two. One might, of course, expect that the relationships between the two aspects of well-being are causal in either direction, i.e. men in poor physical health might experience lower psychological well-being and vice versa.

An overall well-being index combined the above two indices.

FINDINGS

While the main intent of this paper is to examine the influence of job alienation on general well-being, it is worthwhile looking briefly at well-being on-the-job in the form of overall job morale and felt stress. Cross-tabulations indicate that the higher the alienation, of whatever type, the lower the morale (Table 1). The relationships between alienation and stress, however, are more curvilinear in form, with the least alienated men showing the highest percentage feeling stressed. Correlations are highest for subjective alienation and lowest for objective alienation.

Table 1

Job morale and felt stress by job alienation, 780 male workers in Victoria, British Columbia, 1970 (percentages)

Degree of Alienation	Objective Alienation[a]		Perceived Alienation		Subjective Alienation	
	Low Morale	High Stress	Low Morale	High Stress	Low Morale	High Stress
Low (high complexity)	29.2	48.8	14.1	53.5	9.1	60.6
	34.0	41.3	27.6	37.9	25.1	40.3
	43.5	24.3	53.3	24.1	39.0	27.2
	52.9	17.6	61.4	7.1	55.6	12.0
	61.9	22.0	66.0	28.0	72.6	19.2
High (low complexity)	–	–	72.1	20.2	95.7	24.3
eta	.22	.29	.46	.31	.59	.33

[a]Objective alienation on a 5-point index (low to high); perceived and subjective alienation, 6-point indices (low to high).

The relationships between alienation and morale and stress were also calculated, controlling for three possible confounding job variables (prestige,[2] pay, opportunity for promotion) and for educational attainment. Using multiple classification analysis (a close analogue of dummy variable regression) (21), we find the objective alienation/ job morale relationships reduced considerably (from eta = .22 to beta = .07), while the remaining relationships are reduced an average of about 22 percent, i.e. the correlations remain fairly substantial and the pattern of relationships stays the same (data not shown, available on request). In five of the six instances (three alienation measures by morale/job stress), the alienation indices (all except objective alienation/ job morale) have the greatest independent influence on morale/stress of any of the (five) variables included in the analysis.

Overall, then, work perceived as low in control and variety and as less interesting and challenging is associated with lower job morale. Alienated workers do indeed tend to feel unhappy in their work (this in addition to the fact that monotonous work might be judged as inherently deleterious). However, the less alienated workers, while liking their jobs more, are also more likely to feel job stress. Workers at both ends of the job complexity continuum thus show some deleterious on-the-job consequences.

Turning to well-being off-the-job, we find that the three alienation measures correlate at best only weakly with the indices of general well-being (Table 2). Perceived and subjective alienation are more highly related to psychological well-being than to physical well-being, while objective alienation shows the opposite trend. Again, subjective alienation is the most powerful predictor of well-being, objective alienation the weakest.

[2]Job prestige rather than occupational prestige was used because it was a much stronger predictor of well-being. The question was "Would you say the people you know think of you as having: An excellent job–to–not too good a job?"

Table 2

Relationships between alienation and well-being among 780 male workers, 1970
(percentages low in well-being)

Degree of Alienation	Objective Alienation			Perceived Alienation[a]			Subjective Alienation		
	PWB[b]	Physwb[c]	No.	PWB	Physwb	No.	PWB	Physwb	No.
Low (high complexity)	13.7	9.5	(161)	10.6	11.3	(142)	8.4	8.4	(128)
	13.3	6.6	(146)	12.1	7.3	(232)	10.1	8.2	(148)
	12.7	11.3	(259)	13.1	11.6	(199)	10.8	11.3	(201)
	14.7	17.6	(65)	11.4	10.0	(70)	14.3	9.8	(129)
	14.4	11.0	(115)	20.0	10.0	(50)	15.1	10.9	(72)
High (low complexity)[d]	–	–	–	20.9	16.3	(86)	35.7	18.6	(68)
eta[d]	.07	.13		.18	.15		.22	.16	

[a] Perceived alienation collapsed from a 1-11 scale. Eta based on the full scale.
[b] PWB = psychological well-being.
[c] Physwb = physical well-being.
[d] eta = the correlation ratio.

It might be claimed that the influence of alienation on health would be evident only among the most alienated workers. Even if, for example, work alienation strongly affected the health of only a few men (that is, the effects of monotonous work are more intensive than extensive), then alienation would have to be considered of importance to the general well-being of workers, particularly in view of the relatively weak predictability in variance-explained terms of other health risk factors (see, for example, the literature on the health effects of recent life changes (22)). Our data indeed show that most of the influence of work on well-being occurs among that minority of men who are high in alienation. These effects are the most pronounced for the subjective alienation measure. Men who feel they are in highly monotonous and unchallenging jobs are over four times as likely to be in poor psychological health (36 percent compared to 8 percent) and over twice as likely to be in poor physical health (19 percent compared to 8 percent) as men who feel their jobs are interesting and challenging.

Do the alienation indices have additive effects, or is the model one in which objectively alienative work → perceived alienation → subjective alienation → lowered well-being as previous research suggests? The cumulative percentage impact of the alienation indices, and the percentage variance explained, both indicate a process rather than a cumulative model. Men fairly high or high on all three types of alienation are not much more likely to be in poor psychological or physical health than men high in subjective alienation alone. The cumulative percentage variance explained by all these alienation indices together also shows only slight improvement over the zero-order correlations.[3]

[3] These results are supported by an analysis (by the author) of data from Caplan et al. (3). On a sample of 318 white- and blue-collar workers, calculation shows a measure of "boredom" correlates .270 with an index of "depression." Adding perceived job complexity increases this correlation to only .276.

In sum, work alienation is indeed associated with unhappiness on the job. Work alienation is also related to lower general well-being, but (a) mainly for a minority of highly alienated men; (b) more so for psychological than for physical health; and (c) more so for subjective than for perceived alienation and more for perceived than for objective alienative work. Although we have found relationships consistent with previous work and with speculation, some of the relationships shown between work and general well-being are not particularly strong and may be due more to possible confounding factors such as the covariation of alienation with low pay or prestige than to alienative work itself. Before examining alternative hypotheses, however, we want to use a somewhat stricter definition of alienation.

One aspect or component of the Marxian version of alienation is the notion that the worker is exploited, that is, that the worker owns neither the product of the work process nor even the tools he uses, and that profit is extracted from the worker in the process of production (surplus value). Thus, in the present analysis we may be comparing not the alienated (those in monotonous work and exploited) with the nonalienated (interesting work and nonexploited) but simply the alienated with those who are somewhat less alienated.

One way of examining this contention and its influence on the alienation/well-being relationship is by using self-employed workers (including employers of others) as more adequately representing the nonexploited worker. Given the above argument, we would expect the self-employed to be less alienated, hence higher in well-being than employed workers at similar job levels (although the self-employed may also be alienated in the sense that the emphasis on consumption values and money as the measure of all things forces everyone, and not only those employed by others, to have an instrumental orientation toward their work).

Comparing the self-employed with employees, the evidence (not presented) shows: (a) the self-employed are, in general, less alienated than the non-self-employed (using the objective and subjective alienation indices as criteria since the self-employed were not asked all of the items comprising the perceived alienation index); (b) the self-employed differ little in well-being from employees; (c) adding self-employment as a criterion of nonalienation to the other indices does not greatly improve our ability to predict well-being, and in only two of the four possible comparisons are the nonalienated self-employed higher in well-being than the nonalienated employed. In any event, self-employed workers form a relatively small portion of the total Canadian labor force and have been rapidly declining as a proportion of the labor force throughout the 20th century.

Are alienated workers lower in well-being because of their job tasks, or because of associated job attributes such as lower job prestige and lower pay, or because men lower in well-being are selected into or drift toward more alienative type jobs? We have already indicated that alienation is probably a process in which objective alienation → perceived alienation → subjective alienation → lower well-being. We now take subjective alienation, the strongest predictor of well-being, and test its relationship to well-being controlling for a number of confounding variables. Three of these variables tap aspects of the job (job prestige, pay, opportunity for promotion) and four other variables measure individual current or pre-job characteristics (age, education, self-assessed health in childhood, an index of stressful childhood events).

Whether taking the control variables singly (partial gammas) or simultaneously (multiple classification analysis),[4] the data show that subjective alienation retains a substantial (and statistically significant) relationship with all three well-being indices (Table 3). This is also the case for all of the components of the well-being indices except for disability days.

Carrying out the same analyses for the objective and perceived alienation indices produces weaker, and, in the case of objective alienation, more inconsistent, results. In fact, after the control variables are introduced, the relationship between alienative job conditions and psychological well-being is in the opposite direction to that hypothesized. The control variables most strongly influencing the alienation/well-being associations are those related to aspects of the job (rather than those referring to various worker background characteristics).

To summarize, controlling for seven possible confounding variables, men feeling they are in uninteresting and unchallenging jobs and men perceiving their jobs as low in control and variety remain the groups lowest in psychological and physical well-being. These findings support the thesis that work perceived as repetitive and routine affects general well-being. They also support the proposition previously mentioned that well-being is best predicted by taking into account worker characteristics (as reflected in perceptions of and reactions to work) as well as characteristics of the work environment itself. While objectively repetitive work is harmful for some

Table 3

Well-being by subjective alienation: zero-order and controlled
on seven variables among 780 male workers, 1970
(multiple classification analysis: mean scores, 1 = high well-being)

Indices of Well-Being	Subjective Alienation						eta/beta[a]
	Low	2	3	4	5	High	
Psychological well-being							
Zero-order	2.35	2.54	2.54	2.60	2.72	3.16	eta = .23
Controlled	2.40	2.62	2.56	2.57	2.65	2.95	beta = .15[b]
Physical well-being							
Zero-order	2.16	2.12	2.39	2.50	2.43	2.60	eta = .17
Controlled	2.27	2.17	2.37	2.46	2.37	2.48	beta = .11
Overall well-being							
Zero-order	3.50	3.66	3.93	4.00	4.14	4.77	eta = .23
Controlled	3.67	3.79	3.94	4.03	4.01	4.42	beta = .14

[a] Beta equivalent to the standardized partial regression coefficient.
[b] All relationships significant at $P < .001$.

[4] Multiple classification analysis gives the correlation ratio of each variable with a dependent variable plus a standardized partial regression coefficient (beta) of each variable, controlling for all the other independent variables. The technique shows the mean of each category of each independent variable both before and after controlling for all the other independent variables (see reference 21).

workers, others appear either not to perceive it as monotonous and/or to accommodate to it with few obvious effects on their general state of well-being.

We began the paper by mentioning the changes produced by the Industrial Revolution and the fragmentation and routinization of work brought about by new technologies and modes of organizing work. But the technological innovations introduced during the 18th and 19th centuries can be viewed as simply the initial impetus in a continuing sequence of rapid change which has not yet run its course. Since the time of the Industrial Revolution, increased mechanization, the application of "scientific management" techniques, rationalization of work tasks and organization, the introduction of mass production methods, and, lately, automation, have brought additional profound modifications in the nature of work. The rise of large-scale industrial organizations and the swift reduction in self-employment have made most men, and not only industrial workers, small cogs in massive machines.

While, on the one hand, these processes have spread fragmented work through both manual and nonmanual occupations, on the other hand, increasing specialization and occupational complexity have produced more demanding jobs. Among manual workers, for example, Blauner (15) sees a U-shaped progression from nonalienative craft work to alienative assembly-line production to less alienative continuous process production (such as in a chemical refinery). This is not to say that the majority of the working population is now faced with the prospect of work which is much more complex than their abilities. As Braverman (23) has pointed out, much of the supposed increase in complexity may be attributed more to artifacts of job definitions and redefinitions than to basic changes to more complex work. Furthermore, most workers now have white-collar or service jobs rather than industrial work. Many, if not most, of these jobs are as highly repetitive and rigidly controlled as low-level manual work. The only overall examination of changes in job complexity I am familiar with shows only a very slight overall increase in job complexity in Canada in the 1941 to 1961 period (24).

Whether or not work is becoming more complex for the majority, however, it certainly is for a minority. At the more complex end of the work continuum, a man's job has been tied to his health and well-being via the concept of stress rather than alienation. As the present data indicate, interesting work may be accompanied by stress. How can a concern with the health effects of complex work be tied in with the influence on well-being of monotonous, repetitive jobs? This can perhaps be done through a redefinition of alienation which conforms to at least one aspect of the alienation concept but which also closely follows the Person times Environment or congruence-incongruence model mentioned earlier.

In its broadest sense, work alienation refers to estrangement from the job, i.e. engagement in work tasks which are uninteresting and which do not express the capacities of the worker. Productive life, its nature and form, exist for profit, not for the expression of the needs of the worker.

Estrangement from work can be conceived as resulting from a mismatching of a person's capacities with the content of the job. In this sense, one problematique of capitalist societies (or all industrial societies) is that the social structural conditions of capitalism and the capitalist value system produce (not only a situation in which much of work life is alienative but also) a job-person mismatching. People are compelled to work in order to make a living; the class structure dictates that some will develop their abilities more than will others and that the person-job selection mechanisms are related more to social class origins and to educational or other qualifications or characteristics than to innate capacities, interests, or needs. The emphasis on educational credentials by productive enterprises operates in favor of artificial barriers to the development of capacities by those barred, for one reason or another, from the higher reaches of the educational system (it is also now the case that many highly educated workers cannot find jobs suited to their talents). The capitalist emphasis on production for profit (and on a high degree of consumption as a necessary condition) as opposed to production values and on money as the (neutral) system of exchange also produces an extrinsic orientation to work, one in which status, pay, or other instrumental considerations rather than (or in addition to) job content factors are involved in career or job choice, where choice is indeed possible. These processes not only place some workers in jobs which are below their capacities (underload) but also ensure that many take jobs which are, in job content terms, above their capacities or which are not suited to their interests (overload.).

In this conception of alienation the alienated worker is one who is in work not suited to his talents either because his work is too simple (the traditional conception of alienation) or because his work is too complex. The nonalienated worker is one who is in work which he finds intrinsically interesting and involving, work suited to his talents or abilities. (Note again that we are referring here only to job task alienation, one aspect of the alienation syndrome.)

Workers were classed either as alienated (underload or overload) or as nonalienated (worker-job incongruence). At the underload end of the continuum (the equivalent of the traditional concept of subjective alienation), workers were assigned a score of 1 if they felt both that their jobs were pretty dull and monotonous or worse and that their jobs were not very much or not at all challenging. They were given a score of 2 if they indicated either one of these. At the overload end, workers were given a score of 4 if they felt either that their jobs were sometimes or frequently more than they could handle or that their jobs were extremely mentally tiring, and a score of 5 if both of these. The remaining workers were classed as congruent or nonalienated (score of 3). The congruents are men who find their jobs at least moderately interesting/challenging yet who do not feel that their jobs are beyond their capacities. Given the above criteria, 17.6 percent were underload, 60.5 percent were congruent, and 21.9 percent were overload.

The underload-overload index was cross-tabulated with measures of well-being on-the-job (job morale, job stress). Figure 1 shows that the vast majority of underload men are low in morale and low in stress while the converse is true for overload men. The men highest in morale, however, are those in jobs somewhat but not greatly beyond their capacities. Controlling for three job variables (prestige, pay, opportunity for promotion) and education leaves the job-morale stress pattern unchanged, although the job congruence-morale relationship is reduced from eta = .42 to beta = .29 (for stress, eta = .44, beta = .40).

Regarding general well-being, the relationships of job underload-overload to psychological, physical, and overall well-being are curvilinear, with workers at both alienation extremes showing lower well-being than the nonalienated (Table 4). To test

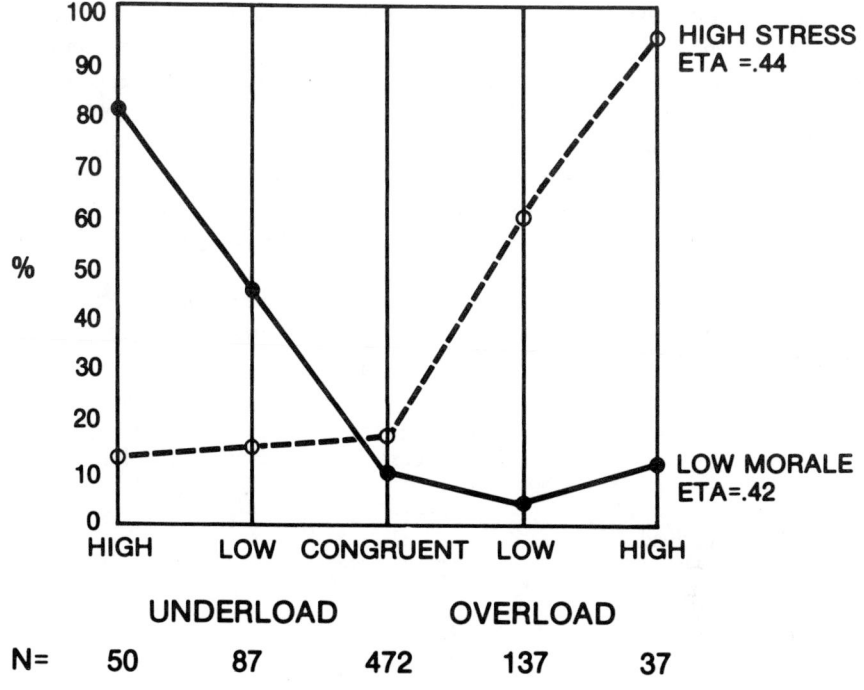

Figure 1. Low job morale and stress by job under-overload.

Table 4

General well-being by job underload-overload index among 780 male workers, 1970
(percentages low in well-being)

Indices of Well-Being	(Alienated) Underload		(Nonalienated) Congruent		(Alienated) Overload	
	1	2	3	4	5	eta
Low in psychological well-being	34.0	18.4	7.4	17.2	37.8	.28
Low in physical well-being	14.0	12.6	9.1	10.4	18.9	.11
Low in overall well-being	24.0	20.6	8.5	12.6	37.8	.22
No.	50	87	472	134	37	

for possible spurious relationships, the congruency index was examined in relation to well-being both before and after introducing the seven control variables mentioned earlier. In each instance but one, the curvilinear pattern remains even after controlling for three job (prestige, pay, opportunity for promotion) and four nonjob variables (age, education, childhood health, index of stressful childhood events) (Table 5). The exception is disability days, in which the main feature is the relatively high number of disability days of the overload men. And, regarding overall physical well-being, it is the slightly overload men rather than the strictly congruent who show the highest well-being.

Finally, looking at the percentage scoring 6 or over on the 9-point index of overall well-being (1 = good health, 9 = low on all four components of the index), we find the following:

	Zero Order %	Controlled on Seven Variables %
High underload	25	19
Low underload	22	20
Congruent	9	9
Low overload	11	11
High overload	37	39
	eta = .22	beta = .21

Table 5

General well-being by job underload-overload: Zero-order and controlled for seven variables among 780 male workers, 1970 (mean values, 1 = high well-being)

	Underload		Congruent	Overload		eta/beta[a]
	1	2	3	4	5	
Psychological well-being	3.08	2.79	2.41	2.73	3.20	eta = .27
	2.84	2.73	2.44	2.74	3.23	beta = .22
Physical well-being	2.53	2.42	2.31	2.20	2.69	eta = .12
	2.34	2.37	2.32	2.27	2.75	beta = .10
Overall well-being	4.65	4.20	3.73	3.93	4.89	eta = .22
	4.18	4.09	3.77	4.01	4.98	beta = .19
Happiness	2.13	1.95	1.79	1.80	2.00	eta = .19
	2.01	1.92	1.80	1.83	2.01	beta = .13
Psychological symptoms	1.97	1.83	1.62	1.93	2.19	eta = .27
	1.86	1.80	1.64	1.92	2.22	beta = .24
Self-assessed health	1.89	1.76	1.62	1.59	1.72	eta = .13
	1.73	1.72	1.63	1.63	1.77	beta = .07
Disability days	2.11	2.28	2.23	1.96	2.75	eta = .12
	2.02	2.24	2.23	2.03	2.81	beta = .12

[a] Beta equivalent to the standardized partial regression coefficient.

Men in jobs which do not allow them to express their abilities are more than twice as likely to be low in well-being than men better suited to their work. The men whose jobs exceed their capacities are over four times as likely as the congruents to be in relatively poor health.

SUMMARY AND CONCLUSIONS

Using traditional measures of work alienation (work as repetitive and monotonous), we found that alienative work is disliked, while bringing with it low or moderate degrees of stress. At the other end of the continuum, nonalienative or interesting and complex work was regarded positively, yet was also stressful. Alienative work was related to lower general psychological and physical well-being, but the relationships were weak and correlations were higher for psychological rather than for physical well-being and for perceived and subjective alienation rather than for objectively alienative work.

When alienation was defined as job-worker incongruence, men in overly simple jobs (perceived underload) tended to dislike their work while also being low in stress; the (perceived) overloads, on the other hand, were high in morale and high in stress. (We should point out, however, that there are elements of tautology in correlations between an index (under-overload) including items such as "How often do you feel your job is more than you can handle?" and an item asking "How much stress or pressure would you say there is in your work?".) Thus, workers' reactions to their work are multidimensional. Insofar as well-being is concerned, a separate focus on satisfaction or on stress oversimplifies the relationship of a man to his job.

The relationships between alienation under-overload and general well-being are curvilinear and consistent although weak in variance-explained terms. The relationships are, however, robust in the sense of holding their shape and strength even after possible confounding variables are introduced into the analysis. In percentage terms, and compared to most findings in the health and illness area, the work/well-being relationships are fairly substantial.

The answer to the question "Does work alienation produce lower general well-being?" must thus be a somewhat equivocal "yes." Yes because work alienation, whether conceived as repetitive monotonous work or as person-job mismatch, is associated with lowered psychological and physical well-being even taking into account a wide variety of possible confounding variables. Equivocal because the relationships did not hold for objectively repetitive work and because, with the present data, we cannot definitely prove that (perceived) alienation leads to lowered well-being rather than the reverse. The causal interpretation is supported by data showing slight curvilinear relationships between a rough measure of objective job times person incongruence (using objective alienation times education),[5] by the *pattern* of relationships which make it seem unlikely that lowered psychological well-being would lead to perceptions of both under and overload, by data (25, p. 429) indicating that men whose job perceptions coincide with objective measures of job type show the expected work/well-being relationships, and by research pointing to a

---

[5] The incongruents are those low in education and high in job complexity and vice versa.

link between objective job monotony and various indicators of psycho-physiological stress such as adrenaline secretion (10).

The findings that perceived and subjective alienation and alienation as (perceived) person-job incongruence are much better predictors of well-being than is objectively alienative work lead to the conclusions, first, that the determinants of general well-being include not only facets of the objective situation but also variables influencing worker perceptions of the job, and, second, that overly complex as well as overly simple work has health consequences. Part of the reason that workers in repetitive, monotonous jobs did not show even larger contrasts in well-being with workers in more complex jobs was that many of the latter are also, in one sense, alienated from their work.

The importance of workers' perceptions is not to deny the ultimate impact of objective job characteristics. Our findings do not imply that objective job conditions can be ignored and workers' well-being manipulated simply by instituting better worker selection processes. First, workers' perceptions of and reactions to their jobs are not independent of objective job conditions. Perceived and subjective alienation, job morale, and felt stress are all related to objective job conditions. And job-worker misfit is not independent of job conditions. While we found between 46-66 percent of the men at various levels of job complexity showing job-worker congruence, it is the case that those in the underload category are predominantly grouped in objectively simple work while those in the overload category are much more likely to be in objectively complex work environments. Part of the influence of job-worker incongruence is thus due to the effect of the job conditions themselves, with incongruence simply adding to the explanatory power of job factors alone. We should also reemphasize the relatively weak nature of our measures of objective job alienation and objective job-worker incongruence. Second, the more extreme the objective job conditions, the more likely the worker to perceive these accurately or to react to them as expected (regarding both job feelings and general well-being). It can be assumed, then, that worker (or person) characteristics are of importance only within certain objective job condition parameters.

It can be understood why Marx (insofar as job tasks are concerned) was chiefly interested in alienation as monotonous, uninteresting work. That component of the alienation syndrome obviously reflected the job conditions of the epoch in which they were formulated. While the factory conditions of the Industrial Revolution (characterized by extreme repetition and monotony) which gave rise to the work alienation concept do have their counterparts in modern occupational structures (Braverman (23) might insist a predominant part), they certainly do not reflect the work experiences of all workers and ignore the potentially deleterious influence of highly complex work. But alienation in the sense of work not suited to one's capacities or preferences is an even more widespread phenomenon than alienation as work monotony in the sense of including, in addition to those in monotonous work, those in work which exceeds their capabilities. And job-worker incongruence does have the anticipated health or well-being consequences.

There does seem to be a widespread need, as the alienation tradition suggests, for workers to use whatever skills and abilities they possess. To put it another way, if well-being is to be preserved or enhanced, workers need to do what they are capable of doing.[6] While the need to use one's skills is widespread, levels of skill and ability vary widely, producing somewhat differing perceptions and evaluations of objectively similar situations.

As we pointed out earlier, in Canada jobs are chosen or workers are selected into jobs subject to a number of constraints and demands. Many, perhaps most, have little choice of jobs or a choice limited to particular levels of complexity and control. Jobs may also be chosen not for reasons of interest but more because of their concomitant attributes of prestige or pay. The facts that 40 percent of the present sample could be described as job incongruent and that nearly 50 percent of the sample state that they would not take the same type of work if they could begin their working lives again are probably low estimates of person-job mismatching.

Whether men can obviate the effects of work monotony by finding outlets for the use of skills outside the work environment is unlikely. Research to date indicates that the relationships between work and nonwork are more carry-over than compensatory in nature, i.e. monotonous, highly directed work may produce workers less capable of creativity off-the-job (28). However, if work was to become much less central both in hours worked and as a place where most men receive their status, income, and self-esteem, then leisure time might replace work as the arena in which to utilize capabilities and abilities. If the above conditions were fulfilled, there seems no theoretical reason why the use or nonuse of abilities in life off-the-job would not have consequences for worker well-being (as indeed they may have already) insofar as these activities were undertaken for reasons other than the performance of the activities themselves.

One question not examined here relates to the possibility of giving man's work meaning and interest by embedding work within a social structure having significance for the individual. Could workers' perceptions of work and their subsequent health experience change if there were increased participation in decision making in the work organization, or on the shop floor itself? Can workers in jobs far below their potential find interest even in routine work if that work contributes to a valued end, such as perhaps in postrevolutionary Cuba, in an Israeli kibbutz, and in utopian or communal settings? Or is job monotony and job complexity/individual capacity matching an important determinant of health regardless of societal setting or prevalent value systems? Affective and physiological reactions to objective situations are conditioned by individual and group cognition. Which is to say that the precise determinants and consequences of alienation are influenced not only by the immediate sociotechnical setting of work but also by the larger social structure of which work is a part. As Israel (29) puts it in another context, "It is not alienation which makes the worker 'class conscious' (and therefore socialist) but rather it is, above all, 'class-conscious' workers who experience alienation." The fact that productive life is largely accepted as a means to an end rather than an end in itself is a precondition in our society for alienative work life. The consideration of social structural characteristics also underscores the focus in this paper on only the job task aspect of the alienation

---

[6]This is close to Maslow's conceptualization (26) of a need for self-actualization or the "full use and exploitation of talents, capacities, potentialities, etc. . ." and Nobel Prize Laureate Szent-Gyorgyi's statement "Ability brings with it the need to use that ability" (quoted in Selye (27)).

syndrome. As Archibald (30) notes, "The very existence of commodity production, of having to produce for others through some such impersonal mechanism as the market—probably promotes alienation by imposing purposes other than their own upon producers' work."

While these questions are largely unanswered, we are still faced with the consequences for Canadian society and for Canadian workers of the unanticipated consequences of past and present social arrangements for production, distribution, and consumption. It is quite obvious that segmental examination of life areas is inadequate if we are to fully account even for the causes and effects located in one analytically separate human activity, that of work. Only now we are beginning to realize the costs of social structures based on the primacy of capital accumulation and economic growth rather than on the needs of men. The real debate now lies in assessment of the magnitude of the benefits versus the dis-ease produced by the existing social organization. In truth the internal contradictions in our societies may indeed be working themselves out.

Acknowledgments—Thanks are owed to Dr. C. R. Pope for his collaboration and support and to Dr. Peter Archibald for his comments, and to Wendy Peace and Rita Dias for aid in preparation of this paper.

APPENDIX
Index Construction

Indices were formed through inclusion of items of similar face meaning and/or factor analysis and/or examination of interitem correlations. Items of differing numbers of response categories were recoded before summation.

Variety
How much variety is there in what you do at your work?
How often do you encounter new situations or new types of problems in your work?

Control
How often are you asked for your own comments or suggestions about your work?
How much influence do you think you and people in your type of position have on how your company or place of employment is run?
How much can you vary the pace at which you work if you want to?
Do you have much freedom in the way you go about doing your job?
Is decision-making an important part of your job?
To what extent do you yourself decide on the way you do things in your job?

Supervision
How closely are you supervised on your job?
To what extent is your work checked by supervisory personnel?

Subjective Alienation
How much challenge do you find in your work?
My job is interesting nearly all the time.
My job is completely dull and monotonous.

Stress
How much stress or pressure would you say there is in your work?
How often do you get the feeling that your job is more than you can handle?
How mentally tiring is your job?

Happiness
In general, how happy are you these days?

Psychological Symptoms
The ten "psychological" items from the Langner index.

Self-assessed Health
What would you say is the state of your health in general?

Disability Days
An index constructed from questions concerning days hospitalized in the past year, days away from work because of illness, days ill in bed without calling a doctor.

Stressful Childhood Events
An index constructed from self-reports of childhood events, e.g. How happy would you say your childhood was? How did your parents seem to get along while you were growing up? Would you say their marriage was: One of the happiest . . . to . . . very unhappy.

REFERENCES

1. Marx, K. *Economic and Philosophic Manuscripts of 1844,* edited by D. J. Struik and translated by M. Milligan. International Publishers, New York, 1964.
2. Report of a Special Task Force to the Secretary of H.E.W. *Work in America.* M.I.T. Press, Cambridge, Mass., 1973.
3. Caplan, R. D., Cobb, S., French, J. R. P., Jr., Von Harrison, R., and Pinneau, S. R., Jr. *Job Demands and Worker Health.* U.S. Government Printing Office, Washington, D.C., 1975.
4. Portigal, A. H., editor. *Measuring the Quality of Working Life.* Labour Canada, Ottawa, 1973.
5. Canada Department of Manpower and Immigration. *Canadian Work Values.* Information Canada, Ottawa, 1975.
6. Gardell, B. Alienation and mental health in the modern industrial environment. In *Society, Stress and Disease,* edited by L. Levi. Oxford University Press, London, 1971.
7. Kornhauser, A. W. *Mental Health of the Industrial Worker.* John Wiley & Sons, New York, 1965.
8. Doll, R. E., and Jones, A. F. *Occupational Factors in the Aetiology of Gastric and Duodenal Ulcers.* Medical Research Council Special Report Series No. 276. His Majesty's Stationery Office, London, 1951.
9. Fraser, R. *The Incidence of Neurosis Among Factory Workers.* Industrial Health Research Board Report No. 90. His Majesty's Stationery Office, London, 1947.
10. Frankenhaeuser, M., and Gardell, B. Underload and overload in working life. *Journal of Human Stress* 2: 35-46, 1976.
11. French, J. R. P., Jr., and Kahn, R. L. A programmatic approach to studying the industrial environment and mental health. *Journal of Social Issues* 18: 1-47, 1962.
12. Selye, H. *The Stress of Life.* McGraw-Hill Book Company, New York, 1956.
13. Levi, L., editor. *Society, Stress and Disease,* Vol. 1. Oxford University Press, London, 1971.
14. Etzioni, A. *The Active Society.* The Free Press, New York, 1968.
15. Blauner, R. *Alienation and Freedom.* University of Chicago Press, Chicago, 1964.
16. Seeman, M. On the meaning of alienation. *American Sociological Review* 24: 783-791, 1959.
17. Seeman, M. On the personal consequences of alienation in work. *American Sociological Review* 32: 273-285, 1967.

18. *Dictionary of Occupational Titles,* Ed. 3, Vols. 1 and Supplement (1966). United States Department of Labor, Washington, D.C., 1963.
19. Langner, T. S. A twenty-two item screening score of psychosomatic symptoms indicating impairment. *Journal of Health and Human Behaviour* 3: 269-276, 1962.
20. Crandell, D. L., and Dohrenwend, B. P. Some relations among psychiatric symptoms, organic illness and social class. *Am. J. Psychiatry* 123: 1527-1538, 1967.
21. Andrews, F., Morgan, J., and Sonquist, J. *Multiple Classification Analysis.* University of Michigan Institute for Social Research, Ann Arbor, 1967.
22. Rahe, R. H. Life change and subsequent illness reports. In *Life Stress and Illness,* edited by E. K. E. Gunderson and R. H. Rahe. Charles C. Thomas, Springfield, Ill., 1974.
23. Braverman, H. *Labor and Monopoly Capital.* Monthly Review Press, New York and London, 1974.
24. Scoville, J. G. *The Job Content of the Canadian Economy 1941-61.* Special Labor Force Studies No. 3. Dominion Bureau of Statistics, Ottawa, 1967.
25. Coburn, D. Work and general psychological and physical well-being. *Int. J. Health Serv.* 8(3): 415-435, 1978.
26. Maslow, A. H. *Motivation and Personality,* second edition. Harper and Row, New York, 1970.
27. Selye, H. *Stress without Distress.* New American Library of Canada Ltd., Toronto, 1975.
28. Kohn, R. M. L. *Class and Conformity.* Dorsey Press, Homewood, Ill., 1969.
29. Israel, J. *Alienation: From Marx to Modern Sociology,* p. 254. Allyn and Bacon, Inc., Boston, 1971.
30. Archibald, W. P. *Social Psychology as Political Economy,* p. 131. McGraw-Hill Ryerson, Ltd., Toronto, 1978.

CHAPTER 6

The Use and Health Consequences
of Shift Work

Dean Baker

As our knowledge and sophistication in the field of occupational health have grown, it has become clear that work is dangerous in many different ways. The worker encounters various physical, chemical, and biological hazards in the workplace which can lead to ill health. Most of the effort in occupational health has been directed toward the technical evaluation and control of these problems. Besides these concrete factors, we now realize that the social organization of work can affect the health of workers and their families.

The social organization of work refers to the way work is structured within the plant and, more generally, how the requirements and organization of the work process affect the community and social environment. In virtually every work setting, people perform their particular jobs in relation to other people doing their jobs. In a sense, the aggregate of these relations constitutes the social organization of the workplace. These relations are not generally random. In the modern workplace, products are not conceived, designed, and built by the individual worker. Rather, through a technical division of labor, each worker contributes one part to the production of many products. This form of production requires that the contribution or job of each worker be defined in relation to other workers' jobs. The nature of these relations is determined by the requirements of the production process and represents the social organization of the work.

With the flowering of capitalism and the development of industrialization over the past two centuries, the social organization of work has become increasingly complex. The essential determinant of the organization of work under capitalism is that its goal is to maximize the creation of surplus value and, thus, profits (1). A characteristic of this organization is that it is structured not by the workers themselves, but by their employers. Braverman and others have written about how the owners of capital have altered the nature of the work process in their drive for greater efficiency and profits (2, 3). Major factors in the organization of work under capitalism have included the collection of workers in one location or plant, scientific management or "Taylorism," the assembly line, and the increasing domination of the worker's health and life away from work. In the effort to maximize profits, essentially all aspects of the productive process have been examined and restructured, from the individual motions of the production process to the overall organization of the plant and the workday. Shift work is a clear example of this phenomenon: the entire workday has been redefined in an effort to increase productivity and profits. This paper will explore the use and health consequences of shift work as a method of the social organization of work.

In order to understand the application and consequences of shift work, one must evaluate it as a manifestation of the development of work under capitalism. Two fundamental trends in the evolution of the work process during this century are (a) the increasing control over workers, and (b) the increasing productivity of workers through technological and organizational changes (2). Control over workers is necessary because the surplus value they create through labor accrues not to them, but to the owners of the enterprise. Therefore, the workers have no intrinsic need to produce ever greater value. Because of competition and the need to maximize profits to survive, the owners must institute practices to control the independence of workers and make them produce ever more products and profits. The basic principle of this control has been to separate the execution of the labor from its conceptualization (2, 3). Rather than having each worker design how she/he will perform the job, each procedure is predetermined and dictated for the worker. Control is achieved not only through social factors such as increased supervision, but also through the technical design of the machinery and workplace. An example of the latter is automation, where workers are restricted to a few prescribed actions, often intervening only when a feeding system is empty or the machine malfunctions. The result of this increasing control has been the increasing alienation of workers from the work process and their evolution into little more than human machines. Consideration of the worker's well-being has become only a minor factor in the design of machinery and production processes.

Increasing productivity, and thus profits, has also been accomplished through social and technical innovations. During the early phase of capitalism, the fight over production concerned mainly the number of work hours in the week. More hours for the same pay meant more profits for the owners (4). In fact, the first labor laws in Italy fixed the maximum for salaries and the minimum for hours of work (5)! The history of labor is replete with stories about the fight for a shorter work week (6). During this century, increased productivity has been achieved primarily through technological change and the reorganization of the work process to make each worker's time more productive (3). Supervision, "scientific management," speed-up, and other methods have been used to intensify work. The technical division of work tasks, the assembly line, and automation have increased the productive capabilities of workers. These changes have virtually completely altered the nature of work. Traditional jobs have been redesigned and adapted to the automated machines, and new occupations have arisen based on the needs of the automated processes. In many cases, the social reorganization of work has followed from technological changes. An example is the development of the large factory based on the assembly line. As we shall see below, the spread of shift work has followed the expansion of automation and the development of continuous production processes. Thus, the growth of shift work can be understood as one facet of the technical and social reorganization of work within the workplace that has been used to increase productivity and profits.

In a more general sense, the social organization of work also refers to the impact of the work process on the community and social environment. Workers do not exist solely within the plant. Many times the requirements of production affect the workers at home and their families and communities. Depression, exhaustion, injuries, and illness due to work affect both the worker and his/her family. Required overtime and night work force the worker and her/his community to adapt to the needs of the plant. Thus, the organization of work within the plant affects the social environment beyond the plant. The requirements of the production process play a central role in the social organization of a worker's life (3). These full social and health effects must be considered in evaluating the impact of the social organization of work.

SHIFT WORK–SOME DEFINITIONS

Shift work exists when a plant or service facility has working periods other than the normal day shift (7, 8). These shifts make it possible for the establishment to operate on an extended or continuous basis. There are many systems of shift work, including two shifts with or without night work, three shifts without weekends, and continuous shifts including nights and weekends (8). The most common pattern is two shifts: early morning and late afternoon. Workers may stay on fixed shifts or rotate through the shifts. The number of days on the same shift is called the rotation period; it may vary from one day up to several weeks. The most common rotation period is one week. The rotation direction is the sequence of shifts in subsequent rotation periods. The usual direction is "day, evening, night." A less common, reverse rotation is "day, night, evening." The length of the rotation cycle is the length of time it takes for a worker to return to the same starting time and day. These cycles vary from two to twenty weeks. Finally, the starting times for each shift vary between establishments. In general, the day shift in the United States begins between 6 and 8 a.m., while in Europe it begins between 4 and 6 a.m. The type of shift system used is influenced by production needs, but most times it is selected by the owner/manager of a plant based on custom, whim, or past experience (8). On the other hand, as shown below, the shift schedule selected does determine the level of disruption of the worker's life and influence his/her health and attitudes.

HISTORICAL DEVELOPMENT

Historically, night work was virtually non-existent until the onset of capitalism and the subsequent rise of industrialization (7). It became more prevalent after the establishment of corporations in England in the early 1790s. Due to pressure from labor, laws were enacted in the 1800s to control shift work. By the turn of the century, England, Germany, France, and Switzerland had created governmental agencies to control the working conditions of shift workers.

During this century, economic competition has increasingly forced the owners of industry to maximize productivity through investment in new machines and automated production processes. Consolidation into large corporations and the development of modern transportation have led to more fierce competition on an ever larger scale. Shift work has expanded as industries have sought competitive advantage through mass production in the shortest possible time. In established industries such as textiles, shift work has increased with automation and competition on a national and international scale. In new industries, such as electronics and automobile manufacturing, the use of shift work and other organizational schemes was incorporated into the initial production designs. As these newer industries grew, so did the amount of shift work.

The prevalence of shift work steadily increased after 1900, making large gains during and after World War II. In France, where data collection methods have remained constant, the amount of shift work increased from 10.3 percent in 1957 to 21.9 percent in 1974 (9). In 1975, the Organization for Economic Cooperation and Development (OECD) estimated that shift work had doubled during the preceding ten years in northwest Europe (10). In the United Kingdom and France, the two-shift system has increased more than the three-shift system. Some authors feel that the rate in the growth of shift work may decline; however, virtually all agree that the amount of shift work will continue to expand over time (8, 11).

EXTENT AND DISTRIBUTION

The prevalence of shift work varies among countries. The proportion of workers doing shift work was 21.9 percent in France in 1974, 26.8 percent in the United States in 1975, 20.4 percent in the Netherlands in 1969, and 13.3 percent in Japan in 1971 (9). This variation is due to differences in cultures, the laws regulating shift work, and the relative development of the industries which use shift work. For example, in 1968 in Japan, about 37 percent of the workers were on shift work in establishments where shift work had been adopted; however, these constituted only 20 percent of the total number of establishments (8). Actually, because there are many families where one of two or more working members does shift work, greater than one-quarter of the working population is likely affected in most industrialized nations.

Surveys have revealed a wide variation in shift work among industries. Among manufacturing industries in France, the proportion of workers doing shift work is 71 percent in metal processing, 58.3 percent in auto manufacturing, 50.2 percent in textiles, and 46.6 percent in plastics (9). In Italy, metallurgy, chemicals, paper, and plastics have the highest proportion of shift workers. In the United Kingdom, auto manufacturing, paper, and textiles have the most shift workers (8). The amount of shift work in some United States industries is shown in Table 1. Both internationally and in the United States, several trends have become clear. Manufacturing industries requiring large-scale or continuous production, such as the manufacture of metal or glass, have the highest proportion of shift workers. Service industries also employ very large numbers of shift workers, providing both essential and non-essential services. As shown in Table 2, the proportion of shift workers increases with the size of the establishment (9). This trend is consistent both within and between industries. Finally, the number of shift workers seems to be growing in the majority of the industries in all industrialized nations.

Within these overall trends, shift work can vary with market or technological conditions. In many industries, the extent of shift work fluctuates with demand for the product. In times of high demand, second or third shifts are added to increase production. When demand drops off, these workers are laid off. Establishments producing a new product or using a newer, more inexpensive production process use shift work to take advantage of their competitive edge. The national figures also obscure regional variation. While the overall proportion of shift workers in manufacturing in

Table 1

Shift work in selected United States industries, 1975[a]

Industry[b]	Number of Shift Workers (1,000s)	Percent of Shift Workers
Hospitals	1,117	36.9
Education	1,115	17.0
Food and kindred products	593	42.7
Private household	507	40.7
Primary metal industries	402	37.5
Machinery (except electrical)	363	18.9
Printing and publishing	327	28.5
Postal	277	45.8
Textile mill products	216	34.4
Chemical and allied products	199	19.7
Paper and allied products	176	32.4
Lumber and wood products	130	25.4
Instruments and related products	56	5.2
Petroleum and coal products	42	17.7
Furniture and fixture	33	7.7
Tobacco	20	32.8

[a] Source, reference 7.
[b] Refer to reference 7 for a more complete listing.

Table 2

Percent of shift workers by size of establishment, France, 1975[a]

Number of Employees	Percent of Workers Doing Shift Work
10-49	5.6
50-199	12.1
200-499	25.1
Over 500	43.1

[a] Source, reference 9.

the United States is 30 percent, it ranges from 10.5 percent in Miami to 43.2 percent in Detroit (10). The proportion of shift workers is highest in industrial areas and large cities where the demand for night services is high.

The distribution of shift workers by race and sex is not easily available. A 1975 National Institute of Occupational Safety and Health (NIOSH) survey discovered that trade associations do not keep information on shift workers (7). A study of food processors did show that, compared to whites, Hispanic workers were heavily and significantly overrepresented on the rotating shifts (12). While there are no general reports of the distribution by race for different shifts, seniority is an important criterion for the assignment to shifts (8). Clearly, minority workers with generally less seniority would be concentrated in the night and rotating shifts. These differences may not be apparent from aggregated data because most workplaces in the United States remain largely non-integrated.

A few European countries have adopted regulations concerning night work which apply equally to women and men. However, in many countries employment of women during evening or night shifts is restricted or illegal (11). From a physiological point of view, some researchers have suggested that an interaction between the 24-hour circadian rhythms and the 28-day ovarian cycle could lead to periods of excessive fatigue or decreased resistance to noxious agents such as noise, heat, or chemicals (11). However, no studies have shown that these differences are significant. Carpentier and Cazamian (11) concluded that they do not constitute a contraindication for night work for women in particular. Other studies have demonstrated that women and men do not differ in the amount of nervous or digestive disorders associated with shift work. After studying the reasons for the laws affecting women only, an International Labor Office (ILO) report (13) concluded that the legislator's prime concern about women workers was "to protect their function of reproduction." Until more laws can be enacted which protect both women and men, the present laws will tend to accentuate the traditional absence of fathers from their family roles and effectively bar women from many jobs available in shift work industries.

JUSTIFICATION

The spread of shift work has been justified for technical, social, and economic reasons. Technical considerations were the earliest and are still an important impetus for the use of shift work. The continuous nature of some physical or chemical processes, e.g. iron founding or steel production, requires having workers present throughout the 24 hours of a day. Many furnaces do not have to be used continuously, but could collapse or crack if allowed to cool down when not in use. In other industries, time and cost would increase substantially with intermittent close-down and start-up of the production process. In many cases, whole establishments go on shift work when only one component of the production process requires continuous production. The rest of the plant operates through the night only to prevent bottlenecks or stockpiling. As the use of shift work has spread and become accepted in industry, more processes have been designed based on the availability of workers around the clock. The apparent technical requirement for shift work merely follows from the assumptions made in the engineering design of the production process. Carpentier and Cazamian concluded in a recent review that in most cases continuous production is not required and, even in continuous production industries, certain operations could be stopped momentarily without any great damage, except that the stoppage would lead to increased production costs (11).

Essential social services, such as hospitals or fire protection, have to be provided continuously. On the other hand, Table 1 reveals that most of the service industries with the highest number of shift workers provide non-essential services. With urbanization, we have been turned into a 24-hour-a-day society. Industries like food and transportation must cater their services around the clock. In New York City, even trash collection occurs throughout the day and night. The demand for diversion and entertainment has also increased. The proportion of the Gross National Product allocated to recreation has more than doubled since World War II and, as a result, an ever larger number of people must work while others take their leisure (10). Finally, as more and more families have two working parents or a single working parent, the need has increased for services outside the normal working hours. The need for shift work in most of these cases is not intrinsic; rather, it has developed from the social conditions and demands of our urban, working environment.

Economic considerations have been and still are the most important stimulus for the use of shift work. Only a small proportion of the industries using shift work require it for technical reasons. It has been most widely used in capital-intensive industries. In these industries, the use of modern technology and automation to increase productivity has led to a substitution of fixed or constant capital for labor. Where the cost of labor has become low relative to capital costs, industry uses labor more intensively to maximize the return on their capital investments. By increasing the daily rate of production, the cost of fixed capital is spread out over more units of output (8). Examples of industries with relatively high ratios of capital investment to labor costs are basic iron and steel, industrial chemicals, pulp, paper and paperboard, and synthetic fibers (7). These industries employ large numbers of shift workers.

With the pressure to increase productivity, there has been an acceleration of technological innovation such that many plants and machines now become obsolete before being worn out. Thus, owners must consider not only the impact of the initial capital investment, but also the technical and social lifetimes of the machines or plants. It is essential that the maximum technical use be extracted from a machine before it becomes competitively obsolete. Shift work provides a constant supply of workers to operate these machines as intensively as possible. The taxation system reinforces this trend by allowing savings on capital investments through higher rates of depreciation. Unfortunately, the intense use of fixed capital also tends to increase the rate of obsolescence, in that new "generations" of the machines are constantly being designed in anticipation of replacing the current machines. A vicious cycle is established between faster obsolescence of fixed capital and the intensification of work. A result of this cycle is the ever increasing demand for shift workers.

Thus, in capital-intensive industries where the cost of labor is low relative to fixed capital costs and the effective use of machines has become critical, shift work is used to increase productivity and profits within the work process. Shift work can also increase profits in both capital-intensive and other industries by increasing the turnover rate for capital investments. The turnover time is the amount of time from capital investment—including plant, machines, raw materials, and labor—until realization of whatever profits will be made. For a constant cost of production and return in profit per unit of output, increasing the rate of turnover of capital puts more commodities onto the market in a given time and thus increases the total amount of profit realized. Therefore, shift work can be used generally to decrease turnover time and increase the absolute amount of profits.

Note that shift work in capital-intensive industries increases profits by both decreasing the cost per unit of output and decreasing the turnover time in the marketplace. In some establishments, the costs of production increase with shift work and can offset the increased profits due to the decreased turnover time of capital. Increased costs occur where the cost of night labor is high, the demand for the product is uneven, and the cost of storage is high, and where supervisory functions are not easily split up over multiple shifts. Establishments tend not to use shift work under these circumstances. Because the costs of storage and supervision are more problematic in smaller establishments with marginal operating costs, small plants use shift work less. The economic profitability of shift work is greatest among large-scale and capital-intensive industries. This trend is seen clearly in Table 2.

On a macro-economic level, shift work is sometimes necessary to effectively use scarce resources. In economically developing societies, where there is a shortage of fixed capital and an excess of labor power, shift work has been used to increase employment. On the other hand, in more competitive societies like the United States, where high levels of unemployment are part of the national economic policy, many workers hold two jobs while others remain unemployed.

Overall then, shift work is used to maximize profits in multiple ways both within the productive process and through higher turnover in the market. Due to competition, the owners of capital have been forced to use shift work to increase their margins of profit. On the other hand, it provides added benefits, particularly for the owners of the large, capital-intensive industries. It creates additional pressure for the elimination of the smaller plants of the competitive sector and an evolution toward large-scale, capital-intensive industries. It is one component of the increasingly complex social organization of work which derives from the need to maximize profits, yet in turn, functions as a pressure in changing the basic nature of work.

ATTITUDES

Surveys of workers' attitudes indicate that they generally do not like shift work (9, 14). A 1977 NIOSH survey of twenty national labor unions revealed that in none of their workers' industries was shift work completely voluntary (7). It was partially voluntary among only 15 percent of industries, and, for the rest, it was involuntary or based on seniority. In another study, Maurice and Monteil asked continuous shift workers in France if they would like to stay on shift work in the future (15). Only 32 percent said yes, without reservations; 35 percent said yes, with reservations; and 33 percent said no. The reasons given for continuing shift work were "free time" and "habit." On the assumption that economic motives were comparatively important in deciding to do shift work, they then asked the workers if they would prefer to do day work if their wages and work remained the same; 65 percent responded affirmatively. Additionally, the authors found that the major use of the so-called "free time" was for working a second job. Among workers doing a rotating three-shift job, 33 percent were working second jobs. They concluded that workers generally do not wish to do shift work. When they do choose shift work, they are motivated by the need for the shift work pay differential and the free time it gives them during the day to work a second job.

In the United States, most research on workers' attitudes has emphasized the individual characteristics of the worker (14, 16). Mott points out that adjustment to shift work is influenced by the following factors: perceived role difficulty caused by the worker's shift, personality factors such as self-esteem and anxiety, general health factors, and marital integration and happiness (16). The attitude toward shift work is also related to the availability of recreation and services during non-work hours in the worker's community. A major problem with this approach is that these factors are essentially considered independent variables. While these factors represent resources available to mediate the impact of shift work, they are also personal reflections of social and environmental factors affecting the worker. For example, Tasto et al. found among food processors that more full-time jobs were held by rotating shift workers' spouses than was the case for other shifts (12). Night-shift workers had the lowest frequency of work schedules that matched their spouses'. Finally, the trend to dissimilar work hours from day to night shift work was paralleled by the trend of reported dissatisfaction by the shift worker's spouse. The impact of shift work itself on these "resources" must be considered when discussing individual attitudes about shift work.

In establishments that do have shift work, the shift workers are ambivalent about their schedules, but generally prefer their current schedule to alternatives (8). This attitude reflects a natural tendency to maintain established habits. They do consistently prefer fixed shifts over rotating shifts. Despite a recent tendency toward shorter rotation periods, workers prefer their present periods—usually a week—or even longer ones. Shorter overall rotation cycles are preferred so that there is less variation in the starting days and times in each rotation period. In general, these attitudes reflect workers' desire to minimize the disruption caused by a constantly changing work schedule.

HEALTH AND SOCIAL EFFECTS

The validity of workers' concerns about shift work has been amply confirmed by a large number of studies on the health effects of night and shift work (8, 9, 11, 17). The major complaints reported by shift workers include disturbances in sleep, nervous troubles, and disturbances of the alimentary tract (9). They also complain of disruptions in their family and social lives. Studies have examined these and other factors, including absenteeism, performance, and accidents. Knowledge about the impact of shift work has come from experimental laboratory studies of animals and human volunteers and from controlled epidemiological studies.

Most of the research on the physiological impact of shift work has focused on the effects of circadian rhythms—rhythms which vary in regular cycles over a 24-hour period (17, 18). Most bodily functions, such as heart rate, body temperature, and the secretion of hormones, display a 24-hour periodicity. Each of these functions has a unique cycle with different peaks and troughs. They are synchronized by certain external cues (19). In animals, light is the dominant synchronizer. However, in humans, the social environment and awareness of clock time are more important (20). When a person must work at night and sleep during the day, her/his bodily rhythms attempt to adapt to the new schedule. It was found that the rate and extent of adjustment of circadian rhythms depend, in part, on the individual (18). The ability to adjust decreases with age. Under optimal experimental conditions, cycles take one to two weeks to adapt to an inversion of the sleep-wake cycle (21). However, under conditions of actual shift work, where the cues from the social environment do not invert, virtually no cycles ever completely adjust to night activity (21, 22). Furthermore, the many circadian functions of the body are interrelated, but independent in their ability to adjust to changes. With a disturbance, they adjust at different rates, causing a desynchronization of bodily functions (19). Incomplete adjustment and desynchronization of cycles are responsible for many of the negative physiological effects of shift work.

The overall mortality of shift workers does not seem to be higher than for day workers, but no long-term or prospective studies have been done (23, 24). In experimental studies, animals live shorter life spans when subjected to inversion of the day-night cycle (18). A study by Aanonsen comparing day workers, shift workers, and day workers who were former shift workers found twice as many symptoms of nervous and digestive disorders among former shift workers as among the others (23). He and others have concluded that about 20 percent of workers are unable to continue shift work because of possible health risks (9, 11).

Dyspeptic disorders and bowel problems are significantly more common among shift workers (8, 12). In a study of factory workers in Copenhagen, Andersen found gastric symptoms were present in 43 percent of shift workers and 17 percent of day workers. Intestinal symptoms, including constipation, "irritable colon," and diarrhea, were present in 30 percent of shift workers and only 9 percent of day workers (25). Studies looking for ulcers have had mixed results, but suggest that there may be a positive association (11). Disrupted eating habits are felt to be an important factor. Additionally, night workers have increased consumption of caffeine and tobacco (26).

Disturbances of sleep are the most common complaint of shift workers. In several surveys, 60 percent to 85 percent of workers complained of sleep disturbances while on rotating shifts, compared to rates of 10 percent to 16 percent among day workers (24, 25, 27, 28). Night workers sleep up to two hours less and their sleep patterns are more disrupted, with a decrease in R.E.M. sleep and frequent awakenings (21, 22, 24). These disturbances are caused by spontaneous awakenings due to incompletely adjusted diurnal rhythms and by noise in the home due to children, traffic, and the telephone (11, 24). Caillot showed that sleep disturbances increase significantly with increasing number of children in the family and with decreasing number of rooms in the house (29). This decreased sleep leads to increased fatigue and higher rates of neurotic complaints.

A poorly studied but important factor mediating the medical effect of shift work is the circadian rhythms in the body's ability to metabolize toxic chemicals and drugs (30, 31). For example, it has been shown that the same dose of digoxin, a common heart medication, will have a greater biological effect if taken in the evening than in the morning. Similarly, the effects of other drugs and toxic agents in the workplace may have a greater effect on a worker at night. More research is required on this problem.

Experimental studies have shown a decrease in sensory-motor performance at night; however, in factory studies, the results have been mixed due to the very different work conditions during the day and night (8, 9). Overall accident rates are comparable in both periods, but significantly more serious accidents occur during night shifts (32). Absenteeism is the same or less for shift workers compared to day workers (10).

The impact of shift work on family and social relations is hard to define clearly, but may be the most important effect. In United States and European studies, shift workers reported significant disruptions of family life (9). Sixty six percent of shift workers in a French study felt that there was greater interference with their family life than in any other area (15). The amount of disruption increased going from two shifts, to semi-continuous three shifts, and finally to continuous three shifts. The disruption also increases with the size of the family at home (29). The impact differs whether the worker is on the evening or night shift and is affected by the frequency of rotation between shifts (8). Evening shifts are particularly bad for social and family contacts, but best for working a second job. Night workers have the most sexual problems. In general, though, all shift workers complain more frequently about perturbations in their sex lives than non-shift workers (9). Rotating shift workers experience the problems of each shift, plus suffer additional isolation from family and friends due to a constantly changing schedule. The shift worker must miss family meals or break-up her/his major period of sleep to be present. Workers are generally less able to take part in raising the children, and family members feel limited in their activities by the presence of the sleeping worker during the day (29).

Socially, Andersen found that 75 percent of workers felt night shifts limited their contact with friends or leisure activities (25). Conceptually, one can divide social time into unstructured time, such as visiting friends or working in the garden, or structured time, such as sports, trade union, or cultural activities (8, 11). Studies have found that the unstructured activities of shift workers are comparable to day workers, except that their circle of friends is smaller—usually other shift workers. On the other hand, shift workers participate and contribute much less in structured community activities. Most shift workers report a sense of social isolation due to their work.

ERGONOMIC APPROACHES

During recent years, many investigators have suggested alternative work schedules to decrease the adverse effects of shift work. These suggestions have primarily been based on the research of the circadian rhythms of the body (17). Areas studied have included differences in types of shifts, length of the rotation period, starting times for shifts, and the timing of breaks. Most experts recommend rotating shifts with short rotation periods of two or three days (11). A few still advocate long rotation periods in the hope that some workers will physiologically adjust to the night work. It is now accepted that in rotating shifts, the rotation direction should be reversed, rather than forward (11). By rotating from day to night to evening, a worker would get more time off between rotation periods than if she/he rotated from day to evening to night. In the usual forward rotation, many workers are required to work double shifts at the change over between rotation periods. Many researchers recommend different shift lengths and starting times depending upon the biorhythms of efficiency and mental performance. No consistent trends have emerged from this work (8).

While the research has focused on the physiological and performance effects of shift work, most workers are also concerned with the associated social problems. Although the experimental evidence suggests a role for very short rotation periods, virtually all workers prefer the usual length of a week or even longer. The disruption caused by a rapidly changing schedule is an important consideration to the workers. When evaluating the shift length and starting times, workers are more concerned with the availability of facilities for eating and public transportation than with the diurnal variation in their production efficiency. Viable solutions to the problems of shift work must not only consider the physiological consequences of circadian rhythms; they must also incorporate the psychological and social needs of the workers.

Because up to 20 percent of workers may not be able to do shift work due to digestive or nervous disorders, some investigators have examined the individual variability in the worker's response to shift work. Two major factors have been suggested. Ostberg and others have posited the existence of "morning" and "evening" people based on physiological differences in sleep patterns and body temperature curves (33). Evening-type individuals should be more suited for night work. Testing for these characteristics in each worker could be rather expensive. Other researchers have focused on psychosomatic factors and concluded that workers intolerant of night work may be more depressed or have early neurotic abnormalities which make them more susceptible to the effects of shift work (11, 24, 25). These conclusions, however, are based on questionnaires of workers where the correlations were not strong and the diagnoses were constructed from a number of only loosely related factors. While it is important to identify workers less able to do shift work, these approaches have emphasized vague personality characteristics that could be used indiscriminately.

Without more clear, objective measures of the ability to tolerate night work, these suggestions could evolve into little more than blaming the victims of shift work.

DISCUSSION AND RECOMMENDATIONS

Minimizing the adverse consequences of shift work ultimately must involve a multi-faceted approach both within the workplace and on the societal level. Most of the research on shift work has concerned its impact on workers' health and the differential effects of various shift schedules. It is now accepted that shift workers suffer from excess sleep disturbances, nervous conditions, and digestive disorders. In addition, their family and social lives are significantly disrupted by their work. Because many of the adverse health effects are associated with disruptions in the body's circadian rhythms, investigators have attempted to design shift systems which minimize the impact of night work on bodily functions. On the other hand, epidemiological research has revealed that the adverse effects are due to social, as well as physiological, disruptions in the workers' lives. Dyspeptic and gastric disorders are related to a lack of adequate eating facilities at night. Sleep disturbances are highly correlated with the amount of noise at home. Family and social problems arise when the missing shift worker is unable to fulfill her/his expected social role. Therefore, selection of shift schedules should be based on both social and physiological considerations. The effects of shift work can also be reduced by providing adequate facilities for the workers during the evening and night shifts.

The shift cycle must be regular so the worker's family and friends will know when the worker will be home. Starting times should be set considering the availability of public transportation and eating facilities. A reverse rotation direction allows more time off between rotation periods than the usual "day, evening, night" pattern. Workers should be able to select the rotation periods and length of cycle, unless clear physiological evidence suggests an undeniable advantage for one particular system. Wherever feasible, workers must have maximum flexibility in determing their hours of work. For night workers, hot, decent meals should be available at or near the plant. Since more serious accidents occur at night, more health and medical protection must be available to night workers. More frequent breaks may be necessary to reduce the accident rate.

Because a substantial proportion of workers may not be able to do shift work, they should be screened for conditions which put them at high risk. Multiple studies have shown that up to 20 percent of shift workers have to transfer to days because of digestive or nervous disorders. Research into high risk personality characteristics has generally been unproductive. Nevertheless, there are many workers at high risk because of medical or social factors (9). Epileptics have increased numbers of seizures with decreased sleep and should not work at night. People with medical conditions, such as diabetes or hyperthyroidism, requiring specific meals or medications are at risk. Finally, workers with known digestive or nervous disorders are likely to worsen on shift work. Older workers do not adapt as well as younger ones to sleep-wake inversion and may have more trouble with night work. Socially, workers with large families or documented small or noisy homes should not have to do night work. Screening for medical or social contraindications to shift work must be used to identify workers at risk, not to punish or exclude those who desire to do shift work. Where contracts exist, language should insure that screening will be used to protect, not hurt the workers.

Physiological research should go beyond the effects of sleep-wake inversion. The toxicology of chemicals must be evaluated during all periods of the day and night. Exposure standards should be based on periods of minimum resistance to noxious agents. Prospective or long-term studies are needed to examine the effects of shift work over time. Sociological investigations should more fully explore the resources available in the community to lessen the impact of shift work. Finally, since all shift work seems to have some adverse effect, industrial research should be oriented toward developing a technology to decrease or eliminate the need for night workers and to allow for discontinuity of production processes.

Although these recommendations could help substantially, if implemented, they remain inadequate because they do not address the basic issue in understanding the role of shift work. While the use of specific shift schedules has often been arbitrary and could be changed with better information, the overall spread of shift work clearly has been based on conscious economic choices. Historically, the spread of shift work began during the early rise of capitalism and increased dramatically with the growth of technology and large corporations. It represents one facet of the complex social and technical organization of work necessary for the owners of industry to maximize their profits. The social cost of those increased profits is the ill-health of the shift workers. As Zalusky concluded in his review (34):

> As long as attention is paid to a company's cost-benefit ratio rather than the whole social, economic and physiological cost, analyses of shift work will be directed at only making the best of a poor situation. There is a great deal of evidence that shift work is not socially or, in the long term, economically desirable.

The solutions to this basic conflict are not easy to resolve. Extensive reviews by Maurice and by Carpentier and Cazamian for the International Labor Office emphasized the need for legislation to limit or eliminate shift work wherever it is not essential for technical reasons (8, 11). In several countries, including Sweden, Denmark, Norway, Belgium, and Poland, regulations prohibit night work altogether, except in establishments specified by law. West Germany, France, Italy, and the United Kingdom prohibit women from working at night, with specific exceptions. In the United States and these latter countries, unnecessary night work should be prohibited for all workers. In all countries, the regulations must be enforced and the number of excepted industries kept to an absolute minimum. Taxation laws should be changed to prevent rapid depreciation when machines are used more than a normal working day. By allowing more rapid rates of depreciation, governments are condoning the use of unnecessary shift work. Since it is the time at work and the disruption of sleep that is basically pathological, shift workers should work less hours for the same wages. Already at some factories in Norway and Sweden, the number of hours worked by shift workers has been reduced to 28 per week, while maintaining the same wages (11). In France and England, national unions are demanding less work for the same pay and a lowering of retirement age without a reduction in the pension for shift workers. The

Confédération Française Démocratique du Travail (CFDT) has also demanded paid rest days in compensation for working on public holidays, prior medical examinations with periodic follow-up for workers assigned to shift work, and an automatic return to normal schedules after ten years of shift work or after 50 years of age for any worker who so requests, at a guaranteed rate of pay without downgrading (8). In areas where shift work is necessary or common, local entertainment, services, and even television programming should be made more available to night workers.

Finally, in the trade-off between the profits of the owners of industry and the health of the workers, it has become clear historically that benefits to workers have been gained only through unification and stuggle. Nevertheless, only one in five workers in the United States belongs to a union. Unionizing to work together for better working conditions and health is key in the effort to control shift work. In addition, most of the above recommendations for more healthful laws could have been implemented long ago. At this point, the Government of the United States remains largely unresponsive to the needs of workers. Labor unions must enter the political arena and fight for laws to restrict shift work. Since shift work and other methods of restructuring work will continually be forced on workers in the drive to maximize profits, workers must ultimately act together to gain control over their working conditions.

REFERENCES

1. Marx, K. *Capital*, Volume 1, Chapter 4. International Publishers, New York, 1967.
2. Braverman, H. *Labor and Monopoly Capital*. Monthly Review Press, New York, 1974.
3. Laurell, A. C. Work and health in Mexico. *Int. J. Health Serv.* 9(4): 543-568, 1979.
4. Marx, K. *Capital*, Volume 1, Chapter 8. International Publishers, New York, 1967.
5. Berlinguer, G. Work and health in capitalist societies: Some Italian experiences. *HMO Packet* 5-VI, 1979.
6. Foner, P. S. *History of the Labor Movement in the United States*. International Publishers, New York, 1947.
7. Tasto, D., and Colligan, M. *Shift Work Practices in the United States*. U.S. Department of Health, Education, and Welfare (Publication number 77-148), Washington, D.C., 1977.
8. Maurice, M. *Shift Work*. International Labour Office, Geneva, 1975.
9. Rutenfranz, J., Colquhoun, W., Knauth, P., and Ghata, J. Biomedical and psychosocial aspects of shift work: A review. *Scand. J. Work Environ. Health* 3: 165-182, 1977.
10. Owen, J. D. The economics of shift work and absenteeism. In *Shift Work and Health*. U.S. Department of Health, Education, and Welfare (Publication number 76-203), Washington, D.C., 1976.
11. Carpentier, J., and Cazamian, P. *Night Work*. International Labour Office, Geneva, 1977.
12. Tasto, D., Colligan, M., Skjei, E., and Polly, S. *Health Consequences of Shift Work*. U.S. Department of Health, Education, and Welfare (Publication number 75-154), Washington, D.C., 1978.
13. International Labour Office. *Médecine du travail, protection de la maternité et santé de la famille*. Occupational safety and health series No. 29, Geneva, 1975.
14. Tasto, D. Social and psychological adjustment to shift work (Discussion I). In *Shift Work and Health*, pp. 151-153. U.S. Department of Health, Education, and Welfare (Publication number 76-203), Washington, D.C., 1976.
15. Maurice, M., and Monteil, C. Le travail continue en équipes successives. *Revue Française du Travail* 18: 5-31, 1964.
16. Mott, P. E. Social and psychological adjustment to shift work. In *Shift Work and Health*, pp. 145-150. U.S. Department of Health, Education, and Welfare (Publication number 76-203), Washington, D.C., 1976.

17. U.S. Department of Health, Education, and Welfare. *Shift Work and Health* (Publication number 76-203), Washington, D.C., 1976.
18. Halberg, F. Some aspects of chronobiology relating to the optimization of shift work. In *Shift Work and Health,* pp. 13-47. U.S. Department of Health, Education, and Welfare (Publication number 76-203), Washington, D.C., 1976.
19. Scheving, L. E. Chronobiology and how it might apply to the problems of shift work. In *Shift Work and Health,* pp. 118-139. U.S. Department of Health, Education, and Welfare (Publication number 76-203), Washington, D.C., 1976.
20. Aschoff, J., Hoffmann, K., Pohl, H., and Wever, R. Re-entrainment of circadian rhythms after phase-shifts of the Zeitgeber. *Chronobiologia* 2: 23-78, 1975.
21. Weitzman, E. D. Circadian rhythms. In *Shift Work and Health,* pp. 51-56. U.S. Department of Health, Education, and Welfare (Publication number 76-203), Washington, D.C., 1976.
22. Weitzman, E. D., Kripke, D. F., Goldmacher, D., McGregor, P., and Nogeire, C. Acute reversal of sleep-working cycle in man. *A.M.A. Archives of Neurology* 22: 483-489, 1970.
23. Aanonsen, A. Medical problems of shift-work. *Ind. Med. Surg.* 28: 422-427, 1959.
24. Thiis-Evensen, E. Shift work and health. *Ind. Med. Surg.* 27: 493-497, 1958.
25. Andersen, J. E. *Three Shift Work. A Socio-Medical Survey.* The Danish National Institute of Social Research (Publication number 42), Copenhagen, 1970.
26. Metz, B. Principes physiologiques d'organisation du travail en zone saharienne. In Ier congrés de physiologie sararienne. *J. Méd. de Dakar,* December 1960.
27. Andersen, E. J. The main results of the Danish medico-psycho-social investigation of shift-workers. In *Proceedings of the XII International Congress on Occupational Health, Helsinki,* pp. 135-136. Helsinki, 1958.
28. Aanonsen, A. *Shift Work and Health.* Norwegian Monograph on Medical Science, Oslo, 1964.
29. Caillot, R. Consequences sociales du travail a feu continu. *Econ. Hum.* 122: 62-72, 1959.
30. Reinberg, A., and Halberg, F. Circadian chronopharmacology. *Ann. Rev. Pharmacol.* 11: 455-492, 1971.
31. Ede, M. C. Circadian rhythms in drug effectiveness and toxicity in shift workers. In *Shift Work and Health,* pp. 140-141. U.S. Department of Health, Education, and Welfare (Publication number 76-203), Washington, D.C., 1976.
32. Andlauer, P., and Metz, B. Le travail en équipes alternantes. In *Physiologie du travail – Ergonomie,* edited by J. Scherrer. Masson, Paris, 1967.
33. Ostberg, O. Interindividual differences in circadian fatigue patterns in shift workers. *Br. J. Ind. Med.* 30: 341-351, 1974.
34. Zalusky, J. Shiftwork–A complex of problems. *AFL-CIO American Federationist,* pp. 1-6, May 1978.

CHAPTER 7

Impending Proliferation of Asbestos

Barry I. Castleman and Manuel J. Vera Vera

"During 1949 I made the first official governmental radiological and clinical survey of the asbestos industry in the North Eastern Transvaal. At that time industrial hygiene in one of these mines and asbestos works was simply deplorable. Exposures were crude and unchecked. I found young [Bantu] children, completely included within large shipping bags, trampling down fluffy amosite asbestos, which all day long came cascading down over their heads. They were kept stepping lively by a burly supervisor with a hefty whip. I believe these children to have had the ultimate of asbestos dust exposure. X-ray revealed several to have radiologic asbestosis with cor pulmonale before the age of 12. Why Dr. Sluis-Cremer did not see them in his survey 10 years later is fairly evident. There was probably not one of them still alive. . . .

"Nor did [Dr. Cremer] say how many of the pickaninnies, who were strapped on their mother's backs, while their mothers worked along the sorting belts, developed asbestosis. However, he did furnish the statistic that the average duration of exposure before asbestosis is recognized is between five and six years. This is ghastly in comparison with what is currently regarded as a reasonable prospect [of survival in health] for an asbestos worker in an enlightened industry. In the North Eastern Transvaal some of the alleged nonindustrial persons who were found to have asbestosis may be children who had formerly been exposed in an unregulated manner within the industry. . . .

This paper was presented at a conference on The Exportation of Hazardous Industries to Developing Countries, held in New York on November 2, 1979.

"In the valley where the mill was located asbestos dust rolled through like the morning mist, and I had a hard time keeping my staff in working trim because of itching skins caused by asbestos adhering to our clothes. Even food at the local hotel was gritty with dust."

> Account provided by Dr. G. W. H. Schepers (1) of South African asbestos mine and mill of the British concern, Cape Asbestos, 17 years after regulations were issued in Great Britain for the control of asbestos dust in Cape's U.K. factories

As the first century of the modern asbestos industry drew to a close, the "magic mineral" was proclaimed the largest single cause of environmental human cancer in the United States. The Secretary of Health, Education, and Welfare announced in 1978 that for the remainder of this century and part of the next, 17 percent of all U.S. cancer deaths (over 50,000 per year) would be attributable to asbestos (2).

Despite the best efforts of U.S. health experts to predict the toll, there is still uncertainty about these figures. Both high-concentration exposure for brief periods (hours or days) and far lower exposure for long periods are associated with some as yet undetermined cancer risk (3). Asbestos dust inhalation has been linked to increased risk of cancer of the lungs, esophagus, stomach, colon, rectum, kidneys, pleura, and peritoneum (3, 4). It has been the otherwise-rare occurrence of mesotheliomas of the pleura and peritoneum that has revealed the extent of the danger.

In shipyards and other places where asbestos products were extensively used, mesothelioma has occurred not only in all the trades that worked around the asbestos, but also among secretaries and psychologists. Neighbors of shipyards and factories have contracted mesothelioma from ambient air pollution. Family members of asbestos workers and general shipyard workers have developed mesothelioma; and although many with household-contact mesothelioma from the dust taken home on workers' clothes have chest X-ray abnormalities consistent with asbestos exposure, some do not (5).

Physicians at Britain's Department of Employment reported a number of "non-occupational asbestos exposure histories obtained in cases of mesothelioma." Included among these were the following three cases (6):

Duration of Exposure	Nature of Exposure
Unknown	Lived in a house largely composed of asbestos-cement sheeting
4 years	Worked on and lived adjacent to chicken farm composed of asbestos-cement buildings
1 day	Sawed up asbestos-cement sheets to construct two sheds

It is, of course, impossible to know for certain whether these three individuals actually contracted mesothelioma from the above exposures. They may have had other unrecognized or forgotten asbestos exposures, and maybe one or two of these cancers were not even caused by asbestos. On the other hand, it is certainly consistent with what is known about the carcinogenicity of asbestos that such environmental exposures would entail a mesothelioma risk. Chrysotile asbestos air pollution has been detected during dry, windy weather, emanating from asbestos-cement roofing tiles (7).

The widespread public recognition of the threat of asbestos in the United States has had a number of favorable results. Workers and their unions have insisted that employers adhere to the workplace regulations, pay premium rates for this hazardous work, and stop using asbestos. Insurance carriers have raised their worker's compensation insurance rates for employers who continue to use asbestos and have all but ceased to insure U.S. manufacturers of asbestos products for product liability suits brought by injured consumers (8). And the U.S. Government has been stimulated to continue efforts to reduce consumer and environmental exposure to asbestos (9-17).

In the courts, several thousand victims of asbestosis and cancer have so far sued the industry for knowingly marketing deadly products while making no effort to inform product users of the time-bomb danger of breathing asbestos dust. These lawsuits, which grow more numerous each day, may eventually cost the Johns-Manville Corporation, Owens-Corning, Armstrong, and a dozen other manufacturers and their insurance carriers several billion dollars in damages. The litigation has uncovered proof that the industry was not only well aware of the developing medical literature on asbestos, but also, the industry was actively tampering with the "scientific" reports of studies it supported as long ago as 1934 and suppressing reports of other studies it supported through the 1940s and 50s (18, 19).

One sequel to these revelations and others linking industrial suppression of internal knowledge to the deaths of employees and others has been a move in the U.S. Congress to declare such acts federal crimes. A bill just introduced by Congressman George Miller and 40 co-sponsors would confront corporate executives who suppress deadly dangers from their employees and customers with the penalty of a minimum two-year jail term.

Though asbestos continues to be used in the United States in many hazardous and unnecessary applications, the combined pressures on the industry have resulted in a decline in total consumption since the peak year of 1974. However, asbestos use is soaring in many other parts of the world, and there is good reason to fear that the tragedies already recorded in scientific literature are being ignored—and repeated—today.

Previously it has been shown that asbestos textile producers were manufacturing in developing countries and supplying U.S. markets; this practice increased throughout the 1970s. Employees in two Mexican border towns of the U.S. firm, Amatex, first learned about the hazards of asbestos from news accounts, not from their employer (20). Extremely hazardous conditions have also been described in the oldest asbestos-cement plant in Mexico, which produces water storage tanks for homes in Mexico City (21).

INDUSTRY VIEWS AND PRACTICES

Before getting into a detailed case study of asbestos-cement products, it is appropriate to consider the broad-based attitudes of the asbestos industry. The industry's marketing approach unquestionably has the potential to vastly limit the extent of the public hazard involved in the manufacture, fabrication, and use of its products.

Of fundamental importance is the issue of notifying those who will work around asbestos of its lethal potential. Not only should workers be apprised of this, but they should also be instructed in detail about the use of available engineering controls (e.g. enclosure, ventilation), housekeeping practices (e.g. wet mopping instead of dry sweeping of debris), and the use and maintenance of respiratory protection that can limit their exposure to asbestos dust. The most basic, minimal means of notifying people that a product is dangerous is through the use of a warning label. Courts in the United States (where at least some asbestos products bore warning labels starting in 1964) have affirmed that the label should be comprehensible, prominently displayed, and not couched in misleadingly mild terms.

The international asbestos industry's own view of its responsibility to label its products as potentially lethal was recently revealed by the disclosure of an internal memorandum of the Asbestos International Association dated July 7, 1978 (22). The industry members generally agreed that it would be best to get by with as little warning labeling as their various markets would bear:

> Most participants were in favour of an action in various stages, the switching over from one stage to a further less favourable one, depending on outside pressure.

The British asbestos industry's approach to the labeling problem was regarded by many observers as worthy of imitation. This is because the British firms have been able to get their government off their backs with a warning label (Fig. 1) that reads, "Take care with asbestos." The memorandum goes on to note:

> Many of the participants were of the opinion that it was advisable to adopt the U.K. label as such *if the use of a label was unavoidable. Rediscussing the wording could bring along the risk of having to include the word "cancer"* in it. The fact that this label had been found satisfactory to the U.K. authorities was also seen as a good argument for avoiding the EEC [European Economic Community] to press for a less favourable one (such as the skull-and-crossbones used for "toxic substances"). (Emphasis added)

The industry appeared unanimous, however, in the view that the best warning label is none at all:

> *In those countries where it was felt still too early to start voluntary labeling, in fear of a negative influence on sales,* steps should be taken in order to prepare commercial people for the idea, making clear that in the absence of an industry's initiative we could run the risk of being imposed the "skull-and-crossbones" symbol for our products. It should also be pointed out to them that the fact to agree on a kind of label did not imply the agreement of starting to use it right now. (Emphasis added)

The spread of asbestos-cement products is particularly worrisome in view of industry attitudes and the low initial cost of installing these products. Asarco, Incorporated,

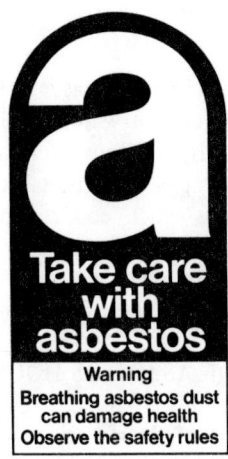

Figure 1. "Warning label" adopted by the British asbestos industry.

is a U.S.-based multinational corporation with asbestos mines in Quebec. The corporation's chief officers opened the 1978 Annual Report by proclaiming that "the outpouring of costly regulations issued in the name of health, safety and environment continues out of control. . . ." The report continued:

> For 1979, asbestos producers face regulatory uncertainties in a number of industrialized countries that could affect the market for both asbestos and manufactured products containing asbestos. However, demand from developing countries for asbestos-cement sheet, a cost-effective building material, remains strong.

ASBESTOS-CEMENT PRODUCTS IN THE UNITED STATES

The incorporation of asbestos as a binder in cement products began in 1900 in Europe. Asbestos-cement sheet products are widely used today in building construction, as is asbestos-cement pipe in water and sewerage systems. In the United States, asbestos-cement sheet and pipe accounted for 29,000 and 146,000 metric tons of asbestos fiber in 1978, respectively, for a total of 41 percent of the nation's asbestos consumption (23).

Hazardous exposures to asbestos commonly occur in the manufacture and fabrication of asbestos-cement sheet and pipe. Asbestos air and water pollution frequently results from the use, maintenance, and disposal of asbestos-cement products. Mixing the ingredients and sawing asbestos-cement products releases dense clouds of visible asbestos dust, with exposures as high as several hundred million asbestos fibers per cubic meter of air (24, 25). Though portable, high velocity, local exhaust ventilation cutting machines are available for sawing asbestos-cement sheet, the use of such devices is not standard practice in the construction industry. Recently, construction workers in Utah developed obstructive respiratory impairment shortly after five months of sawing asbestos-cement panels inside a new building (26). None of the deflection shrouds tested by industry in the United States for cutting asbestos-cement pipe are equipped with dust collection devices, though they do reduce operator exposures (27).

Drinking water is widely contaminated by asbestos from conduits and asbestos tile roofing. With asbestos-cement pipes, the water conditions favoring leaching of fiber from pipe walls are acidity (low pH) and low calcium saturation. Drilling and cutting for installation and maintenance pose additional contamination threats. Cisterns in St. Croix, U.S. Virgin Islands, which collect drinking water from asbestos tile roofing material, have been shown to have contamination levels of over 500 million fibers per liter. High fiber concentrations have also been reported in cisterns in Ohio and Kentucky by the U.S. Environmental Protection Agency (28, 29).

THE RISE AND FALL OF ASBESTOS HOUSING IN PUERTO RICO

Around 1973, the government of Puerto Rico was looking for safe, sturdy, and resistant materials which could be used in developing housing alternatives for the poor people of the island. It was accepted that the construction of houses using wood and zinc roofing was inappropriate, due to the climatological conditions on this tropical island. At the time, asbestos-cement looked like the answer. Over 500 asbestos-cement schools had been built in the late 1950s and early 60s. So beginning in 1975, nearly 2,000 houses of asbestos-cement were built throughout the island by the Housing Department. The houses were bought from Eternit Pacifico, S.A., a Colombian manufacturer, and delivered to Puerto Rico for assembly. This company is a subsidiary of the large European Eternit multinational. The original government investment was supposed to be around $6 million, but as a result of some problems with shipping and delivery, it was closer to $11 million. In the summer of 1978, the construction and sale of the houses was stopped because of public outcry against the asbestos and its health hazard. Meanwhile, the asbestos-cement classrooms continue to be used by nearly 50,000 children.

Servicios Legales de Puerto Rico, Inc. had been working with one of the asbestos-cement communities in San Sebastian, a small town in western Puerto Rico, since 1977. The community's concern at that time was the physical condition of the houses. They were plagued by defects such as broken and cracked asbestos-cement roofing, wall panels, and ceiling panels and malfunctioning electrical systems and plumbing. The floors were unleveled, and moisture would collect on them during rainy days.

Except for the concrete floors, the houses in this community (as in the others in Puerto Rico) were totally built of asbestos-cement. Since the majority of the floors were unleveled, the asbestos-cement panels were forced into place and secured by the use of bolts and nuts. The result of this construction method was that soon after the houses were built, the upper corners of the asbestos sheets cracked under the stress on the materials. At the same time, the lateral panels (inside and outside) started to crack under the pressure created by the unleveled floors and by the blows of children playing and other normal living conditions.

In most of the houses, the wind blowing through the ceiling space between the corrugated roofing and the layer of ceiling panels below jostled the ceiling panels, even breaking some of them, leaving the corrugated asbestos roofing exposed in the inside of the home. There was considerable dust caused by wind shaking the ceiling panels. Some of the residents replaced the asbestos-cement with decorative wood panels.

Another major construction problem of the houses was that most of their plumbing was deficient and inadequate to sustain the water pressure. As a result, the lines broke in the bathrooms and the kitchen. The residents were then forced to break the asbestos sheets, using hammers and saws to expose the plumbing. There was no other way to get to it, since the plumbing was sealed behind the asbestos-cement sheets.

Some residents made major renovations, e.g. knocking out an archway in a wall. They had not been warned that the dust was a mortal danger. In one home where the infants had developed breathing difficulties, an archway stood with threads of asbestos hanging along the cut edges of the asbestos-cement wall panels.

After a year of vain efforts with the Housing Department, Servicios Legales, representing 27 families, filed a suit in July 1978 against the Housing Department claiming for damages resulting from the construction defects and for breach of contract. At that time, Servicios Legales and its clients were totally unaware of the health hazards of asbestos. That was the reason for claiming damages only for the construction defects.

Around September 1978, the U.S. Social Security Administration circulated among the Social Security beneficiaries in the community a publication of the U.S. Department of Health, Education, and Welfare related to asbestos and asbestos exposure. It was then that the members of the community asked for information about possible health problems in their homes. At this point, Servicios Legales started a complete investigation of the subject and, after analysis and consultation, amended the suit in December 1978 to include the health issue and the implicit warranty of habitability.

The main legal problem then, and now, was that the Colombian manufacturer and its parent European multinational, Eternit, which sold the asbestos houses to the government of Puerto Rico, were out of the residents' reach for a legal claim. The company, which had made millions of dollars and was responsible for the importation to Puerto Rico of the asbestos housing, could not be made legally responsible for the health harm that the product causes in Puerto Rico. (There appear to be no specific regulations for workplace exposure to asbestos and asbestos pollution in Colombia, which is another aspect of the overall problem.)

The only alternative available to the residents was to file suit against the government, which had sold them the houses after assembly in Puerto Rico. Since then, the government has denied that the asbestos schools or houses are dangerous. But in the summer of 1978, after a study was issued by Dr. William Nicholson of the Mount Sinai School of Medicine, New York, on the asbestos concentrations in schools and houses, the government decided to discontinue the use of the schools and start a replacement program under the excuse that the facilities were old and obsolete. The authorities also discontinued the construction and sale of the houses because they were "structurally unfit and dangerous."

This study by Dr. Nicholson was prepared under a contract with the Consumer Product Safety Commission following a request in June 1977 for a survey and air samples of the asbestos-cement schools and housing by Rafael Ramos Lacen, a Puerto

Rican industrial consultant (30, 31). The findings were highly "criticized" by the asbestos manufacturers in and out of Puerto Rico, and additional air samples were taken to add to the data base. The results of that second sampling have not yet been reported.

In his analysis of the initial house samples, Dr. Nicholson found:

> ... air concentrations somewhat higher than those normally encountered in urban settings. . . .[T] he possibility exists that a contribution to asbestos levels may result from the erosion and washing of fibers from the roof and concomitant dissemination into the air. . . .

His findings in the schools were more illustrative of the extent of the asbestos contamination:

> Uniformly high air concentrations of asbestos were seen in seven samples taken in or about schools constructed of asbestos-cement panels, including one (4,500 ng/m^3) of a degree rarely seen in environmental circumstances, even near known asbestos sources.

The report contained one photograph of elementary school children napping on an asbestos-cement schoolroom floor.

Following the Nicholson study and the filing of the amended claim in the Superior Court, the local press started an investigation of the issues, and the problem was given wide coverage in the media. The asbestos communities in Puerto Rico were represented in two press conferences calling for the attention of the Governor, the Housing Department Secretary, and the Legislature. Servicios Legales started a campaign to locate all the asbestos-cement communities and schools in Puerto Rico and to start a census on the construction and health problems that had already started to appear (e.g. respiratory problems, allergies, rashes, and a peculiar type of skin ulcer on the lower limbs, mainly of children).

The official position of the government at first was that Nicholson's study did not find any abnormal concentrations of asbestos in the houses' air samples and that it was only a political issue since there was no scientific evidence relating low levels of airborne asbestos to any health problems. For this reason, no public warnings or instructions were given as to the need for great care in repairing or renovating the asbestos houses.

The issue was finally taken up by the government, and three legislative measures were submitted for the substitution of the asbestos houses and schools. Most significant was House Bill No. 2654, which pointed out in its Exposition of Motives that not only had studies made by the Housing Department found the houses to be unsafe and vulnerable structurally, but also—and even more alarming—scientific studies showed that asbestos was highly associated with cancer.

This was the most unambiguous acknowledgment by the Puerto Rican government of the health risks of asbestos in the schools and houses. At legislative hearings in March 1979, Servicios Legales de Puerto Rico presented a scientific analysis of the asbestos issue. Servicios Legales also criticized Bill 2654, because even though it considered the health issue, its wording tended to encourage the home owners to do their own repairs and renovations, failing to provide any warnings to the public about ways to handle and dispose of asbestos materials in compliance with the standards of the U.S. Occupational Safety and Health Administration (OSHA) and the Environmental Protection Agency (EPA). Bill 2654 suffered some amendments, including the elimination of the reference to cancer, which was requested by the Justice Department because of "its possible legal repercussions" in the future, and ultimately was substituted by Bill 1109. Bill 1109 was finally approved as Law No. 125 in July 1979, and $16.4 million was provided for the substitution of the asbestos houses in a two-year plan.

Before the law was approved, the Superior Court of Puerto Rico certified the residents' suit as a class action. This decision was appealed by the Housing Department, the defendant in the case. The apparent intention of this is to delay the court action until the houses are substituted and to let the issue subside. In the meanwhile, the National Association of Asbestos House Owners, established in the summer of 1979 with representation of the majority of the asbestos-cement house communities on the island, is active in the supervision of all contracts, rules, and regulations under which the houses are to be substituted, especially the ways in which the Housing Department contractors are going to dispose of the asbestos-cement materials in compliance with EPA and OSHA regulations, practically unknown in Puerto Rico.

It has been three years since the San Sebastian community first made its complaints to the Housing Department because of the construction defects, and over one year since the issue went to court. Only $16.4 million has been provided to replace nearly 1,391 houses and relocate over 5,000 human beings in a slow and bureaucratic process. Many of the asbestos-cement schools are still in use. The resulting chronic health effects are impossible to predict or prevent.

ASBESTOS-CEMENT SUBSTITUTES

Corrugated and flat fiber-cement roofing can be made without asbestos. The fiber can be something that is locally available, e.g. human hair cuttings, common grasses, crop wastes from bananas or coconuts. The roofing panels made with these harmless fibers cost one-third as much as asbestos-cement sheets, can be made in 20 minutes, and require no special equipment or skill to manufacture (32). Another product that shows promise as a substitute for asbestos-cement is glass-reinforced, stabilized clay. A full and competent evaluation of available substitutes would certainly be of value at this time.

The Economic and Social Committee of the European Economic Community considered the problems of asbestos and made a number of recommendations early in 1979. Among these was a ban on asbestos "in manufacturing processes where substitutes are available which do not have the hazardous properties of asbestos"; and "where liquids are processed for human consumption." (33)

Sweden has banned the manufacture of asbestos-cement, mainly because of occupational hazards, and imports of asbestos fiber have declined from 20,000 tons per year to only a few thousand tons per year (34).

U.S. Environmental Protection Agency researchers have finally concluded that asbestos contamination of water supplies from asbestos-cement pipe constitutes a carcinogenic hazard to the public (28). In Seattle, Washington, where the water supply is aggressive and quite capable of entraining asbestos from the walls of asbestos-cement conduits, local authorities have moved to ban further installations of such pipe for water supplies (29). There has also been considerable controversy over the use of asbestos-cement water pipe in Virginia; the city of Chesapeake has halted its use, following City Council hearings on the subject in which citizens, industry, and an environmental group participated.

In light of available information, the use of asbestos-cement in the construction industry worldwide ought to be drastically curtailed, if not altogether eliminated.

SUBSTITUTION OF OTHER ASBESTOS PRODUCTS

Recent advances elsewhere in the commercial substitution of asbestos warrant mention here.

By far the largest toll of asbestos disease is attributable to one class of products: insulation. Although only a small fraction of shipyard and construction workers actually installed asbestos-containing pipe and boiler insulation, the dust created exposed millions of workers in other trades to severe hazards of cancer and asbestosis. The spraying of asbestos in British naval ships, which started in 1944, was abandoned in 1963 (35). The use of sprayed and molded asbestos insulation in the United States continued into the 1970s. Following state and local action, in 1973 the U.S. Environmental Protection Agency issued rules to curtail the use of sprayed asbestos, and in 1975 banned the use of asbestos in molded pipe insulation (12). Safer substitutes had long been available (36, 37).

Despite the fact that the epidemic of disease caused by asbestos insulation has been thoroughly documented worldwide, the Novex Foreign Trade Company of Hungary announced in 1977 that it was going to market an asbestos-containing material for use in spray, molded, and sheet form (38). This material, Asket, vividly illustrates how a marginal byproduct (short-fiber asbestos) can be converted into a major cancer hazard. The continuing use of asbestos insulation in ships today assures the needless perpetuation of the threat of asbestos disease to ship repair workers all over the world beyond the year 2000.

One of the most prominent uses of asbestos today is in automotive friction products: brakes and clutch facings. On September 7, 1979, General Motors announced to the EPA that approximately 60 percent of all passenger car disc brakes manufactured and used by GM had non-asbestos friction materials. It was projected that all GM 1983-model passenger cars with disc brakes would have asbestos-free brakes, and all cars with drum brakes and light trucks would have asbestos-free brakes by the 1985 model year (39).

The largest U.S. manufacturer of friction materials, Raybestos-Manhattan Corporation, already faces product liability suits brought by brake mechanics for failure to warn of asbestos dangers in the past. In its 1978 Annual Report, this firm announced: "We are planning to eliminate asbestos from our friction materials by 1982 in order to minimize the effect of any further government regulations in this area." One would presume from a liability standpoint alone that the substitutes must entail substantially less health hazard than the old asbestos formulations.

The friction products industry was described in a 1976 industry report as the employer of nearly 20 percent of the asbestos plant workers in the United States, the largest employer of nine primary asbestos industries with a work force of 7,304 employees (40). In addition, an estimated 900,000 auto mechanics and garage workers are deemed "potentially exposed to asbestos" in the servicing of brakes and clutches, according to a warning circulated by the National Institute for Occupational Safety and Health (41). Thousands more are exposed occupationally in mining, milling, and transporting 80,000 metric tons of asbestos a year for the U.S. friction products industry (23). The rest of us are exposed to asbestos air and water pollution from all the mining, milling, manufacturing, brake repair, and brake decomposition in both remote regions and towns. Brake linings have been an asbestos industry advertising symbol of life-saving value based on irreplaceability.

It is thus a matter of tremendous significance that friction products are ready to join pipe insulation and others as asbestos-free industries in the 1980s, not only in the United States but worldwide. Whether this life-saving advance will take place, however, remains to be seen.

REFERENCES

1. Schepers, G. W. H. Discussion. *Ann. N.Y. Acad. Sci.* 132: 246-247, 1965.
2. Bridbord, K., et al. Estimates of the Fraction of Cancer in the United States Related to Occupational Factors. U.S. Department of Health, Education, and Welfare, Washington, D.C., September 15, 1978.
3. International Agency for Research on Cancer. *Monographs on the Evaluation of the Carcinogenic Risk of Chemicals to Man: Asbestos,* Volume 14. Lyon, France, 1977.
4. Selikoff, I. J., Hammond, E. C., and Seidman, H. Mortality experience of insulation workers in the United States and Canada, 1943-1976. *Ann. N.Y. Acad. Sci.* 330: 91-116, 1979.
5. Anderson, H. A., et al. Household contact neoplastic risk. *Ann. N.Y. Acad. Sci.* 271: 311-323, 1976.
6. Greenberg, M., and Davies, T. A. L. Mesothelioma register 1967-68. *Br. J. Ind. Med.* 31: 91-104, 1974.
7. Spurny, K. R., et al. On the evaluation of fibrous particles in remote ambient air. *Sci. Total Environ.* 11: 1-40, 1979.
8. Solomon, S. The asbestos fallout at Johns-Manville. *Fortune,* May 7, 1979, pp. 196-206.
9. Standard for exposure to asbestos dust. *Federal Register* 37: 11318-22, June 7, 1972.
10. Occupational exposure to asbestos/Notice of proposed rulemaking. *Federal Register* 40: 47652-65, October 9, 1975.
11. Finklea, J. Evaluation of Data on Health Effects of Asbestos Exposure and Revised Recommended Numerical Environmental Limits. Memorandum from National Institute for Occupational Safety and Health to Occupational Safety and Health Administration, December 15, 1976.
12. National emission standards for hazardous air pollutants/Amendments to standards for asbestos and mercury. *Federal Register* 40: 48292-311, October 14, 1975.
13. Commercial and industrial use of asbestos fibers and consumer products containing asbestos. *Federal Register* 44: 60056, October 17, 1979.
14. Asbestos-form particles in drugs for parenteral injection. *Federal Register* 40: 11865-69, March 14, 1975.
15. Electrolytic diaphragm process for salt; revocation. *Federal Register* 41, January 22, 1976.
16. Consumer patching compounds and artificial emberizing materials (embers and ash) containing respirable free-form asbestos/Banned hazardous products. *Federal Register* 42: 63354-65, December 15, 1977.

17. U.S. Environmental Protection Agency. Federal Register Citations Pertaining to the Regulation of Asbestos. In-house report, April 1979.
18. *Asbestos-related Occupational Diseases.* Hearings before the Subcommittee on Compensation, Health and Safety of the Committee on Education and Labor/House of Representatives. U.S. Government Printing Office, Washington, D.C., 1979.
19. Castleman, B. How the asbestos industry avoids its victims. *Business and Society Review,* Fall 1979, pp. 33-38.
20. Castleman, B. The export of hazardous factories to developing nations. *Int. J. Health Serv.* 9(4): 569-606, 1979.
21. North American Congress on Latin America. Occupational health and asbestos. *NACLA Report on the Americas,* Volume 12. New York, 1978.
22. Asbestos International Association. 8th Executive Committee Meeting, Agenda Item 6: Labelling. July 7, 1978.
23. Clifton, R. A. *Asbestos.* U.S. Bureau of Mines, Washington, D.C., 1979.
24. Cross, A. A., et al. Practical methods for protection of men working with asbestos materials in shipyards. In *Safety and Health in Shipbuilding,* pp. 93-101. International Labour Office, Geneva, 1972.
25. Remarks by Milt Trosper/Johns-Manville Corporation. In *Third Annual Industry-Government Conference,* pp. 109-115. Asbestos Information Association, Arlington, Va., 1976.
26. Harless, K. W., Watanabe, S., and Renzetti, Jr., A.D. The acute effects of chrysotile asbestos exposure on lung function. *Environ. Res.* 16: 360-372, 1978.
27. Asbestos Exposures During the Cutting and Machining of Asbestos Cement Pipe; and Separate Report of Additional Studies. Report prepared for Asbestos-Cement Pipe Producers Association, Arlington, Va., 1977.
28. McCabe, L. J., and Millette, J. R. Health Effects and Prevalence of Asbestos Fibers in Drinking Water. Proceedings of American Water Works Association Conference, San Francisco, June 24-29, 1979.
29. Environmental Defense Fund. Comments before Senate Subcommittee Studying Asbestos Pipes, Arlington, Va., September 18, 1979.
30. Harmful asbestos found in units in Puerto Rico. *Washington Post,* June 18, 1977.
31. Nicholson, W. J. *Chrysotile Asbestos in Air Samples Collected in Puerto Rico.* Report to Consumer Product Safety Commission, March 16, 1978.
32. *Low-Cost Handmade Roof Sheets of Strong Fibre Reinforced Cement.* Available from J. M. Parry and Associates, Ltd., Corngreaves Trading Estate, Overend Road, Warley, West Midlands B64 7DD, U.K. (associated with Intermediate Technology Development Group).
33. European Economic Community. *Study of the Economic and Social Committee on Health and Environmental Hazards Arising from the Use of Asbestos.* Brussels, 1979.
34. *Asbestos and Asbestos Substitutes.* International Metalworkers Federation Bulletin on Occupational Health and Safety No. 5, 1979.
35. Harries, P. G. Asbestos dust concentrations in ship repairing; A practical approach to improving asbestos hygiene in naval dockyards. *Ann. Occup. Hyg.* 14: 241, 1971.
36. Kalousek, G. L. Calcium Silicate of Microcrystalline Lathlike Structure. United States Patent Number 2,547,127, April 3, 1951.
37. Bowles, O. *The Asbestos Industry.* Bulletin 552, U.S. Bureau of Mines, Washington, D.C., 1955.
38. New Insulation from Hungary. *Asbestos* 12, Sept. 1977.
39. General Motors Programs on Non-Asbestos Friction Materials for Brake Systems. September 7, 1979.
40. Table 3-1. *Technological Feasibility and Economic Impact of OSHA Proposed Revision to the Asbestos Standard.* Prepared by Weston Environmental Consultants–Designers for Asbestos Information Association, March 29, 1976.
41. National Institute for Occupational Safety and Health. Alert on Asbestos Hazards of Brake Repair. Rockville, Md., August 8, 1975.

APPENDIX

INTERVIEW WITH A FORMER EMPLOYEE OF HINDUSTAN FERODO, LTD.

Hindustan Ferodo, Ltd. manufactures a number of asbestos products at its factory in Bombay, India. The plant was built in 1956. Turner and Newall Ltd. of Manchester, England—the largest asbestos enterprise in Western Europe—owns 74 percent of the share capital of Hindustan Ferodo. The interview which follows, conducted in March 1980, describes working conditions and business practices in the Bombay plant.

Q: What products are produced and how much?

A: There are two divisions to the plant. One produces about 250 tons a month of brake and clutch linings. The other manufactures a wide variety of asbestos textiles, from heavy webbing mat to finer yarns (about 125 tons a month).

Q: Which were exported to where, and how much?

A: Production has been held to less than full capacity, despite ample demand. Domestic and export markets are strong, but there is a shortage of asbestos, which must be imported. Hindustan Ferodo imports about 95 percent of its asbestos, predominantly from Canada and, until recently, from Rhodesia. Most of the products are consumed domestically; about 5 to 10 percent are exported, with the major destinations being Sri Lanka and South Asia. Until two or three months ago, both textile and friction materials were shipped to the United Kingdom. However, this has stopped because of capacity problems and objections about inadequate packaging at British docks.

Q: Are the products labeled as to possible health hazards?

A: There's no indication on any product that it may be hazardous to health.

Q: I've been told that the products must be shipped in unmarked containers, as there have been problems unloading these shipments in the West. Is this true?

A: It is true that the company has been having problems, particularly with webbing and friction materials sent to the U.K., where there are very stringent packaging requirements. The products must be triple-packed in polyethylene so that there will be no leaks due to container damage during shipment. They weren't packaging it this well, and as a result several consignments were returned. They stopped exporting to the U.K. two or three months ago, for this reason [it increases the cost], and because they have such a domestic demand that they don't need to export to the United Kingdom. They haven't had any such problems in Southeast Asia and Sri Lanka, so they're not triple-packaging any shipments to those areas.

Q: Are the workers informed of the nature of the hazard and, if so, are they told of preventive measures?

A: No, they're not told at all. Virtually no one is told, in fact. Not only are the workers not told, but even management personnel are not informed about any work-place hazard. Ventilation systems are poorly maintained. Dust on the floors is just swept up dry with a broom, instead of a wet mop. The workers even have the idea, which management does nothing to dispel, that if you drink alcoholic drinks, the asbestos won't do you any harm. A lot of the workers are heavy drinkers.

Q: Are there workplace standards for asbestos fibers? If so, what are they and what is the penalty for non-compliance? Are the workplaces monitored regularly and how?

A: [He has no idea what standards there are or what the penalty is for non-compliance.] They do take dust counts on a relatively regular basis. The dust levels in many spots in the factory are easily visible, with much dust in the air in some of the operations. Hence, although there is some air monitoring, there appear to be no hygiene standards maintained.

Q: What protection is given to the workers?

A: The workers are given uniforms, which they leave at the shop and which are laundered every two to three days. The same locker is used for work clothes and street clothes, however. The fluffing and the carding operations are the most dusty. It's very visible, as dense as the dust in the air behind a bus on a dirt road in dry season. These areas are enclosed, and workers are supposed to wear respirators of the cannister type. However, they generally avoid this, because they're not given any indication that this dust is extremely hazardous. As far as they know, it's just very unpleasant to breathe because it's so thick. So the workers often avoid the respirators because of the discomfort of wearing the face masks for hours. It's only in these two operations, the fluffing and carding, that cannister-type respirators are provided. The rest of the workers in the plant are given cloths that resemble surgical masks—a piece of cloth tied around the head with strings. Except for top management officials who wear them every time they go into the work area, few employees use these devices. Generally, unless the dust is really a nuisance, clogging up the nose and so forth, no face mask is worn. There are no notices anywhere in the plant warning against the dangers of excessive dust inhalation.

There is also a sort of hazard pay scheme in effect. Workers in the fluffing opera-tion and in the carding operation get a 5 percent "inconvenience allowance" (this has been in effect for the last two years). It's called an "inconvenience allowance" because they have to put up with the inconvenience of wearing respirators.

Q: What is the medical monitoring program and when was it implemented?

A: They've had medical monitoring since around 1970. Once or twice a year each production worker is screened. There is no screening for office personnel, and no one in the office is ever told anything about what the screening is for. Workers are simply taken off the job for a couple of hours, put in the company van and driven up to the medical building, given an X-ray and sent back. *The workers are not told of the results.* They just view it as a way of getting out of a couple of hours of work. The workers know nothing about the medical records kept by the company.

Q: How is asbestos dust generated, captured, and ultimately disposed of?

A: The plant is a fairly dusty place. Asbestos is received in polyethylene bags, which are cut open with a knife. The sack cutters do not wear dust respirators, though some wear the useless cloth masks. Workers slice the bags open, then they flip them over and empty them. The asbestos comes out like a block, and is tossed onto a conveyor belt which goes a short distance to the machinery. Overwhelmed exhaust ventilation is used in some dusty areas. All the suction ducts lead into a room outside of the plant. This equipment is designed to pack and seal the dust in polyethylene bags; unfortunately, jute bags are used instead, which leak dust profusely. The area is like a dust storm. "Outside" contract laborers are used in this area, and they are given no respiratory protection, no uniforms, no medical check-ups. They are completely covered in dust and look like they work in a flour mill, white from head to toe. The sacks of short-fiber waste dust are taken out by truck and just dumped nearby beside a small stream. In the last couple of months, the municipal council has objected to the dumping, and consequently big piles of pure asbestos wastes are accumulating in the factory yard.

Q: Are there ever visitors at the plant, who observe typical operations?

A: When visitors are expected, extra cleaning workers are hired, and the dustier operations are shut down for awhile to clean up the plant.

PART 3

Occupational Health in Developed Capitalist Countries

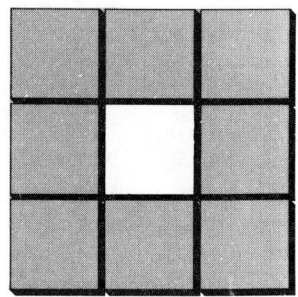

CHAPTER 8

The State of Industrial Ill-Health in the United Kingdom

R. Charles Clutterbuck

Nowadays everyone is concerned about health and safety. Safety committees are popping up like mushrooms all over the United Kingdom. Legislation providing rights for safety representatives came into effect on October 1, 1978. For the first time outside the mines in 150 years of factory legislation, provisions for training and information for worker representatives have been brought into being. Industrial designers are being urged to "think safety." Safety posters, conferences, courses, films, and books are all carrying "the message." Protective equipment is big business. It's the smiling face of capitalism.

This concern comes at a time of continued wage restraints.[1] Phases One, Two, and Three have passed, all set for Phase Four of incomes policy. Productivity deals,

---

[1] This article was prepared in March 1979, and therefore does not reflect changes occurring since the Labor Party lost power in the May election of Prime Minister Margaret Thatcher (Conservative Party).

where increased wages are paid for increased overall productivity, abound as a way of overcoming continued inflation. There have been severe cutbacks in spending among government services, in education, health, and the civil service. There is no extra money for training government safety representatives and no chance of any occupational health facilities being developed in the National Health Service. The fire fighters, in their historic strike for decent pay under extremely dangerous conditions, were smashed by the unemployed and use of the Army and scabs. There are 1.5 million unemployed, and layoffs at British Leyland (auto), Spillers (milling), and Imperial Chemical Industries add to that total daily. It's the chronic crisis of late capitalism.

Are these two aspects of present-day industry as contradictory as they appear? Will the new legislation reduce the appalling toll of industrial ill-health, where each day 50,000 people do not go to work because they have been crippled by an industrial accident or disease? Or will the legislation keep a lot of people happy (except the 50,000 already incapacitated) while making sure everything continues as normal? What was it designed to do? And what is the effect of the continued economic crisis on the organization of health and safety on the shop floor and in the Government? To understand what developments could occur, it is necessary to look at Britain, which has the longest history of safety legislation in the world. Then it will be possible to analyze the role of the trade unions, corporations, and the State, and to assess the impact of the new legislation on the shop floor.

THE 19TH CENTURY

The industrial war started in Britain with the rise of industrial capital at the beginning of the 19th century. Occupational hazards were on a scale previously unimaginable. Long hours, child labor, and appalling conditions soon led to the first factory legislation of 1802. But it was not until 1833 that the Factory Inspectorate was set up. Four inspectors policed 2000 mills to ensure that child labor was not over-exploited. "How could the essential character of the capitalist method of production be better shown than by the need for forcing upon it, by Acts of Parliament, the simplest appliances for maintaining cleanliness and health?" (1)

Following this, regulations were passed in the 1840s concerning machine guarding and, in response to the Chartists' movement, the length of the working day. Although the Chartists campaigned for over ten years to reduce hours for all workers, the law ended up in 1847 being applied only to women and children. This was to be the beginning of "protective" legislation, whereby women are treated differently from men. It has been a source of disagreement within the women's movement ever since as to whether such protection should be extended to men or whether it should be abolished altogether because it is discriminatory. Certainly men felt that their jobs were protected by the new legislation (2).

Although popularly realized, it was not until the 1860s that the medical establishment began to recognize that widespread disease was caused by factory conditions. In 1864 a Royal Commission found an excessively high incidence of pulmonary disease among working people in tin mines in Cornwall and lead mines in the north of

England (3). A survey by Dr. Arnold Knight in Sheffield found that fork-grinders who used grindstones died before they were 30 due to the silica dust (4). Similar reports of pottery workers in the Midlands suffering from phthisis and diseases of the respiratory organs were eventually published in 1875 (5).

In response, liberal reformers in Parliament established the Factory Extension Act of 1864, which required that "every factory to which this Act applies shall be kept in a cleanly state, and be ventilated in such a manner as to render harmless so far as is practicable any Gases, Dust, or other Impurities generated in the Process of Manufacture that may be injurious to Health." (The Factory Act of 1961 was to sound remarkably similar!) These requirements applied to factories making earthenware, matches, cartridges, and staining paper, and contained rules to make sure that ventilation was not impeded by "the wilful Misconduct or wilful Negligence of the Workmen." The emphasis was clearly on *cleaning up.*

Despite the formation of the Trades Union Congress (TUC) in 1868, there seem to have been few advances over the next 20 years, especially regarding control engineering. This was due in part to the impact of the "laissez-faire" attitude of the Government toward both trade and legislation. The laissez-faire economists argued that the control of dangerous occupations would be ensured by market forces—wages would be forced higher to compensate for the dangers. These "voluntaristic" arguments were undoubtedly accepted by most union leaders, who also believed that it was better to rely on union bargaining power than on the law.

The 1890s produced some important developments in health and safety. While the economy was beginning to improve following a long period in which the rate of profit fell (6), conditions in factories did not. Capital was exported to develop foreign markets, with disastrous effects on agriculture and on the development of technology in industry (slow compared to the United States and Germany).

There seems to have been a growing awareness of poor working conditions, due to the publication of the Registrar General's statistics on occupational mortality and the growing confidence in trade union organization. As the Webbs noted, "In the trade union world of today, there is no subject of which workmen of all shades of opinion and all variations of occupation are so unanimous and so ready to take combined action as the prevention of accidents and the provision of healthy workplaces." (7) There was the famous match-girls' strike over wages and conditions in the East End of London. Gertrude Tuckwell publicized the plight of women trade unionists regarding the hazards of lead in the pottery trades, and workers in the coal mines, potteries, and railways managed to force employers to appoint safety representatives—however token they may have been (8).

In response, there was a spate of safety legislation. The Factories and Workshops Act of 1891 stated that factory inspectors had powers to issue notice to employers to improve ventilation, but also insisted that employed people adopt increasingly stringent methods of personal protection (e.g. respirators, head coverings, and overalls). The new twist was pointed out at that time: "This leaves alone the process of production. As long as dangerous processes remain, compulsory provision of a dispensary and free muzzle avails little." (9) In 1896 the first Chief Medical Officer for Factories, Thomas Legge, was appointed (10). Pressure also built up for the separate establishment of women factory inspectors. In later years their greater commitment and more militant reports were met with patronizing derision by Members of Parliament. After World War I they became amalgamated with the rest of the Factory Inspectorate.

Probably the most important piece of legislation was the introduction by the new Conservative Government of the Workmen's Compensation Act of 1897 for accidents at work (to be followed by a 1960 act covering certain diseases). The purpose of this legislation was not primarily to care for workers, or to prevent accidents and diseases, but to help the employers rebut claims for damages (11). For this, company doctors were increasingly employed, which was "an unhappy introduction of medicine to industry." (12) When the 1897 act was first introduced, workers were owed compensation irrespective of negligence. However, the unions preferred to rely not on legislation but on the judicial system to prove negligence in the courts. This was strange, because judges were known to be closely linked with factory managers. It was something that the larger companies did not want either. According to one M.P., "Several large employers said 'Why do you not go in for compensation generally? It is only a matter of insurance. We are sick of litigation as to liability'." (13, p. 430) It seems that British unionists felt that "self-help" was the only effective means of attaining labor reform, whereas French and other European union leaders hoped for permanent improvement of their conditions through legislation and state cooperation (14). The trade unions had no overall policy regarding accident prevention, initiating very little legislation and focusing instead on merely improving existing legislation and getting collective bargaining agreements regarding safety.

THE PRE-WORLD WAR II PERIOD

These confused attitudes reflected themselves in the piecemeal advances up to the start of World War I. There were many Royal Commissions, reports, inquiries, and regulations, especially in the pottery and mining industries, and later in the munitions industry. After the war, the important Whitley Report of 1919 accepted the idea of joint councils of workers and employers, which were then recognized by the Factory Inspectorate as including safety issues within their bounds (15).

It was not until 1924 that there was a unique but significant TUC publication, *The Waste of Capitalism.* It stated categorically that workers should control their own working environment and challenged the value of joint negotiating committees where workers have no real power. "Joint Control is simply employers' control plus workers' advice—which may or may not be taken. The worker cannot be expected to take an interest in production so long as he is denied the elementary right to determine, in cooperation with his fellow workers, the conditions under which he labours." (quoted in 16, p. 330) During the late 1920s and early 30s, the failure of the General Strike and mass unemployment dealt massive blows to union organization. In the ten years between 1921 and 1931, union membership fell from 37.6 percent to 23.9 percent of the total work force. This reduced rank-and-file participation in national union affairs and increased bureaucratization of the leadership. The latter became wary of preventive health and safety schemes for fear that they would increase unemployment, emphasizing instead hazard pay ("dirt money") and increased workers' compensation benefits (17). Compensation had the added bonus that it was a *visible* attack on dangerous working conditions, which was good for recruitment, whereas accident prevention had no such "selling points." (16, p. 342)

Workers probably went into World War II under similar conditions as World War I, except that there was a whole range of new hazards. The asbestos, rubber, motor, and petrochemical industries had all developed enormously during the interwar period, while the unions and the State were still trying to deal with the hazards of the past.

The "Three-Generation Law" was now well established in the mills, potteries, and mines. In one generation a hazard is introduced; in the next the hazard may be recognized; and in the third a law may be introduced to control it. It then may take a fourth generation before the hazard is properly controlled, but whatever the event, the law is always late arriving. Asbestos was in its second generation between the wars. Writing in 1934, Sir Thomas Legge (who had retired from the Factory Inspectorate over the Government's refusal to ratify the Geneva White Lead Convention) said of asbestosis: "Looking back in the light of present knowledge, it is impossible not to feel that opportunities for discovery and prevention were badly missed." (10, p. 191) Many cases of cadmium poisoning had been reported, but it was not to be a recognized occupational disease until 1953 (16, Ch. 22). Beta-naphthylamine was known by Imperial Chemical Industries to cause bladder cancer in rubber workers, but they continued to make it. They were eventually fined £20,000 (18), but even today it is recognized that all the people who were exposed have not been contacted and checked. Polyvinyl chloride (PVC) plastic is another example of a substance which was manufactured without any attention to its potential damage to health.

WORLD WAR II

World War II brought significant changes. The longer hours and increased work load made industrial problems more apparent (19). There were growing demands for integrated welfare services to improve standards of nutrition and education. The Beveridge Report (20) led to changes in workers' compensation and, eventually, to the setting up of the National Health Service. Despite the interest of the Labor Party and TUC in such a service, formation of an Occupational Health Service designed to prevent accidents and diseases was consistently blocked by the Government (16, pp. 385-415).

The need for organized research was recognized with the creation of the Industrial Health Research Board, directed by the Medical Research Council (MRC), which pointed out that "until June 1943 there was no complete organisation for Research in industrial medicine in this country." (21) The MRC established units on pneumoconiosis (1945), toxicology (1947), and pollution (1955). Industrial health and safety departments were set up at a number of universities, although there are now units only at Aston, London, Manchester, Newcastle, and Dundee, those at Glasgow and Durham having been closed.

The idea of integration and organization also became part of the same union policies. According to a 1945 union report, "Unity of foundry interests is given practical form in the Committee on Conditions in Iron Foundries . . . and enquiries into conditions cannot stop in the Iron Foundry with all the attention now being given to questions of health and amenities." (22)

THE POSTWAR SITUATION

With the hopes for a new life and the landslide victory of the Labor Party, it was expected that an integrated attack on work conditions would occur. It did not. Instead, as the economy was rebuilt and expanded in the postwar boom, new processes were introduced and the Conservative Party told us "we've never had it so good." Presumably, it had forgotten about the thousands of people at home crippled by work. Union membership was at its highest level, and hardly a TUC conference passed without health and safety being debated. In 1954 a motion was put forward urging the Government to take steps to introduce an accident prevention organization in every form of industrial and nonindustrial employment by setting up joint commit- tees. The resolution was withdrawn when the General Council argued that it might reduce the employers' liability for accidents and create a mere facade without any real intention of carrying out the necessary work. Motions in 1956 and 1958 also failed to produce advances, until a 1959 TUC report stated the need for more factory inspectors, more inspections, more financing for research, more powers for factory inspectors, and improvements in standards (23). The Council was thus proposing improvements in existing legislation rather than instigating anything new. The result was that while individual unions (e.g. in mines and foundries) fought and gained certain concessions, there was again no unified policy.

Bill Simpson, the general secretary of the Foundry Workers Section of the Amalga- mated Union of Engineering Workers, was the most notable trade-union leader to organize, campaign, and train on safety issues. He is now chairman of the Health and Safety Commission. Probably the most significant enactment during this period was the Mines and Quarries Act of 1954, which consolidated the rights for safety represen- tatives. The Factory Act of 1961 laid down a series of specific regulations relating to cleaning, ventilation, heating, lighting, guarding, and fire procedures. While reasonably comprehensive, it really only pulled together existing legislation and established minimum standards for institutions that were considered to be traditional factories. Although minimal, these standards are still ignored in many factories today.

According to Grayson and Goddard, "Between 1950 and 1973, at least 15,533 workers met their death—two or three every working day. From 1962-69 there was a relentless increase in the Factory Inspectorate's statistics on accidents at work. However dubious these statistics may be, they had an important impact on TUC delegates." (8, p. 2) They may have had an impact on TUC delegates, but whether they had an impact on the TUC itself is another question.

The 1960s saw many changes in trade unionism. Workers, especially those in the automobile industry, were becoming more organized on the job with the establishment of the shop stewards' movement and combined committees throughout certain indus- tries. There was a rapid increase in the number of white-collar and technical workers, following in the wake of the "white heat of the technological revolution," as Harold

Wilson called it. Many of them were becoming unionized into white-collar unions such as the Association of Scientific, Technical and Managerial Staffs (ASTMS) and National Association of Local Government Officers (NALGO). Many more women were coming into industry, so that by the end of the 60s they made up 40 percent of the working population.

There is little evidence that the new laws on health and safety resulted from pressure by elected union officials. Of course there were motions at TUC conferences, but there always had been. For example, there was a call at the 1971 TUC convention for widespread action to force employers to move the Conservative Government toward legislation on compulsory union safety representatives and safety committees (8, p. 4). The TUC's ambivalence may be traceable to the fact that many of the new proposals contradicted its traditional stance in favor of joint management-union safety committees and responsibilities.

It seems more likely that the pressure for new legislation came directly from the shop floor. With the increasing power of shop stewards in plant-level bargaining, there was more and more pressure to remove health and safety hazards rather than to depend on workers' compensation to take care of the injured (24). The increase in unauthorized wildcat strikes may have put additional pressure on the State and Factory Inspectorate to redefine occupational health and safety as a "technical" issue above and beyond politics. The Factory Inspectorate realized that the maze of regulations and government bodies was often self-contradictory, that many new industries were not properly covered, and that its own resources and powers were totally inadequate to maintain any semblance of doing the job it was supposed to do. The fact that occupational health and safety services were being reorganized in several other capitalist countries, particularly the United States, may have had a demonstration effect. Perhaps the interests of the multinationals could be better served by cosmetic changes than by no changes at all.

THE 1970s

The Labor Government set up the Robens Committee in 1970 to look into health and safety organization and to propose changes. Robens's recommendations and philosophy served as the basis of the new Health and Safety at Work Act of 1974 (HASAWA), so his conclusions are important. After receiving 600 pages of evidence from companies, industrial associations, many government departments, some unions, individuals, and a joint submission from the TUC and CBI (the Confederation of British Industry, the employers' association), he concluded that "the single most important reason for accidents at work is apathy." (25) Apathy apparently resulted from too much complicated law. He also believed that there was "less conflict of interest over matters of health and safety than most other areas of industrial relations." After 150 years of maiming and killing, of struggles to improve conditions, to set standards and enforce them, and to organize research, all he could blame for dangerous working conditions was apathy! Robens believed that there was no need for an Occupational Health Service, merely that the law should be simplified and regulations replaced by voluntary codes of practice. Apathy would be overcome as people understood the law and became involved. Joint safety committees were central to this philosophy, so that people would have the chance to discuss the problems and govern themselves by "in-plant voluntary self-regulation." Representatives of workers were to be trained so that they could be better members of the committees, an idea originating from the joint TUC/CBI submission. Robens conveyed no indication that there was any conflict of interest between workers and management. Throughout the report, profits were not mentioned, nor was the conflict between labor and capital that has existed for the past 150 years. Instead of blaming the root cause of the problem—the production process—Robens blamed the crutch (the law) that tried to support the cripple.

Thus, it is not surprising that the 1974 act avoids any substantial and effective intervention on behalf of workers against the needs of production. Every liability on the employers is qualified by the term "as far as is reasonably practicable," which legally means "a quantum of risk is placed on one scale and the sacrifices involved in the measures necessary (whether in money, time, or trouble) is placed on the other." (26) Nowhere in the act is there the right to stop work under dangerous conditions without victimization. The responsibilities of manufacturers are so vaguely defined that it will take 20 years of court action to decide what they mean. There are no regulations making it compulsory to monitor pollutants or give regular medical check-ups to people exposed. Workers will continue to be used as guinea pigs in some vast experiment where the data will not be collected. The act does not challenge the process of production, but merely gives the impression that somebody, somewhere cares.

Since the act came into force, a lot of "improvement" and "prohibition" notices have been served by the Factory Inspectorate. There has also been a reorganization within the government inspection agencies to unify the approach of the Factory, Mines and Quarries, Nuclear, Alkali, Agriculture, and Petroleum Inspectorates within the Health and Safety Executive. With the new premises covered, the ratio of factory inspectors (700) to premises (400,000) is very similar to that in 1833!

Most importantly, the safety representatives regulations came into force on October 1, 1978. It was quite clear during the consultative period that the unions took a much stronger role in drawing up the document as time went along. This was the period following two national miners' strikes which had brought down the Conservative Government, leading to a new Labor Government. The unions were thus able to make changes at that time which previously were unobtainable. They have made sure that worker representatives are not held liable and that there are adequate facilities for training and time off for safety representatives—so much so that some managements are now worried that workers are better educated than their employers. Nevertheless, this still fits the pattern that unions work to improve existing legislation rather than propose new laws.

However, the new powers of safety representatives are greater than those shop stewards ever had. They have the right to inspect plants, to receive information from management and factory inspectors about past conditions and future proposals, to have time off, and to set up safety committees—if they wish. These new powers have not gone unnoticed by the employers' organization, the Confederation of British

Industry. It proposed that there should be a long period of delay between publication of regulations and their becoming law. This was to give its members time to set up safety committees, which were expected to incorporate whatever powers the safety representatives have (27). While the idea of worker representatives having any power is an anathema to more traditional managers, the construction of "concerned" joint safety committees with no teeth fits well with the ideas of the more progressive monopoly capitalists.

THE PRESENT SITUATION

Although there appear to have been dramatic changes in the organization of health and safety, these are changes which could have been made 30 years ago, and they are changes which do not radically alter the conflicts between profits and health and between *cleaning up* the production process or relying on workers to *cover themselves* with protective clothing. The confused attitude toward compensation still exists, as does the lack of a coherent preventive policy on the part of the unions.

In recent years the unions nationally have been involved in a number of issues involving asbestos, PVC, and acrylonitrile, where ASTMS is taking a verbally aggressive stance. It is one of only two unions with a full-time safety officer. The TUC recommended to the Government Advisory Committee on Asbestos in December 1976 that exposures should be reduced to 0.2 fibers/cc and that asbestos should be phased out of use, although it has done little since to encourage that view. The General Municipal Workers Union (GMWU) has pushed strongly for lagging work to be undertaken only by licensed companies, but the Transport and General Workers Union (TGWU) has done nothing but block any initiatives by its Glasgow branch of lagggers, 90 of whose members have died of asbestosis (28). The building workers union (UCATT) conducted a survey of conditions among its members, while the clerical workers union (APEX) called for an inquiry to counter "hysterical public statements, because exaggerated claims were being made by those who wanted to ban asbestos." (29)

On the PVC issue, the unions in the U.K. have been much less active than their U.S. counterparts. TGWU, ASTMS, and GMWU were involved in joint consultation with employers and government officials. So it was impossible to find out what evidence was submitted, what demands were made, and how certain issues were resolved—this being in stark contrast to the U.S. procedure. The result was a 10 ppm level, with the hope that there would be a gradual reduction, as far as is reasonably practicable. What was clear was that, despite all the publicity throughout the world, much of the new information did not get to where it was most needed—the shop floor (30). None of the unions held a conference to explain hazards or produced handouts detailing the dangers of PVC. The GMWU, despite a lot of statements (31), actually provided very little support or help to people trying to get compensation for loss of jobs due to disablement (32).

But there are signs of change on the shop floor. The most striking one is the hunger for information, which is found in courses, conferences, and day schools up and down the country. The interest of workers in technical details and legal intricacies has been intense. The need for information is reflected in the growth of Work Hazards groups of scientists (part of the British Society for Social Responsibility in Science) in six major towns; they help trade unionists and produce the magazine *Hazards Bulletin*. An understanding of preventive measures, a lack of reliance on the factory inspectors, and confidence in a "self-help" approach have been developed, all with enormous potential.

This potential is reflected in many recent actions. There have been hundreds of isolated instances of people refusing to work with asbestos. It's only in the last few years that the general work force has learned of the hazards of asbestos, highlighted by several television programs and by a government report condemning the actions of the Factory Inspectorate at the Cape Asbestos factory at Hebden Bridge (33). On building sites, power stations, hospitals, schools, and even television studios, people have stopped work. There was an 18-week strike by cleaners at North East London Polytechnic, preventing classes until the building was cleaned properly and all those exposed were put on a register (34). There were two long strikes in 1976 at the Isle of Grain power station which involved over 3000 people following the firing of 13 men for refusing to work unless they were supplied with overalls for handling glass fiber. Quite a heavy response for such a limited demand! All 70 employees at British Steel Greenwich went on strike in April 1977 for two weeks when they refused to work an unsafe machine. The employer's response was to make them all redundant, so the workers staged a month-long sit-in. At Rovers, Solihull, 4000 workers voted overwhelmingly to go on strike if night work was introduced, and welders in Sunderland shipyards went on a one-day strike in May 1978 to draw attention to the hazards of their work (35). And at ICI, shop stewards are pressing to have all the Threshold Limit Values reassessed—this time with union involvement (36).

AND THE FUTURE?

Probably the most significant development has been the establishment of area health and safety groups consisting of members from different trade unions. The Coventry Health and Safety Movement (CHASM) was the first, and it established an information center, newsletters, regular meetings, and a delegated structure that keeps it independent of other interests. Following CHASM has come WHAC (Work Hazards Advisory Committee in Southampton), HASSEL (Health and Safety in S.E. London), MASH (Middlesex Action on Safety and Health), LASH (Leeds), HASH (Hull), HASSARD (Doncaster), TUSC (Sheffield Trades Council), MASC (Manchester Advisory Safety Committee, Merseyside Health and Safety Group, and BRUSH (Birmingham Regional Union Safety and Health Campaign). If they are as promising as their names, we can expect much of these groups. They usually work with the Work Hazards groups, and some have links with tenants and community groups fighting pollution. Although each differs in composition and aims, all are based on local trade-union activists, generally apart from the traditional union structures. Much will depend on funding and on continued educational facilities, which will in turn rely on shop stewards maintaining an interest and commitment beyond their own workplaces. These groups will obviously cause concern among full-time officers and national officials, not to mention local employers, but there is no doubt they are going to be the core of any future health and safety movement in the United Kingdom. As more workers turn away from struggling around wage issues because increases are decided by the Government, these groups may provide the basis for the long-awaited organization to intervene on behalf of workers in the industrial war that has been raging for the past 150 years.

REFERENCES

1. Marx, K. *Capital.* Penguin, London, 1976.
2. Hutchins, B. I., and Harrison, A. *A History of Factory Legislation.* King Sons, London, 1926.
3. *Royal Commission on Metalliferous Mines and Quarries.* Second Report. Cmnd 7476. Her Majesty's Stationery Office, London, 1914.
4. Farr, W. *38th Annual Report of Registrar General for 1875.* Her Majesty's Stationery Office, London, 1877.
5. Hunted, D. *Health in Industry,* Chap. 2. Pelican, London, 1959.
6. Mandel, E. *Late Capitalism,* Chap. 4. New Left Books, London, 1975.
7. Webb, S., and Webb B. *Industrial Democracy,* Vol. 1. Longmans, Green & Co., London, 1911.
8. Grayson, J., and Goddard C. Industrial safety and the trade union movement. *Studies for Trade Unionists* 1(4), 1976.
9. Nash, V. *Fortnightly Review.* February 1893.
10. Legge, T. *Industrial Maladies.* Oxford Medical Publishers, Oxford, 1934.
11. Meiklejohn, A. The successful prevention of lead poisoning in the glazing of earthenware in the North Staffordshire potteries. *Brit. J. Ind. Med.* 20: 163-180, 1963.
12. Schilling, R. S. C. *Occupational Health Practice.* Buttersworths, London, 1973.
13. Howell, G. *Labour Legislation, Labour Movement, and Labour Leaders.* 1902.
14. Follows, J. *Antecedents of International Labour Organisation.* 1951.
15. *Chief Inspector's Report of Factory Inspectorate.* Her Majesty's Stationery Office, London, 1920.
16. Williams, J. *Accidents and Ill-health at Work.* Staples Press, London, 1961.
17. Williams, R. Trade Union Activity around Health and Safety at Work: The Foundry Workers Union. MSc Thesis. Dept. of Safety and Hygiene, University of Aston, Birmingham, 1978.
18. Law Report for Nov. 1, 1972, Court of Appeal, Cassidy and Wright v. Imperial Chemical Industries Ltd. *The Times,* Nov. 2, 1972.
19. Fox, A. *A History of NUBSO.* Quoted in A. Calder. *The Peoples' War.* Panther, London, 1971.
20. *Beveridge Committee on Social Insurance.* Cmnd 6404. Her Majesty's Stationery Office, London, 1942.
21. Industrial Health Research Board. *Health Research in Industry.* Her Majesty's Stationery Office, London, 1945.
22. *National Union of Foundry Workers, Journal and Report,* p. 4. October 1945.
23. Trades Union Congress. *Annual Report.* 1959.
24. Royal Commission on Trade Unions and Employers' Associations, 1965-1968. Chairman: Lord Donavon. Cmnd. 3623. Her Majesty's Stationery Office, London, 1969.
25. Robens Committee. *Safety and Health at Work.* Cmnd. 5034. Her Majesty's Stationery Office, London, 1972.
26. Lord Asquith. *Edwards v. NCB.* 1949. Quoted in O. H. Parsons, Safety—A step back, p. 92. *Labour Research,* May 1974.
27. *Hazards Bulletin* 3: 3, 1976.
28. British Society for Social Responsibility in Science. *Asbestos Worker—Community Guide to Hazards and How To Fight Them.* London, 1978.
29. *Guardian.* December 11, 1976.
30. Clutterbuck, C. Death in the plastics industry. *Radical Science Journal* 4: 61-80, 1976.
31. Statement to ICF Conference on vinyl chloride—GMWU. In *The New Multinational Health Hazards,* edited by C. Levinson. ICF. 1975.
32. *Hazards Bulletin* 11: 5 and 12, 1978.
33. *Third Report of the Parliamentary Commission for Administration Session,* pp. 189-211. Her Majesty's Stationery Office, London, 1975-1976.
34. *Hazards Bulletin* 7: 9, 1977.
35. *Hazards Bulletin.* Volumes 1, 3, 6, 9, and 11, 1975-1978.
36. *Mond Mail.* May 12, 1978, p. 6.

CHAPTER 9

Workers' Participation and Control in Italy: The Case of Occupational Medicine

Giorgio Assennato and Vicente Navarro

THE NATURE OF OCCUPATIONAL MEDICINE PRIOR TO WORLD WAR II

It is impossible to understand the evolution of occupational health and medicine in Italy unless one also knows the socioeconomic and political forces which have shaped the overall capitalist development in that country. Thus, let's start by briefly describing the evolution of industry at the beginning of the 20th century.

By 1901, the most important industry was the textile industry, which employed 18 percent of the overall labor force, followed by the metallurgical industry and coal mining. The size of the productive units—that is, the factories—was small and the technologies used were primitive. During this time, no laws existed to protect the worker at the workplace. The only law that could be interpreted as reflecting any concern about the labor force itself was one established in 1902 forbidding children under the age of nine to work in industry and those under the age of ten to work in mining. Otherwise, there was no protection at the workplace, which explains the high figures of death, disease, and accidents among the working population.[1] For example,

This article was prepared with the collaboration and assistance of many Italian colleagues. Thanks are particularly due to Professors Giovanni Berlinguer and Irene Fica Talamanca of the Department of Occupational Medicine at Rome University for very valuable conversations. Needless to say, all opinions and positions expressed in this paper are ours, however.

[1] Very interesting and informative accounts of the health conditions among different sectors of the working class at the beginning of the century can be found in references 1 and 2.

it has been estimated that no less than 10,000 workers were killed in building the famous San Gottardo Tunnel through the Alps. Needless to say, that high mortality at the workplace, and the waste of labor which that high mortality implied, gave concern to the employers. Also, and most importantly, the growing strength of the working class represented a challenge to that picture of death and disease and created a demand for change. It was in 1891 that the trade union councils of Milan and Turin were founded and in 1892 that the Socialist Party was established. Altogether, working-class pressure on the one hand and employers' concern about the cost of labor on the other determined the creation of the first occupational health clinic of Milan, which was built in 1902.

It is interesting to note that the building of the Milan clinic was made possible by a temporary alliance between the Liberal Party and the majority branch of the Socialist Party, usually referred to as the Reformists, who believed that gradual evolution was the best means by which to achieve social justice. The ideological position of the Reformists was that the damage which occurred in the process of capital accumulation could be adjusted and conditions improved gradually. Medical intervention was perceived as part of that adjustment which could repair the damage created by the process of capital accumulation. In opposition to that view, there was a minority group both within the unions and the Socialist Party which was against this gradualism and, instead, demanded that the working class alone be the primary force to direct the overall process of capital accumulation and be the hegemonic force in all the different institutions of the State. To achieve this, a revolutionary rather than evolutionary road was demanded. This group was the one which placed great focus on workers' control of the process of production, indicating that unless the workers controlled the process of work, all occupational health legislation would eventually be turned against the worker, however well intended that legislation might be. This minority position was stated in the Congress of Padova in 1911.

The gradualist approach, however, won over the revolutionary one and became the dominant force in establishing the nature of social (including occupational) legislation in Italy. It was felt that all groups and social classes in society could unite and work for the improvement of working conditions. Dr. Devoto, the first chairman of the occupational health clinic of Milan, reflected that view when he indicated that it was necessary to create a social pact between government, employers, and workers so that occupational health services could be created (3). He stressed that it would be to the benefit of all society that workers be protected at the workplace. Consequently, the first occupational health services were created and an initial network of occupational clinics was established.

Development of that network was discouraged under fascism during the 1922-1943 period. The heightening of the conflict between the working class and the employers' class had determined such social unrest that it threatened the overall fabric of Italian society. Fascism was the response by those in power to stop the gains of the working class. It was therefore not surprising that one of the first things the fascist regime did was to try to slow down the growth of occupational health which had taken place at a time when working-class militancy was at its height. Under fascism, the nature of occupational medicine changed, so that instead of providing services as such, it became an insurance system whereby workers affected by occupational injury and disease were supposed to be compensated. According to the Labor Act of 1927, the function of occupational medicine was to define the nature of damage created at the workplace and the monetary compensation for that damage, rather than to provide services to the damaged workers. In this sense, it was a change from national occupational *services* to national occupational *insurance*. Thus, a public insurance agency was created, Istituto Nazionale Assicurazione per gli Infortuni sul Lavoro (INAIL), which was responsible for compensation for those occupational conditions which had been recognized by the Geneva Convention of 1925. Among them were the hazards created by lead, mercury, phosphorus, and CS2 poisoning. During that period, occupational medicine became a branch of medicine in charge of certifying whether labor was to be compensated or not because of injury and, if so, by how much. Thus, the task of the occupational health doctor was to indicate whether the worker had incurred damage at the workplace and whether he/she or his/her dependents needed to be compensated.[2] Also part of the occupational physician's responsibilities was to make sure that absenteeism was kept down so that the workers would alter only minimally the overall process of production.

OCCUPATIONAL HEALTH AFTER WORLD WAR II

After World War II, the evolution of occupational health policy in Italy followed three periods, which responded to different union strategies.

During the *first period*, from 1945 to 1969, occupational health was not considered to be a very important issue for the unions. There were struggles to reduce the overall working time of the labor force but, outside of this concern, there were not many specific demands about the protection of the worker at the workplace or about changing the nature of work in Italy. It was in the fall of 1969, when a revolt against the social and working conditions in Italy took place, that the picture changed most substantially. The economic boom throughout Europe in the 1960s created a false sense of social stability which was shattered by the May revolts in France in 1968 and by the "hot autumn" of 1969 in Italy (4). In both countries, a clear case of social revolt took place in which the questioning of the nature of work in those societies was very much at the center of that revolt. It is therefore not surprising that after 1969, most of the collective and local contracts contained provisions concerning the protection of the worker against damage created by either the working environment or the nature of work itself.

Consequently, this *second period,* opening after 1969, put occupational health issues at the center of industrial disputes in Italy. It is worth stressing that concern about the relationship between work and health in Italy during that period came more from the working class itself than from the left-wing parties or the unions. Actually, the unions and the major left-wing parties were awakened by the workers

---

[2]It is interesting to note that occupational medicine became a branch of forensic medicine, a characteristic which still prevails in Italy today. Many professors of occupational medicine have backgrounds in forensic medicine.

themselves as to the importance of this subject. And in order to be able to continue on the crest of the rebel wave, those organizations made the issue of work in society and its relationship to health a major part of their political and economic struggles. Struggles around work and health, however, were not always coordinated with other struggles carried out by those forces. On many occasions, the unions' policies aimed at reducing unemployment, for example, conflicted with policies developed by the same unions regarding occupational health.

It was not until 1972—the beginning of the *third period,* in which Italy is now—that the unions attempted to integrate their occupational health strategies and positions on related issues (e.g. piece work, shift work, and the like) with other strategies aimed at transforming society. During this period the unions saw themselves as not only economic but *political* institutions whose objective was to change society. In order to do that, they needed a coordinated strategy where the different demands and struggles would be integrated and directed to that purpose.

Having described the three main periods of occupational health after World War II, let us now backtrack for a moment and explain the relationship between union policies, political parties, and occupational health in the postwar period.

UNIONS, PARTIES, AND OCCUPATIONAL HEALTH

In the 1950s, the unions in Italy were weak because of high unemployment and also because of divisions created in the labor movement in 1950 when the Christian Democrats split from the major Italian union—the Confederazione Generale Italiana del Lavoro (CGIL)— and created the Confederazione Italiana Sindacati Liberi (CISL) (4, pp. 138-139). This split was an outcome of the Cold War and a result of U.S. influence on the Italian scene.[3] The American AFL-CIO and United Automobile Workers Union stimulated the breaking off of Christian Democrats from the CGIL, assumed to be Communist-dominated. The CISL followed a model of bargaining and organization similar to the American United Automobile Workers Union. Its basic ideological assumption was that capital and labor did not intrinsically conflict and thus could benefit from mutual collaboration. Two major unions were thus established following different ideological and political orientations.[4] Out of the nine members of the secretariat of the CISL, five were members of the Christian Democratic Party (CDP). In the CGIL, out of the eleven members of the secretariat, four were members of the Communist Party and the other seven were members of the Socialist and other left-wing parties (6). The primary reason for that split of the labor movement was the desire by the United States and by the leadership of the CDP to isolate the left-wing forces, parties, and unions in Italy.

With labor divided and weakened, the Italian industrialists were able to carry out, in the 1950s and 60s, a most aggressive program of industrial and technological reconversion in such a way that there was a reshaping and remodeling of industrial plants by

[3]There is a very extensive bibliography showing the direct involvement of the United States in Italian politics. See, for example, reference 5.

[4]While there are other unions besides the CGIL and the CISL—e.g. the Social Democratic-Republican UIL—they play a very minor role on the labor scene.

new technology and machinery. These measures were aimed at creating a rapid process of capital accumulation and guiding the overall economic development in Italy toward its integration within the European one. That reconversion was made by replacement of old with new machinery and plants, by an increased use of available manpower (provided by internal migration from southern Italy), and by greater emphasis on increasing productivity. All of these policies led to a dramatic increase in occupational injuries, increasing them from 950,000 in 1956 to 1,400,000 in 1960 (7). This enormous sacrifice could not have been imposed on the working class if it had not been divided in pursuing different and conflictive policies. The CISL, for example—the new trade union created by the Christian Democrats—placed great emphasis on (a) improving the human relations of the workplace; and (b) establishing productivity committees where both management and labor would collaborate in finding ways to increase productivity (8, 9). It put management and labor in collaborative rather than opposing roles. Within that strategy, the major struggle on the labor front was focused on higher wages.

In this respect, the policies of the CISL were aimed at increasing the wage level of the unionized workers, relating that increase to the overall increase of productivity. Damage at the workplace was regarded as unavoidable and as much a part of the compensation as the skill or the physical performance of the worker. Accordingly, the CISL demanded the creation of job evaluations in the industries estimating the workers' salaries and compensation by taking into account the risk of damage at work. In other words, the worker would be compensated depending on his skills, his performance, and the risk to which he would be subjected at the workplace. All the jobs were scored according to a system where risk or damage was a variable in that score. In terms of compensation, 15 percent of the total wages in a productive unit (i.e. a factory or any other center of employment) was set aside for compensation for occupational hazards. According to this strategy, the best prevention for an injury was to choose the right person for the right job in order to avoid mismatching of workers with jobs which could further increase the injury picture. Needless to say, this approach accepted injury as unavoidable and caused by an overall industrialization process which could not be changed. This reflected a view that industrialization was a natural process intrinsically positive and not modifiable. From this approach comes the sequela that accidents are an unavoidable byproduct of this process.

This attitude was very prevalent among the working class and was revealed in the results of a study carried out in Turin in 1959 in which no less than 65 percent of the workers thought that the damage created at the workplace was practically unavoidable (10). This attitude, incidentally, was shared not only by the Christian Democratic and Social Democratic unions, but also by all other political forces and unions in Italy. In the late 1950s, for example, in the congress which took place in Rome at the Gramsci Institute, the main intellectual center of the Communist Party, it was pointed out that the development of automation and mechanization at the workplace would lead to an upgrading of the nature of work and improvement in the workers' qualifications (10). Here again, technological development was regarded as a natural and positive process. The nature of the struggle around the bargaining table, then, had more to do with the distribution of the product of the working process than the redefinition of the working process itself. This ideological position clearly complimented the need for rapid industrialization in the 1950s and 60s, presenting the struggles around the workplace as ones focusing on wages but not on working conditions per se, since the process of work was considered to be unchangeable. From the capitalist point of view, this picture of acceptance of technology as such enabled a rapid process of capital accumulation which led to the economic boom of the 1960s, characterized by heavy investments, high migration from the south to the north of Italy, and the creation of new industries leading to a situation of almost full employment. Needless to say, this boom took place not without cost. It created a collapse in the northern urban areas unable to cope with the migrant population; a severe crisis in the agricultural sector which remained completely underdeveloped in the south; and last, but certainly not least, continuous increase in the rate of occupational injuries which, in 1973, reached the maximum figure of 1,600,000 (11).

In the 1950s, the working class had been divided on the union front by the establishment of the CISL and the CGIL. In the 60s, the left-wing parties were split and the Socialist Party entered into government with the Christian Democrats. The political situation in the 60s in Italy was characterized by a coalition of the Christian Democratic Party with the Socialist Party under the overall rubric of the center-left government carried out under the personal influence of the Christian Democrat Aldo Moro—the same leader who, in the 70s, explored an informal agreement to establish the historical compromise with the Communist Party before being kidnapped and assassinated by the Red Brigades.[5]

Needless to say, this process of intensive capital accumulation with an increased rate of extraction of labor from the working class could not have taken place if the working class had not been divided, with large sectors of it supporting the Christian Democrats, the Socialists, and the Social Democratic Parties (the parties in government) and other sectors supporting the Communist Party. Also, this division relegated the Communist Party to a role of isolation and ghettoization. It was the hope of the capitalist class that the boom and full employment which were created would absorb the working class within the capitalist system, making the Communist Party irrelevant and increasingly less attractive to the workers. Included within this strategy was the hope of the capitalist class that the Socialists and Social Democrats would establish a big Labor Party in Italy, a biparty model similar to the one in Great Britain. Both parties would accept the existence of capitalism as the economic structure of their society, with their differences based on the level of state intervention and on the nature of social reforms demanded. This strategy, if proven successful, would have guaranteed the reproduction and strength of capitalism in Italy. Meanwhile, all the parties which were part of the center-left government had agreed to emphasize the rapid industrialization of Italy and to focus on investments in the south under the overall guidance of the Southern Italy Guvernative Fund, which led to the construction of several large factories, especially steel and chemical plants, which are now being referred to as "cathedrals in the desert."

This was the strategy of the leading groups in Italy. It ran into considerable

---

[5] See reference 12 for a discussion of the split within the Italian left.

problems due to the anarchic nature of capitalist development. Indeed, this chaotic boom, referred to as the Italian "miracle," created as many problems as it solved. And in a somewhat unexpected manner, the student movement in 1968, followed by a mass protest movement in 1969, indicated that the majority of the Italian population was questioning the economic and political assumptions of those leading groups. In several elections in 1969, the parties in government lost considerable support, while the Communist Party reported remarkable gains. The Communist Party, far from being weakened, gained considerable strength.

THE IMPACT OF THE 1969 EVENTS ON OCCUPATIONAL MEDICINE

The nationwide strikes and takeovers by factory workers in 1969 had a most substantial impact on all areas of Italian life, including occupational medicine. It is worth stressing, however, that although 1969 was a key date to explain subsequent changes in Italy, some of those changes had already appeared—although in embryonic form—in the early 1960s. For example, the perception of industrialization as a positive and intrinsically neutral process was questioned in the early 60s when some of the most militant sectors of the working class—such as metal and chemical workers—started perceiving industrialization not as neutral but rather as reflecting a type of control that was contrary to the workers' interests. For the first time, in 1962-1963, struggles took place around the design and control of the work process. Those struggles culminated in the mid-1960s with the provision in collective bargaining that local sections of the unions could negotiate with management at the local and factory levels on three areas: (a) management demands for increased productivity; (b) the design of the work process and division of labor in that process; and (c) the job evaluation or evaluation of the different components of that work process (13). As part of that negotiation process, joint committees were established (following the introduction of such committees in the chemical industry) with union representatives and management discussing conditions of safety at the workplace. For the first time, then, joint committees for prevention and safety were established to deal with issues related to the workplace. These committees (appointed by unions and management) varied considerably, some being meaningful and active while others were merely perfunctory.

After the hot autumn of 1969, a completely different strategy developed. The social upheavals awakened the unions to the profound discontent of the working class with working conditions in Italy. They also showed the power structure in Italy that the majority of the working population was not satisfied with either working conditions or the nature of power in that society. Nationwide strikes took place in 1969 demanding changes not only at the workplace but also in medicine, housing, schools, and in the overall nature of fiscal policies and taxation. The issues of democracy, control of the work process by the workers, and social consumption by communities were very much at the center of those struggles. Several grass-roots committees were established in the factories—Comitato Unitario di Base (CUB)—and also in the communities, committees which grew initially outside the union and political party structures (14). And in all these struggles, the nature of work and of community control became a major issue. In a document prepared by the CUB of the factory

Pirelli, for example, the need to solve the problems of damage at the workplace under the direction of committees directly elected by the workers and not appointed by the unions was established. In quite uncompromising language, it was indicated that the workers' health must not be sold out any longer. The whole system of compensation for injuries was questioned, and harm at the workplace was now considered changeable and avoidable.

As an outcome of this process of social revolt, the organization regarding the protection of the worker at the workplace changed considerably inside the factory. Instead of workers' safety committees which included representatives of management and unions, the members of the new committees were directly elected by the workers. Thus, the newly elected workers' committee appeared in a situation of great conflict. The delegates—delegati—that were elected to those committees were called conflict delegates (*delegati di lotta*) and their duty was reflected in the title given to those workers' committees: conflict and/or agitation committees. As one delegate at Fiat indicated (15, p. 152):

> If you want to reject a certain type of social system, this is not possible with organizational structures . . . which do not have any direct contact with the workers. Thus, if you want to move in this direction, you must necessarily create a different type of organization for yourself which can only take the form of the delegate movement and of the workers committee.

Those delegati were elected from the rank and file according to homogeneous groups, defining homogeneous groups as those consisting of workers having similar working conditions and therefore assumed to have identical interests. A delegate was elected by each homogeneous group, remaining a worker and a representative of the workers at the same time. In other words, when the representative was elected, he/she did not move away from production as had happened before with worker representatives in previous committees. According to earlier structures, the worker representative used to be a union delegate who would leave the production process once elected. It is worth stressing that large sectors of the union movement saw, with great misgiving, the creation of those grass-roots workers' committees and the power they had acquired. Those misgivings were due partially to concern that the decentralization of bargaining power from the central direction of the unions to the shop floor could strengthen the corporate tendencies within the working class, i.e. that each group of factory workers would look to its own specific interests and not to all the interests of the entire working class. The fear expressed by some unions was that the decentralization of the power to bargain could contribute to the division of the working class. Experience, however, showed quite the opposite. The demands that came from those workers' committees included egalitarian demands (such as demands for equalizing wages among white- and blue-collar workers and among all types of workers), democratic demands (such as demands for more equal distribution of power within the factory and within the union), and revolutionary demands (such as demands for transformation of power relations in all of Italy) (16, 17). The workers' committee movement politicized most substantially wage labor and workers such as women, salaried, and migrant workers who have been marginal to most workers' struggles (15). A measure of their success was that the unions had to change their position from one of antagonism to one of support for those committees. According to Censi (15), "They were forced to recognize those new structures, because otherwise they would have lost the remains of their influence and credibility in their work shop."

It is worth stressing that not all sectors of the labor movement opposed the workers' committee movement. Even prior to the 1969 events, sectors of the CGIL had asked for such directly elected committees that would carry forward the struggles of *all* workers at the shop level. And among those struggles, a very important one concerned control of the work process and its implications for workers' health. For example, the metal workers union of the CGIL, in its meeting in Bologna in 1968, made the following demands:

1. The worker in the safety committee should be elected by homogeneous groups.
2. The principle of non-delegation of control should be accepted. By that, it was meant that workers would not delegate to anyone—including physicians, industrial hygienists, or any other professionals or experts—the right to establish the allowable working conditions for workers.
3. The principle of group evaluation should be accepted. According to that principle, the workers would evalute their working conditions themselves, an evaluation which would take place in the workers' assemblies within the homogeneous groups.
4. A book should be established in which each homogeneous group would record the conditions of the working environment. The information would be collected by the workers themselves in assembly meetings.
5. A biostatistical book recording morbidity data for each homogeneous group should be established. It would include data concerning mortality, morbidity, absenteeism, and injuries, and would be prepared by the workers themselves.
6. A book of individual hazards should be kept by each worker, equivalent to the biostatistical data book but on an individual level. It would include data about previous exposures and characteristics of previous and present jobs according to types of hazards on those jobs.
7. Individual health books should be established and kept by each worker, recording the outcome of periodic medical examinations, including laboratory data.
8. Health should be considered as an important outcome of the work process itself. In this sense, each job should be evaluated by the workers themselves, and the damage created to the worker should be grouped according to: (a) physical factors such as radiation, noise, and microclimate; (b) chemical factors; (c) physical load factors; and (d) factors related to the work organization such as piece work, shift work, overtime, and monotonous operation.

The 1969 revolt made all of these proposals possible, and they were taken up by the workers' committees and by the unions in their collective struggles. Since 1969, all collective bargaining has included the demand for all these items. The degree of success in their implementation varies by geographic area (implementation is more advanced in northern Italy); by type of industry (metal and chemical workers are the most politicized); and by industry's size (implementation has been higher in larger factories). Also, in subsequent struggles, the workers have won the right to know what chemicals and substances are used in the work process and the effect that those chemicals may have on them. They have also won the rights to investigate the introduction of new technologies and to carry out their own analyses at the workplace, with the expenses incurred in those analyses and in those studies being paid by management and/or by the occupational health authorities of the regional governments (almost half of them under left-wing control).[6]

Another outcome of those struggles was the establishment in May 1974 of the Workers' Rights Law, which included the right of assembly by workers during working hours, the right of not being dismissed without just cause, and three other articles directly related to occupational health. Those three articles are: (a) that occupational physicians paid by management do not have any power whatsoever inside the factory, and the certification of absenteeism for occupational conditions has to be done not by the factory physician, but by public health physicians under the responsibility of the regional health authorities; (b) that the workers have the right to call on experts of their choice to help them resolve whatever problems they may have; and (c) that the workers have the right to set up in each working place the occupational and related services run by the unions.

Also, the unions have struggled for the occupational health services to be integrated within an overall national health schema, referred to as the national health services project (passed by Parliament in 1979). This demand was aimed at requiring that occupational health services be removed from management control and put into the hands of public authorities. In this respect, the request for a national health service has been one of the major demands. At the Rimini Congress of 1972, the major unions demanded a national health service which would be regionalized and whose basic unit would be the local health center—Unita Sanitaria Locale (USL)—to be controlled by the community and by the workers in that community. Also at that congress, immediate steps were demanded to transform the national health insurance into a regionalized national health service. For example, it was demanded that the national health insurance schema be divided into administrative and political structures which would facilitate the later implementation of the national health service. Within that new structure, it was planned that each social political area, such as Lombardy, be divided into smaller areas in which an occupational health service—Servitio di Medicina nel Ambiente di Lavoro (SMAL)—would be set up.

The functions and responsibilities of those SMAL centers are: (a) to provide technical assistance to the workers when asked by them; (b) to collaborate with the delegati committee, discussing with it the characteristics of the work process and the products used in that process, and the impact that they have on the health of the workers; (c) to prepare, in collaboration and under the direction of the delegati and the homogeneous group, a map of hazards within the factory. The homogeneous groups which meet in assembly are the ones to produce the information to define and evaluate the risks of the working environment, work process, and products used, and to evaluate

---

[6]For an interesting analysis and evaluation of some specific examples of workers' control of occupational services and of the work process, see reference 18.

and accept or refuse the technical information (such as lab tests or epidemiological information) that they had requested; (d) to produce medical, laboratory, and epidemiological information asked for by the assembly of workers; and (e) to assist the delegati in their collective bargaining session with management, providing whatever information on health-related issues those delegati might require. Needless to say, these responsibilities put the occupational doctors working witn SMAL in a role different from the classic one of occupational physicians. No longer is the occupational physician the controller of absenteeism for the employer, but is rather a public officer who, with his knowledge, supports workers in their struggles against management. The physician, therefore, is put in a supportive, not a controlling role, which makes the physician acceptable to the worker, although less acceptable to the management. This evolution of occupational medicine has been clearly linked with the shift of power relations within the overall process of capital accumulation.

The militancy of the working class has indeed shifted the focus of occupational medicine from defending management interests to defending workers' interests. In this new relationship, it is perceived that management and workers do not necessarily have similar or identical interests, but rather, their interests are in conflict. Needless to say, the changed role of occupational health has also been reflected in the training of occupational physicians. An element of the revolt of 1969 further appeared in the universities, where the nature of academic work and for whom that work was established was clearly questioned. As an outcome of those events, the discipline of occupational medicine has changed quite substantially from a branch of forensic medicine working primarily for management to a branch of public health devoted to the service of workers. As indicated in the introductory speech of the 36th Congress of the Italian Occupational Medicine Society given by the chairman of that society, Dr. Casula, the role of occupational physicians is defined today as one of supporting the working class in its struggles (19). Quite a change from the previous understanding of occupational medicine as a neutral instrument in theory but at the service of management in practice. Quite a reversal of roles! As indicated in a paper (20) published in 1973 in the most important journal dealing with occupational medicine in Italy:

> ... the traditional role of occupational medicine has been to consider medicine as a merely scientific method assumingly controlled by the physician, and to consider the factory as a closed and static system which perpetuates itself and considers research and its findings as strictly consistent with the capitalist rationale. Within this framework, it was impossible to understand the impact of the working process on the health of our working population. It was impossible, also, to understand the nature of our socio-economic system based on the extraction of the work aimed at optimizing profit. The factory, however, has to be seen, not as a closed system, but as an open system, part of the overall social system, full of internal contradictions which affect the lives of the workers. Life inside and outside the factory is interdependent. And it is because the worker's life is largely conditioned by the factory and also because outside the factory, the women and men are exposed to a lot of problems which can be indirectly related to the presence of those problems in the factories.

Another interesting experience for those in academia is that one of the rights which the workers have gained from their own struggles is the right to continued education on company time. Specifically, the workers have won, as part of their collective contract, the right to spend 150 hours a year in any learning institution of their choice for their own cultural improvement. Among the courses which the workers take are ones on occupational health or on the medical care system in general.

MODUS OPERANDI OF THE HOMOGENEOUS GROUPS

The experience with homogeneous groups, workers' committees, and worker delegati is extensive by now. And they represent a most interesting development in the history of the labor movement and of occupational health. While rich and varied in experience, a certain pattern of commonality can be observed. The following section will discuss: (a) how these homogeneous groups operate, i.e. how they go about struggling and solving their work-related problems; and (b) how this approach to solving such problems differs from the "experts' " approach.

How the Homogeneous Groups Work

The first step is the establishment of homogeneous groups by the assembly of workers. The workers themselves meet in assembly and establish these groups based on their own perceptions of the different working conditions and environments to which different types of workers are subjected.

Each homogeneous group keeps a work book where all the information regarding the work process, the work environment, and the products used in that process is recorded. That information is produced, discussed, and analyzed by the assembled workers of each homogeneous group. It is of great importance that all the information is analyzed and discussed collectively, not individually. The information collected is based on a guidebook prepared by the Center for Documentation and Research (funded by the three major unions), which groups information into two types: (a) *objective information* on potentially hazardous factors in the workplace, including microclimatic factors such as noise, temperature, and ventilation; chemicals, toxins, and harmful substances; physical position while working, physical effort, and fatigue; and physiological factors such as speed of work, and shifts; and (b) *subjective information,* discussed and analyzed collectively, regarding disease, malaise, stress, and other forms of disease or unease that workers experience while working. The workers discuss while assembled the types of health problems they have that they perceive are related to their work. Besides that collective book, each worker keeps a work health book which includes all of the medical information related to his/her work experience.

The workers' assembly can request from experts of their choice technical assistance and further technical information such as laboratory tests, physical and other types of medical examinations, epidemiological studies, and so forth. When those studies are reported back to the workers' assembly, they are subject to what is called a *mutual validation process.* Those findings are discussed, accepted, or rejected depending on whether the assembled workers feel that they conform with their own feelings or perceptions. In other words, "scientific" information is not automatically accepted at face value, i.e. objective data are made dependent on subjective ones.

Once the problem and its causes are discussed and defined by the workers, the assembly decides on the strategy to solve that problem.

The Experts' vs. the Workers' Approach

Prior to 1969, if management felt that a health problem might exist in a factory, it would call on an expert who would engage in researching the nature of the problem and its solution in the following way. First, he/she would obtain as much information as possible from each individual worker. Through questionnaires, interviews, medical records, and the like, the expert would try to obtain the maximum amount of objective and quantifiable relevant information. Based on that individually collected information, he/she would come up with some hypothesis regarding the possible nature and cause of the problem. He/she would also find out the collective dimensions of the problem by adding up the individual problems. And last but not least, the expert would try to test his/her hypothesis by statistical manipulation of quantifiable (objective) information. During the whole process, the expert tried to be as emotionally distant from the problem as possible, not letting his/her emotions (and those of the workers) interfere with scientific objectivity. Finally, the report with suggestions for solving the problem would be submitted to management for implementation. In that scheme, workers appear as passive subjects of research, in the background, but not in the forefront of the analysis and solution of the problem.

It is not surprising that the workers rebelled in 1969 against that understanding of scientific research and did not want to have any part of it. From the time that workers' committees were established in 1969, workers have refused to allow that type of research to be carried out in their factories. Contrary to the "experts' " approach, the process that they have developed is based on:

1. *Collective, not individual, generation of hypothesis and of all information needed to define and solve the problem.* All information is produced and discussed collectively with the correct understanding that a collective problematique is far more than the mere aggregate of individual problematiques. Moreover, the workers' assemblies have a collective memory and experience that put their perception of reality in a collective and historical perspective. They know what is going on and has been going on in that factory process and environment for a long time. And they have first-hand experience of what that has meant to their collective and individual sense of health and well-being.
2. *Workers' priorities, giving top importance to their own subjective perceptions of what is going on and why.* Subjective feelings, symptoms, unease, and stresses are the primary data that guide all processes of gathering of objective and subjective data.
3. *Healthy skepticism of science, expertise, and objective information.* Workers scrutinize all objective data, and through the process of mutual validation, they accept the value of such data on the basis of how they fit within their own perceptions of reality.
4. *An acceptance of experts only when that expertise is under the direction of workers.* Many years of exposure to occupational medicine have taught workers

the lesson that science is not value-free knowledge, but very value-laden, reflecting the values of the institutions where that science is created and the values of the scientists who create that science.

5. *The workers' understanding that the solution to their problems requires a collective, not an individual response of all the workers, without delegation of responsibility to anyone outside that collective.*

This collective production of knowledge based on collective practice is an alternate form to the individual production of knowledge referred to as scientific knowledge. It is a most important contribution of the workers' committee experience in Italy to have shown the clear interrelationship between democracy and the production of knowledge useful to the working class for the solution of its problems.

PRESENT TRENDS IN OCCUPATIONAL MEDICINE IN ITALY

In January 1979, the National Health Service (NHS) law was approved by the national Parliament. According to the new legislation, the Government delegated the task of organizing health services, including occupational health services, to each region. In some regions, these services are already existing and have been active for some years. The pilot experiences of Lombardy, Tuscany, and Emilia in the occupational health area have been the guideline for the national health service. The peripheral units of the National Health Service (local health units or USL) provide occupational health services both within and outside the factories (minimizing the role played by the pro-industry plant physicians) in a close relationship with the workers' committee in the factories. This "first-level" service is supported by a "second-level service" which consists of industrial hygiene departments and outpatient hospital facilities. Another important aspect of the new legislation (and the aim of union struggles since 1969) is that it is mandatory to use the forementioned individual and collective health and hazards books. Moreover, the NHS law requires management to inform the workers of all chemical products and hazards involved in the industrial process. Last, but not least, the law requires that the Government make a list of threshold limit values for industrial hazards (so far in Italy there has been no such list). Consequently, with the NHS law, all the union demands of the late 1960s and early 70s have been achieved. It is worth stressing, however, that there is a wave of skepticism about its future implementation.

Indeed, a law is valid as long as it can be implemented. And for this, there is a need to have a militant working class prepared to struggle for the law's implementation at local and factory levels. In the last few years, however, the majority of left-wing forces and unions have been focusing their struggles on nationwide issues, such as unemployment, inflation, and other related issues. This shift from a *local* to *national* focus and from *direct* forms of local participation and control to *indirect* forms of struggle, carried out at the level of representative politics, has weakened that impetus for local control.

Moreover, during the last few years and until very recently, the way in which the "historical compromise" was carried out—with an alliance at all levels of government between the largest workers' party, the PCI, and the Christian Democrats (perceived by the majority of the working class as being the bosses' party)—led to a demoralization and demobilization of sectors of the working class, and a weakening of their involvement and participation in the workers' committees.

Also, capital, forced by the local struggles of the 1960s, has shifted a large part of hazardous jobs to small factories and even to workers' homes where the organizations of the working class are weak. By decentralizing hazardous jobs and by having them done in small working units or in people's homes, capital has tried successfully to bypass the powerful workers' committees of the large factories and places of work. Consequently, the movement of the early 70s questioning the division of labor and the nature of work in the factories has been somewhat diluted and slowed down. In this sense, the NHS law raises concern to many, since it gives the illusion (but not the reality) of new relations of power at the workplace. As Gramsci once indicated, the law always reflects relations of power but does not create those relations.

Also, this weakening of struggles at the workplace has had implications in how professionals relate to workers. Indeed, while academic departments of occupational medicine have increased quite considerably in the last few years (both in terms of budgets and staff), and while those departments have become more pro-labor than pro-management, still, the reality is that they see themselves as being the leaders of inquiry, research, and analysis of damage at the workplace. In this respect, instead of seeing the workers' committees as the leaders in the creation of knowledge (as they did in the late 1960s and early 70s), the professionals increasingly see themselves as the primary actors and agents in that creation of knowledge. The dilution of the struggle at the workplace has thus meant the strengthening of the professionals and the weakening of the workers in analyzing, studying, and doing research at the workplace. As a consequence, the "workers' approach to science," as opposed to the "experts' approach," has not, as yet, materialized.

In summary, the workers' committees in Italy—one of the most important developments that occurred since 1969 on the international labor scene—are at a very delicate historical conjuncture. Their weakening would represent a most substantial loss for not only the Italian labor movement but all other labor movements that struggle for the development of health at the workplace.

REFERENCES

1. Berlinguer, G. *Malaria Urbana.* Feltrinelli, Italy, 1976.
2. Berlinguer, G. *Medicine e Politica.* DeDonato Editori, Italy, 1973.
3. Devoto, A. The conditions of work in Italy. *Journal of Occupational Medicine,* 1903 (in Italian).
4. Crouch, C., and Pizzorno, A., editors. *The Resurgence of Class Conflict in Western Europe Since 1968,* Volumes I and II. Macmillan, New York, 1978.
5. Platt, A. A., and Leonardi, R. American foreign policy and the postwar Italian left. *Political Science Journal* 93(2): 197-216, 1978.
6. Ricardo, P. *Los Sindicatos Italianos.* Ediciones Populares, Italy, 1968.
7. Istituto Nazionale Assicurazione per gli Infortuni sul Lavoro. *Notiziario Statistico.* Italy, 1974.
8. Sclavi, M. *Lotta di Classe e Organizzazioni Operaia.* Mazzotta, Italy, 1974.
9. Garavini, S. Strutture della autonomia operaia sul luogo di lavoro. *Rinascita* 7, 1971.
10. Assennato, G. Occupational Medicine in Italy. Unpublished manuscript, 1979.

11. Istituto Nazionale Assicurazione per gli Infortuni sul Lavoro. *Notiziario Statistico.* Italy, 1975.
12. Ingrao, P. *Las Masas al Poder.* Critica, Italy, 1978.
13. Zoll, R. A comparison of union structures at shop floor level in Italy and the Federal Republic of Germany. In C. Crouch and A. Pizzorno, editors. *The Resurgence of Class Conflict in Western Europe Since 1968.* Macmillan, New York, 1978.
14. d'Agostini, F. *La Condizioni Operaia e i Consiglio di Fabbrica.* Reuniti, Italy, 1974.
15. Censi, G. et al. *Delegati e Consiglio di Fabbrica in Italia.* Milan, 1973.
16. Herrmann, U. Gewerkschaft und Egalitarismus in den Arbeitskämpfen in der Italienschen Metalindustrie nach 1968: Ein Analyse der Metallarbeiters Gewerkschaft FIM-CISL. University of Bremen, 1976 (mimeographed).
17. Centro Operaio di Milano. *Consejos de Fabrica y Sindicatos en Italia.* Iniciativas Editoriales, Italy, 1978.
18. Basaglia, F. et al. *La Salute in Fabbrica.* Savelli, Rome, 1974.
19. Casula, D. La Missioni di la Medicine di Lavoro. Unpublished manuscript, 1978.
20. Roseto, R. La salute di operai. *Medicina dei Lavoratori,* 1973.

CHAPTER 10

Why Work Kills

A Brief History of Occupational Safety and Health in the United States

Daniel M. Berman

Marcos Vela began working as a machine tender for the Johns-Manville asbestos factory in Pittsburg, California around 1935. In 1959 the company started a policy of periodic medical examinations concentrating on the detection of lung disease. That year a private physician paid by Johns-Manville obtained a chest x-ray on Vela and noted a finding of occupationally related chest disease. The report contained no recommendation about changing the work environment, and Vela was not informed that he was developing asbestosis.

In 1962 Vela was examined by Dr. Kent D. Wise, another company-paid physician. A chest film taken at his office showed the presence of lung disease. As before, the patient was told nothing. Dr. Wise saw Marcos Vela again in 1965 for another routine examination and sent him to a nearby hospital for another chest x-ray. The radiologist made a diagnosis of work-related pneumoconiosis, which he communicated to Dr. Wise. Vela was told nothing.

This article is an adaptation of the first chapter of the forthcoming *Death on the Job* by the author and is printed with the permission of the publisher, Monthly Review Press.

In February 1968, at his next routine physical by Dr. Wise for Johns-Manville, Marcos Vela complained of coughing and shortness of breath. Though his x-ray showed a "ground glass appearance" (1), Vela was told by the company nurse that "everything was fine." Again he was not informed of the adverse medical findings by Dr. Wise. That August he was hospitalized, unable to catch his breath. He would never return to work.

Thus for ten years doctors under contract to the Johns-Manville Corporation, the world's largest private producer of asbestos, knew that one of their workers was developing asbestosis, and not only refused to tell him, but took no measures to prevent further exposure to the asbestos which was ruining his health. That same company had known since 1931, from research it had sponsored, that asbestos caused lung disease (2).

On the suggestion of his workers' compensation attorney, Marcos Vela sued Dr. Wise for medical malpractice, and personally insisted on taking the case to court. Expert witnesses from both sides testified that the Vela x-rays showed evidence of developing lung disease and that it was the physician's duty to inform the patient of that fact and to take effective action to secure treatment and prevent the disease from developing further. In November 1973, a Contra Costa County jury agreed with the worker-plaintiff that Dr. Wise had committed medical malpractice, and awarded Marcos Vela damages of $351,000 against the doctor, in the only decision so far of its kind. On January 2, 1975 Vela received a check for $208,506.30, and his attorneys collected another $170,596.06 in fees from Dr. Wise's insurance company[1] (3).

Marcos Vela now wears a $100 gold watch inscribed:

> *Marcos A. Vela, presented by Johns-Manville Corporation in appreciation of 25 years of loyal service, October 1960.*

Marcos Vela is a slight, courtly man who has to move about and gesture in slow motion. His lung capacity is down to one-fourth of normal and he stops to take quick shallow breaths when he speaks quickly. He consumes 18 kinds of medicine daily, and has a respirator connected to an oxygen tank in the bedroom. Some of the pills have the effect of eroding the enamel of his teeth, so he takes other pills to counteract that effect. He described his condition this way:

> *I can't run; I have to walk slow, though I'm not crippled completely. I have a bulb of compressed oxygen with me, in case of coughing spells. As soon as I have a cold I have to go to the hospital. Once I had a fever of half a degree and had to stay in the hospital for three weeks. The doctor says I have to be careful about shaking hands with people, because of the germs, and I can't stand smokers or smoggy days, when I have to stay inside with the air filter on. It's hard on my family; with all this money I have I can't get my health back (3).*

How could such an atrocity occur? What system made it possible for a physician to neglect to treat a progressive, disabling, and potentially fatal illness; to refuse to tell the sick man about it; and to avoid taking any steps which would prevent the further development of the disease? Why did a company which knew about the dangers of asbestos for at least three decades allow exposure to lethal levels of asbestos dust?

[1] Quantities add up to more than $351,000 because of accrued interest.

Where were the insurance company and state and federal inspectors who were supposed to ensure healthy conditions on the job? Why did the union allow its members to work under such hazardous conditions? Is Marcos Vela's story being repeated in workplaces throughout the United States, or is his case a rare anomaly caused by wicked managers and a heartless physician? Must the everyday functioning of American capitalism destroy Marcos Velas as inevitably as it produces Chevrolets?

INTRODUCTION

In the first two decades of this century, U.S. corporations in the monopoly sector responded to the movement around occupational safety and health by setting up a business-controlled "compensation-safety establishment" which withheld the issue of working conditions from the public agenda until the late 1960s. The founding of the privately owned workers' compensation system between 1910 and 1920 in most states gave minimal compensation to many workers disabled by work accidents. The skeleton implementation of workers' compensation and state-run industrial inspection programs was enough to create the public impression that working conditions were improving as quickly as possible and that injured workers were being satisfactorily helped.

In fact, the workers' compensation system stabilized compensation costs to employers at one percent of payroll by almost totally ignoring the problems of occupational disease and worker rehabilitation. By setting up a closed compensation bureaucracy, companies avoided the costs and embarrassments of jury trials. The compensation system, in effect, shifted at least 90 percent of the financial burdens of work-related casualties onto workers, their families, and the public, while government and private agencies ostensibly designed to prevent injuries largely ignored such tasks (4, Ch. 4). To minimize financial settlements to workers, companies created the ghettoized institution of company medicine, in which the industrial physician became the company's advocate in compensation claims, backed by an infrastructure of lawyers and corporate-sponsored research findings discounting job hazards.

Only in the last ten years has independent research, often with union support, begun to systematically question the doctrines and practices of the "compensation-safety establishment." The political movement which created the Occupational Safety and Health Act of 1970 has called increasing attention to the importance of preventing casualties. Activists from unions and the professions have questioned "establishment" efforts to blame "accident-prone" workers, and have focussed more on speed-up, sloppy maintenance, worker powerlessness, and faulty industrial design as causes of work injury and disease.

Despite the occurrence of sporadic rank-and-file uprisings over working conditions, it has only been since the late 1960s, during a time of new environmental consciousness and general social unrest, that unions have been strongly involved in the questions of job health and safety. Concern over health and safety has helped provoke radical reform within a few unions. Although the corporate elite, through the "compensation-safety establishment," has been able to dominate the operation of the new federal institutions created by the OSHA law, working conditions are now on the permanent agenda of workers, unions, and the U.S. public.

THE POLITICAL-ECONOMIC CONTEXT OF INDUSTRIAL SAFETY
AT THE TURN OF THE CENTURY

The rapid industrialization of the United States produced a multitude of new dangers for workers. Big business, unable to control "ruinous" competition and confronting a militant working class and growing socialist movement, sought the aid of the federal government. The competitive sector of independent farmers and small business was being squeezed by the relentless advance of the power of big business allied to the banks. The fruits of fabulous productivity increases were being concentrated in fewer and fewer hands, symbolized in 1901 by the organization of the United States Steel Corporation, the nation's first billion dollar business. Smaller manufacturers, unable to raise prices easily, violently fought unionization, while a few leaders from the monopoly sector began to devise sophisticated methods to forestall unionization through token "welfare" policies (5-10).

Farming was becoming more expensive as more machines were used per worker, and small farmers often lost their land, hopelessly in debt (11). In the South most black people were being pushed to the edge of survival by the reimposition of legal segregation, loss of the vote, and systematic expropriation of what little property they had by the combined use of sharecropping and the lynching, jailing, and expropriation of "uppity" blacks (12-14). Indians who had survived the "winning of the West" were locked on reservations, and U.S. troops were now fighting Filipinos in the Philippines in the drive to open new areas to U.S. capitalist exploitation.

Large corporations and sweatshops were employing millions of hopeful immigrants in dirty new jobs which still paid better than peasant work in Southern and Eastern Europe. Giant corporations, led by the railroads, usually learned to use regulatory commissions as a facade behind which they could consolidate their control of markets and public opinion. In 1893, six years after the formation of the Interstate Commerce Commission, Richard Olney, former U.S. Attorney-General, wrote (11, pp. 178-179):

> The Commission . . . can be . . . of great use to the railroads. It satisfies the popular clamor for government supervision of the railroads at the same time that that supervision is almost entirely nominal. . . . It thus becomes a . . . barrier between the railroads and the people and a sort of protection against hasty and crude legislation hostile to railroad interests.

The Congress and presidency were finally secured for big business by the election of William McKinley over the ragtag Democratic-Populist coalition in 1896 (11, Chs. 1-3).

Labor, badly beaten in a series of strikes in the late '80s and early '90s, was on the ascendancy by 1900, but unions were making little progress in organizing the new mass production industries in the monopoly sector. Unions had been practically eliminated in the steel industry. There were bloody struggles in both coal and hard rock mines and in the garment industry, some of the few sectors where industrial [2] unions had managed to make permanent inroads. Between 1890 and 1914 the few

---

[2] Industrial unions organize all workers in a workplace into one union, rather than dividing them according to craft. The Carpenters Union is a craft union; the United Auto Workers Union is an industrial one.

unionized craft workers and the unorganized majority saw their wage increases negated by inflation, and many of their efforts to organize stymied by the open-shop campaign of the National Association of Manufacturers, representing smaller manufacturers in the competitive sector (8, pp. 376-387). It is no wonder that the Industrial Workers of the World (the famous "Wobblies") won a couple of spectacular strikes, that strenuous attempts to organize unions resulted in the enlistment of thousands of workers and that millions of voters turned to the Socialist Party (15, 16).

Work in those days was hard and dangerous for most; hours were extremely long, and nonunionized workers were largely unable to fight back against employers' attempts to extract more production (17, 18). A report in the labor press in 1904 estimated that 27,000 workers were killed on the job annually (9, p. 21), and a 1907 Bureau of Labor report put the annual death toll at 15,000 to 17,500 of 26 million male workers (19, p. 418). Though the figures are difficult to interpret (20, Ch. 2), it is likely that the work accident death rate at the turn of the century was at least double the present rate. An idea of just how dangerous work was is reflected in such contemporary accounts as that by Mack Sennett, the inventor of the Keystone Kops, who started working at 17 for the American Iron Works in East Berlin, Connecticut.

> In my day it was common for four men to hoist a four-hundred pound rail, place it on the shoulders of a single man, and expect him to tote it a hundred yards.
> I . . . loathed a "bucker-upper" named Smith, who caught white-hot rivets in a bucket as fast as he could—he was a pieceworker . . . and ordered me to slam them home at high speed with a ten-pound sledge hammer. The faster I slammed, the more money Mr. Smith made.
> An ironworks is a hot place. Iron is produced from ores, hematite, magnetite, limestone, and siderite. This is heated in smelters, some of them one hundred feet tall, and poured in a molten liquid often as hot as 3500 degrees. When you ladle the slag of a pool of iron it sometimes sputters like fat on the stove. My hands are scarred with white marks from doing that when I was seventeen (21, p. 19).

Women's work was lower paid than men's, and was often more dangerous, particularly in the garment industry sweatshops. On March 25, 1911 the upper three stories of a ten-story building in New York City, where the Triangle Waist Company was located, caught fire. Most of the doors were blocked, locked, or opened inward, trapping the workers inside. There were no fire escapes. One-hundred and forty-five of the 500 employees, mostly young Jewish and Italian immigrant women, were burned to death or died jumping from the building. The New York State Factory Investigating Commission was formed in the aftermath of the fire (9, pp. 20-24).

Children often did dirty work now done by machines. One reporter who tried manning a "coal breaker" where children crouched to clean slate and other refuse from the coal, mangling their hands and permanently hunching their backs like old men, describes this setting where twelve-year-old boys worked ten hours a day, for sixty cents a day (22):

> Within the breaker there was blackness, clouds of deadly dust enfolded everything, the harsh, grinding roar of the machinery and the ceaseless rushing of coal through the chutes filled the ears. I tried to pick out the pieces of slate . . . my hands were bruised and cut in a few minutes; I was covered from head to foot with coal dust and for many hours afterwards I was expectorating some of the small particles. . . I had swallowed.

William Z. Foster, leader of the great steel strike of 1919 and an early leader of the U.S. Communist Party, almost lost his life to industry as a young man (23, p. 12):

> From 1901 to 1904 my revolutionary development suffered a rude interruption. The two and a half years I had worked with lead in the type foundry as a child worker had undermined my health. The three years following in the fertilizer industry, where we usually toiled totally unprotected, in dense clouds of poisonous dusts, broke me so that the doctors pronounced me a consumptive. I was in a fair way to go to an untimely grave, grinding out profits for employers, as vast armies of workers had done before me. So I quit my job, pulled up stakes and headed for the West. I hoboed my way.

UNION-BUSTING AND WORKING CONDITIONS IN STEEL

The steel industry was the most dynamic sector in the economy from 1890 through 1910. What happened in steel had a great effect on the rest of the economy, both because of the economic power it represented and by force of example. After 1890, the rapid reorganization of productive techniques, the huge investment in new equipment, and the gigantic increases in productivity per worker were accomplished only at a tremendous cost in human suffering. Steel owners found that they would have to break worker control over the flow of production in order to implement their new plans, and they did so with a vengeance. Unions were smashed, labor activists purged, and the workweek almost doubled in many cases.

The work pace, no longer under the control of skilled steelworkers, was speeded up mercilessly, and, as a result, injury and death rates in steel became a national scandal. Accidents were so frequent that they interfered with production, and owners feared that safety and health issues might become the basis for union organizing drives. The response of the industry, led by the newly organized U.S. Steel Corporation, was to begin to implement safety programs to reduce the number of accidents, and to use programs borrowed from Germany and Great Britain to compensate workers disabled on the job. It is important to understand the situation of the steel industry around the turn of the century because steel's safety and compensation programs became the model for the rest of the nation.

Prior to 1890 most steel was produced on contract by skilled steelworkers and laborers operating equipment owned by the capitalists. Workers would bargain with the mill-owners to decide what price they would receive, though their share could fall no lower than a certain amount per ton. This revenue would then be divided up among the crew producing the steel, depending on their status within the production team. These arrangements were assured by the Amalgamated Association of Iron, Steel, and Tin Workers, which reached the height of its membership and power in the late '80s and early '90s. The Amalgamated Association was a craft union, enrolling only skilled workers. The Homestead, Pennsylvania mill was the Amalgamated Association's biggest local. It was also the biggest mill of Carnegie Steel, the largest U.S. steelmaker (17, pp. 64, 65; 24).

At Homestead about 25 percent of the 4000 workers were in the union, where they controlled all aspects of production. This situation was unsatisfactory to Carnegie Steel for two reasons: workers got a constant share of the increasing sales of the mill and had the power to prevent the introduction of labor-saving technology if it didn't benefit them. Carnegie resolved to break the Amalgamated Association's power at Homestead in a definitive test of strength. Before the contract expired in 1892, the management built a 3-mile-long fence around the plant, with rifle-holes every 25 feet at shoulder level. The workers were told that Carnegie would deal with them only as individuals after June 24. On July 2 most unionized workers were locked out. The union, backed by all the workers, responded by shutting down the mill, renting a steamboat to patrol the Monongahela River, and organizing the whole town for resistance. When bargeloads of 300 armed Pinkerton men were brought up to force open the mill and bring in scabs, an open gun battle resulted in which 16 were killed, including 7 Pinkerton agents. The rest surrendered to the workers and their families and were beaten and run out of town. But Carnegie finally won the Homestead war after a four-month strike, with the help of the Pennsylvania militia, and the plant resumed production without the union. Loss of its most important outpost was the beginning of a rapid decline for the Amalgamated Association. After another disastrous strike in 1902, the union was completely uprooted from basic steel in the United States (8; 25, Ch. 3).

The steel bosses, who now had total administrative control of steelmaking, set out to reorganize the industry as they wished. In the 20 years following 1892, productive techniques were revolutionized. Much physical labor was replaced by huge electrical cranes and intricate intraplant railway systems. Gigantic new furnaces and heaters were built, and formerly separate operations were integrated into single complexes. Production was increasingly carried out under orders, military style, according to a strict chain of command. Skilled workers who had been in charge of organizing production in their work gangs were demoted to semi-skilled status, with their pay cut. Union activists were fired and political conformity was enforced in small "company towns" by blacklisting known socialists and driving the rest underground (24, p. 216). Finally, the dirtiest and most unpleasant jobs were often filled by blacks and immigrants, with the result of higher casualty rates than among native-born whites (26, p. 100), and a hindrance to labor's overall ability to unite against a steel industry now more centralized than ever.

Management efforts to increase production were awe-inspiring, and the pace of work was speeded up almost beyond belief. Production doubled every 10 years or less, under the stimulus of an apparently inexhaustible demand for steel. The work week, which had averaged 8 hours per day 6 days a week, was increased to 7 days a week for a third of the U.S. Steel employees in blast furnaces and rolling mills. Twenty percent of those 153,000 employees worked an 84-hour week (27). The effect on working conditions was disastrous. John A. Fitch wrote in *The Steel Workers*, published in 1911 (24):

> ... there is always a fine dust in the air of a steel mill ... not very noticeable at first, but after being in a mill or around the furnaces for a time, I always found my coat covered with minute shining grains. A visitor experiences no ill effect after a few hours in the mill, but the steel workers notice it and they declare that it gives rise to throat trouble....

Fitch thought that heavy physical work had been decreased by the new technology, but believed that the dangerous responsibilities for tons of molten steel and other materials had increased the "nervous strain" associated with being a steelworker. In most mills there were "no heat reducers," no fans, and no noise dampers. Men walked into the winter cold directly from the furnace heat, and washed up in troughs used to cool tools. A comparable study of British conditions at the time, published in 1902, showed that iron and steel workers had a "mortality figure 37 percent above that of the standard of occupied males. . . ." (28, p. 141). Evidence collected from the death benefits fund of the Amalgamated Association of Iron, Steel, and Tin Workers suggested that injuries and "diseases caused by dust, heat conditions, and sudden changes of temperature . . . [such as] tuberculosis and pneumonia" were very important causes of death. But Fitch called attention to the 12-hour day as "by far the greatest menace to health in the steel industry" (24, Ch. 7):

> When the mills are running full the men are chronically tired. The upsetting of all the natural customs of life every second week when the men change to the night shift is in itself inimical to health. It takes until the end of the week, the men say, to grow sufficiently accustomed to the change to be able to sleep more than four or five hours during the day. And then they change back. . . . If this is true, it must be trebly so at the end of the twenty-four hour shift, which is experienced fortnightly in Allegheny County [where Pittsburgh is located] by nearly 6,000 blast furnace men . . . it is a rare man who can keep his mental faculties alert . . . for twelve consecutive hours . . . in any accident case the long workday enters as a factor. . . .

As a result of the capital improvements, speed-ups, and long workdays, the steel industry was able to beat labor costs down from 22.5 to 16.5 percent of the total cost of making steel between 1890 and 1910 (29).

To counter the appeal of socialism and unionism, many steel companies instituted "welfare" programs to make life more pleasant for workers, without giving them any additional control over their lives. As Judge Gary, the head of U.S. Steel, told his chief executives (30, p. 78):

> Don't let the families go hungry or cold; give them playgrounds and parks and schools and churches, pure water to drink and recreation, treating the whole thing as a business proposition, drawing the line so that you are just and generous and yet . . . keeping the whole thing in your own hands.

Given the pressure of muckraking journalists (31), rising lawsuit costs, worker discontent over working conditions, and the costs of lost production, the steel industry led the way in the "voluntary" safety movement, financed and controlled by industry, with no outside intervention from government or labor. As early as 1907, U.S. Steel began to look for ways to reduce its casualty rates. The approach combined impressive engineering hardware with slogans and some on-the-job instruction in safety techniques (32, 33). A glance at books such as George Alvin Cowee's *Practical Safety Methods and Devices* published in 1916 (34) constitutes persuasive evidence of the ingenuity of early safety engineers, and of the large resources placed at their disposal by the steel companies. Not surprisingly, the role of the steel worker in safety in this nonunion industry was a passive one, largely limited to looking at occasional safety posters and handbills, listening to rare safety lectures, and obeying regulations made by management. The effect of this highly praised safety "education" was to blame workers and absolve the company of responsibility for accidents, as illustrated by the following case, taken from a safety publication of the time (35, pp. 176, 177):

> A workman in a foundry was wheeling a barrow and while passing by a crane the chain broke, the load dropped on him and he was killed.

The safety publication called this a clear case of "disobeying safety orders," rather than equipment failure, even though existing knowledge showed conclusively that "there are defects in structure and use of chains which can be removed by engineering attention" (35, p. 177). In its safety literature and studies the steel industry paid no attention to speedup and long hours as possible accident causes, and the 12-hour day in steel was only ended in the early '20s.

In 1910 U.S. Steel inaugurated the Voluntary Accident Relief Plan, based on models developed in Bismarckian Germany by a conservative capitalist class under challenge from the fastest-growing socialist movement in Europe (36, pp. 325-330). This program, soon superseded by state workers' compensation laws, was "the first of its kind in the United States," and paid workers or their families fixed amounts for job-related injuries causing disability or death. The plan, for all its purported liberality, stated explicitly that: "No relief will be paid to any employee or his family if suit is brought against the company," and workers who received "relief" from the plan were required to sign away any further rights to sue U.S. Steel (17, p. 76). U.S. Steel's experiments in safety and compensation would soon serve as models for the rest of the United States.

THE CORPORATE ELITE AND THE ORIGINS OF WORKERS' COMPENSATION AND THE "COMPENSATION-SAFETY ESTABLISHMENT"

The "compensation-safety establishment" (37) is the complex of mostly private (4, Ch. 3, Tables 5, 6) corporate-dominated organizations which are concerned with compensation, workplace inspection, standards-setting, research, and education in occupational health and safety. It is called the *"compensation-safety* establishment" because it emphasizes compensation over prevention and safety over health in its activities. It is an *establishment* in that it is a self-selecting closed group which has operated until recently as the only organized constituency in occupational health and safety, carrying out the policies of the corporate elite. Only in the last 10 years has its dominance come under challenge by unions and progressive worker-oriented organizations (4, Chs. 3-6).

Although Massachusetts passed the first factory inspection law in 1867 (37, p. 47) and Illinois passed one in the '90s, these pioneering efforts were in fact unenforceable (38, p. 644):

> In Illinois, when Mrs. Florence Kelley was appointed factory inspector by Governor John P. Altgelt, not a lawyer or prosecuting attorney would handle the violations that she quickly detected. It was necessary for her to study law, gain admittance to the bar, and try such cases herself.

The issues of safety and compensation did not reach widespread legislative expression until the corporate elite from the monopoly sector (5, pp. 13-18) felt pressured enough to create its own policies to deal with the problem and quiet the public outcry over carnage in the workplace.

At the turn of the century new organizations sprang up among the corporate elite to help coordinate political activities, deal with labor, mold public opinion in favorable paths, and plan for the future. The National Civic Federation (NCF) was organized in 1900, and the American Association for Labor Legislation (AALL) in 1906. Their principal support came from the large corporations and banks. The policies of NCF and AALL often opposed those of smaller producers in the competitive sector, whose interests were represented by the National Association of Manufacturers. The first NCF president was "Dollar Mark" Hanna, wealthy banker and mine owner, U.S. Senator, and the manager of William McKinley's successful Republican presidential campaign against William Jennings Bryan in 1896. The NCF also gained solid backing from men such as Andrew Carnegie and Judge Elbert H. Gary from the steel industry and Cyrus McCormack and George W. Perkins of International Harvester. Of the biggest capitalists, only the Rockefellers stayed aloof from active participation (7, 36, 39, Ch. 6).

In the first five or six years of its life, the National Civic Federation preached the mutuality of interests of capital and labor and the importance of dealing with organized labor through collective bargaining and a written contract. The NCF theorized that there was no such thing as class conflict, and tried to make arbitration substitute for strikes where unions did manage to organize. The National Association of Manufacturers opposed this theoretical acceptance of labor unions, as they later initially opposed workers' compensation laws. Though most of the NCF's chief corporate supporters bitterly resisted unions in their own factories, the NCF was in principle pro-union. In practice this meant trying to "channelize the labor movement into conservative avenues" wherever possible (7, pp. 11, 12; quotation by Ralph M. Easley, founder of NCF, as cited in 8, p. 384).

Samuel Gompers, founder of the American Federation of Labor, had decided in the late 1890s that bread-and-butter trade unions had to work with the trusts, and eventually became a vice-president of the NCF (8, pp. 376-378). Both he and John Mitchell of the United Mine Workers were personal friends of big business leaders of the NCF, hunting and dining with them and consulting them for investment advice. The American Association for Labor Legislation (AALL) was active in promoting uniform legislation on a state-by-state basis throughout the United States, on the theory that this would prevent companies from moving their operations to states with less restrictive laws. The AALL made particular efforts in the areas of industrial diseases, industrial accident inspection, and workers' compensation. In dealing with industrial diseases, its major success was passing federal legislation banning the use of white phosphorus in making matches, thus eliminating "phossy jaw," a disease which caused the victims' jaws to stink and rot away (39, p. 168).

The achievements of Dr. Alice Hamilton, the founder of occupational medicine in the U.S., were due more to her personal knowledge and prestige than to the creation of strong institutions which carried out her work. Her famed "Illinois Survey" of health conditions in the lead industry was carried out on a "completely informal" basis with "no authority to enter workplaces." Since her "Illinois Survey" couldn't mention dangerous workplaces by name and since her recommendations were unenforceable, she ". . . made it a rule to try to bring before the responsible man at the top the dangers [she] had discovered in his plant and to persuade him to take the simple steps . . . that were needed" (40, pp. 8-11). Where top management was uninterested in cleaning up, there was no recourse. Interestingly enough, one of her prime success stories, the National Lead Corporation, has recently attracted attention for poisoning a large number of workers in Indianapolis, then compounding the problem by "curing" them of the lead intoxication with a medicine that ruins their kidneys (40, pp. 9-11; 41). State laws regarding industrial inspection and occupational diseases which were passed in the first two decades of this century proved to be almost universally ineffectual in preventing accidents or industrial disease (4, Ch. 3; 42, Chs. 3, 4).

In addition to advocating specific programs for companies and governments at the state and federal level, both the NCF and the AALL were concerned with more general "ideological and social problems," especially the threat of socialism, which was understood as the "only serious ideological alternative to . . . policies of social responsibility" (7, p. 117). A long letter from an executive of the Lackawanna Steel Company to his vice president in 1912 suggested that he contribute to the National Civic Federation because "the socialists and extreme radicals are very distrustful of it;" because it gives lawmakers "a sought-for excuse" to resist anti-business legislation; and because it projects an aura of civic-minded impartiality onto its programs. Though it sometimes looked like the NCF got involved in programs which many employers would criticize, the executive wrote (36, p. 332) that it

> . . . only takes up a subject after it has assumed an important national aspect and it appears . . . that it . . . will be fought to an unfair conclusion. . . . Also there are many big men on the inside of the [NCF] who are able to inform and influence the action of legislators even after the [NCF] has been obliged to yield to popular clamor and let some subjects get away from them. . . .

The attitudes and actions of Theodore Roosevelt, President from 1901 to 1909, well expressed the anxieties of the corporate elite which shaped the country's legal and private response to the unrest over job health and safety. As New York City's police commissioner and as governor of New York, his first impulse had been to use troops against workers during strikes (43, p. 219). Roosevelt considered socialism to be the most serious threat to capitalism, and fretted about how muckraking literature was "building up a revolutionary feeling" (43, Ch. 9). As President his closest advisors were "almost exclusively representatives of industrial and finance capital" (43, p. 222), and he believed in the benefits of monopoly. In key crises his artfully created and totally undeserved reputation as a "trust-buster" (11, p. 246) was utilized to convince the public that the government was impartial. In handling the great 1902 anthracite coal strike (11, pp. 236, 237), he heeded Mark Hanna's and J. P. Morgan's push toward mediation, once he understood the strength of the union, its public backing, and the disorder and "socialistic action" which could result from an attempt to break it:

> I was anxious to save the great coal operators and all of the class of big propertied men, of which they were members, from the dreadful punishment which their own folly would have brought on them if I had not acted (43, p. 223).

The image of a President who could take "strong and independent" actions was of the highest symbolic importance in conferring legitimacy on the new economic order being brought about by the corporate elite (11, p. 235; 44, Ch. 2).

Public consciousness of workplace casualties in the giant monopolies was a constant reproach to the consensus of "thoughtful men of all classes" which the corporate elite was trying to forge. The popular and socialist media were full of stories about atrocities at work, which directly or by implication questioned the legitimacy of capitalism. Novels such as Upton Sinclair's *The Jungle* (1906) aroused vast resevoirs of sympathy for workers, socialists, and unions where none had existed. A third of the members of the American Federation of Labor (AFL) were socialists (36, p. 132); and unions, beaten down by the open shop drive of the National Association of Manufacturers, only regained their 1904 membership levels by 1910 (8, p. 384). Thousands of workers joined radical unions such as the Western Federation of Miners, or took part in strikes led by the "Wobblies" (7, 9, 15, 16).

By 1908 the questions of workers' compensation and job accidents had become major items on corporate agendas. Existing common law doctrines made it almost impossible for workers to collect damages for injuries suffered on the job because the worker had to prove the employer was at fault. This was particularly difficult for severely injured workers or for the families of workers killed on the job, who had to depend on the testimony of supervisors or of coworkers subject to employer pressure. The employer could argue in his own defense that: (a) the accident had resulted from the worker's own carelessness; (b) the worker "assumed the risks" of the job in taking it; or that (c) a fellow employee of the injured worker had caused the accident. These defenses were usually enough to prevent successful worker suits (42, Ch. 3).

The reaction of reformers in some states was to pass laws weakening the common law defenses of employers. In states where these "employers' liability" laws were passed, workers began to win more and larger settlements. As costs spiraled and open jury trials became a public embarrassment, the NCF began to lobby for a workers' compensation system which would "substitute a fixed, but limited charge for a variable, potentially ruinous one" (45, pp. 259, 260). Soon corporate and government money started to flow for studies. The federal Bureau of Labor began to make careful estimates of the number of industrial casualties (19), and the new $10 million Russell Sage Foundation financed the Pittsburgh Survey, which paid a great deal of attention to working conditions. A whole book in the Pittsburgh Survey, Crystal Eastman's *Work-Accidents and the Law* (1910), was devoted to the wrongs of common law and "employers' liability" practices and the necessity for replacing them with a system of workers' compensation. The NCF led the forces for reform.

Speakers on workers' compensation at the 1908 meeting of the National Civic Federation included leading bankers, lawyers, insurance company executives, and Russell Sage Foundation experts; everyone but workers and their unions seemed to be represented. By 1909 the NCF's "Department of Compensation for Industrial Accidents and Their Prevention" had become the center for lobbying and publicity.

Experts from England and Germany (including a Major Piorkowski from Krupp) came to address the Federation, and model compensation laws written by both the NCF and the AALL began to be requested by states all over the country. Occupational diseases never merited much attention in the model laws (7, Ch. 2; 39, Ch. 6), and so it remained until the late 1960s (4, Chs. 4, 5). By the time government and foundation studies were completed and groups such as the National Civic Federation and the American Association for Labor Legislation had finished their conferences and come to their conclusions, the only question left to be answered was whether or not compensation insurance would be carried by private or state-run companies (7, p. 51; 39, Ch. 6). Theodore Roosevelt's address to the National Civic Federation in 1911 included workers' compensation as a major theme. Conservative court opposition was overcome within the next near, and with active promotion by the NCF's reorganized "Compensation Department" and the AALL all but six states had some kind of workers' compensation law by 1920 (7, Ch. 2).

The private workers' compensation systems and the unenforced industrial safety laws which were passed in most states proved to be everything their corporate sponsors had hoped for. Both management and insurance interests benefited by the shift from chancy jury trials to controllable administrative agencies whose employees could be bought off or co-opted. Since it took a long time for a bar of plaintiffs' lawyers to develop, the first two decades of workers' compensation were "largely a period of unilateral advocacy" by an "expert, specialized, full-time ... bar" to defend the interests of insurance companies and corporations. Amendments to compensation laws by state legislatures followed the same pattern (46). Costs to companies were stable and averaged around one percent of payroll (47); occupational disease payments were almost nonexistent; and companies were protected from negligence suits at common law. Physicians were hired to deal with work injuries and to represent employers within the compensation bureaucracy, creating that peculiar institutional ghetto called "industrial medicine" (48).

The corporate response to the problem of preventing injuries (industrial diseases were mostly ignored) took two forms: the founding of the "voluntary" industrial safety movement and the passage of ineffective and unenforced industrial inspection laws in most states. Of these responses, the "voluntary" safety movement was by far the most important, because its doctrines and practices, under the leadership of the National Safety Council, were to dominate the field of occupational safety and health unquestionably for over half a century.

The organization which would become the National Safety Council was conceived in 1911 at a meeting of the Association of Iron and Steel Electrical Engineers, and finally saw light the next year in Milwaukee to the sacred incantations of Dr. Edwin A. Steiner, Professor of Applied Christianity at Grinnell College. Judge Gary, of U.S. Steel and the National Civic Federation, was a guiding light of the new group, and the sixteen charter members of the "Committee on Permanent Organization" were rather broad-based: five from different federal agencies; four from the steel industry; two each from state governments and the National Association of Manufacturers; and one each representing the railroads, the insurance industry, and the Red Cross. No unions were involved (32).

The National Safety Council was conceived of as a "separate safety organization, national in scope, that could better serve as a coordinating agency and general clearing house for all phases of accident prevention" (33). Several features of the steel industry's experience became permanent aspects of the "voluntary" safety movement: it was undertaken without government compulsion; accidents were blamed largely on workers' carelessness; workers and unions were left out of decision making (except for some later tokenism); occupational diseases were ignored or suppressed from public view; and speedup and long working hours were not considered to be within the realm of industrial health and safety (4, Ch. 6; 42, Chs. 4, 5).

This corporate-financed and corporate-controlled "compensation-safety establishment" dominated occupational safety and health policy without serious dissent from the early 1900s until the late 1960s. In 1926 a major summing-up of corporate experience in the field (in which unions were barely mentioned) revealed a self-satisfied tone and a sense that the main challenges had been met and overcome and that the field had nothing new to offer (49). The silly safety posters workers have come to expect today in place of a real program had already begun to make their appearance. One plant newspaper sponsored a "safety first limerick contest." The winner, accompanied by a cartoon of a guy heels over head in the air, went like this (50):

> A grouchy guy, Isaac Maloney
> Said "Safety first—bah—that's bologney!"
> 'Til he once looped the loop
> When he stepped on a hoop
> *'Tis "Ikee" not "safetee" that's phoney*

In "putting safety across to the worker," "safety contests" began to acquire the form of athletic events, with injuries a test of team spirit, if we are to believe one oil industry editor (50):

> A young man in one of the large industrial plants in Philadelphia had the end of his finger torn off . . . the other day. His department had been striving for a 100 per cent no-lost-time record for that month, and up to his injury its record was perfect. Although his accident was mighty painful, and he was advised to go home and remain there for a few days after the doctor dressed it, this young man was so anxious to keep that 100 per cent record perfect that he refused to leave, and insisted on going on with his work. The *morale* of his department did it.

Increasingly, the engineers' focus on redesigning and guarding machines and on regularizing and smoothing the traffic of workers and materials were being replaced with an emphasis on the psychological defects of workers, as if the safety establishment were beginning to believe its own propaganda. Studies by the British Industrial Fatigue Research Board made during the First World War became the basis for a whole new area of research. The "accident-proneness" concept was coined in 1926 and picked up by a whole wave of industrial psychologists in the United States, who searched for the causes of accidents in characteristics of individual workers. Some of these studies also examined factors such as lighting and rate of production; but most of the studies had the effect of blaming the victim of the accident rather than seeking to modify the conditions which produced it. If accidents were caused by workers' "carelessness," "light-heartedness," "excitability," "psychomotor retardation," or "deficiency of English" (37, pp. 108-110), why bother about workplace design?

As late as 1966 the *American Handbook of Psychiatry* article on "Industrial and Occupational Psychiatry" found that "accident syndrome" might be associated with a diagnosis of "impulsive character" or "anxiety reaction"; and that "pulmonary insufficiency ('pneumoconiosis,' 'emphysema,' or 'chronic bronchitis')" could be caused by "depressive reaction, anxiety reaction, or psychophysiological reaction (asthma)." The authors made no plea for cautious examination of the real conditions of work before making use of their outlandish labels. Apparently there were no problems which couldn't be traced to the mental disease or personality defects of workers if a clever psychiatrist looked hard enough (51). The emphasis was now on "blaming the victim" (52, pp. 28, 29) rather than examining the details of the job or even the nature of work under monopoly capitalism (17, 53).

The nit-picking approach of the "accident-proneness" school was in sharp contrast to the boldness characteristic of early engineering work in industrial safety, and exemplified the decline of corporate interest, once the obvious problems which cost the corporations a great deal of money in lost production and compensation were solved. Sincere occupational safety and health specialists were caught between their desire to actively promote better conditions and a lack of corporate interest. One "president of a large corporation" told his "safety man": "You know I am very busy and have little time to give to safety, but keep me in touch with your work. It is a non-controversial subject. I can make train conversation of it" (54).

In the absence of strong unions or a national movement around health and safety, progressive specialists in this field had nowhere to go outside the corporations. They were left to plead for recognition of the importance of their mission "from the men that control the destinies of business life" (54). By 1926 W. H. Cameron, director of the National Safety Council and an astute analyst of the decline of the corporate-backed safety establishment, wrote (54):

> It must ... be admitted that there is a lack of leadership in the safety movement. Because the economic stake in many industries is small, small men are given the responsibility. The minds of the major executives are occupied by the major problems of production, distribution, finance.

By the mid-'20s the big names from government and business were no longer thinking and speaking and writing about occupational safety and workers' compensation. With the outside agitation under control, the field was turned over to the not-so-well trained specialists of the "compensation-safety establishment."

ATTITUDES OF UNIONS AND WORKERS

The struggle for humane working conditions has a long history and has taken many forms. Sometimes it has meant fighting for shorter hours of work. When the first unions were organized in the United States they brought pressure to shorten the workday. In June 1835 the ten thousand workers of the Trades' Union of the City and County of Philadelphia, two years after its founding, organized what was probably the first successful general strike in America. The shoemakers, followed by the workers in the building trades, the cigarmakers, carters, saddlers and harness makers, smiths, plumbers, bakers, printers, and even by the unskilled workers on the docks, struck for a 10-hour day. After a mass meeting of citizens endorsed the demands of the union, "the city council agreed to a 10-hour day for all municipal employees." Between 1834 and 1857 the demand for a 10-hour workday swept through New York City, Boston, Baltimore, Washington, D. C., Newark, St. Louis, and other cities, until the collapse of the unions in the panic of 1837 (55, pp. 30-35). In 1847, after agitation from labor, New Hampshire became the first state to pass a law making 10 hours the legal workday, "unless otherwise agreed to by the parties." New Hampshire's lead was followed by Pennsylvania, New Jersey, Ohio, and Rhode Island by 1853, but "it was one thing to write a statute and another to enforce it" (55, pp. 52-54).

Unions did not become common until the growth of the Knights of Labor in the 1880s. Agitation and organization for the 8-hour day was the basic issue in the mass strikes begun on May 1, 1886, which brought out 80,000 strikers in Chicago and scores of thousands in other cities, creating May Day, the international workers' holiday. The Haymarket bombing in Chicago three days later and its subsequent show trials constituted the employers' mostly successful attempt to destroy the 8-hour movement and the union organizing which proceeded around it (25, Ch. 2).

In the earliest period of lobbying and public relations around workers' compensation, organized labor was conspicuous by its absence. In 1906 unions had less than two million members, and many of them were fighting for their very survival (8, pp. 376-387). As unions were liquidated from the steel industry after the Homestead strike, the workweek for some workers nearly doubled, to 84 hours. Unions still had little success in penetrating meatpacking, oil, and most of the other big new industries. Clearly the first task for workers who wanted to reduce working hours and improve working conditions was to organize.

Union reluctance to join the National Civic League's rush to write compensation laws is understandable. After all, the basic models for "workers' compensation" and "industrial safety" in the U.S. were first tried out by the steel industry, in a context of union-busting and a corporate welfare paternalism designed to keep unions out. Furthermore, the compensation programs were being propounded at a time when workers were beginning to win larger and more frequent negligence judgments against employers, as traditional common law defenses were weakened and juries became more sympathetic.

> Compensation laws, in contrast, could be expected only to pension off the worker during his period of disablement at something less than his regular wages. In addition, almost all unionists, conservative or socialist, opposed government regulation of working conditions on the theory, often only implicit, that government was controlled by business, either directly or through conservative politicians or judges (7, p. 43).

Later on, when Samuel Gompers, head of the American Federation of Labor, had reluctantly endorsed the concept of workers' compensation under pressure from his big business friends and from the belief in the inevitability of some kind of legislation, the labor movement and the Socialists each developed their own positions on the issue of workers' compensation. Business dominance over the political process in a culture basically favorable to private enterprise had made it very difficult for organized labor or the Socialists to come up with workable alternatives. The programs of both labor and the Socialists usually called for compensation levels of 100 percent of lost wages (as opposed to 50 or 66-2/3 percent); retention of the right to sue at common law before a jury; and state-owned insurance companies, to prevent the diversion of most premiums to insurance interests rather than injured workers. Crystal Eastman, for example, had found in 1910 that only 24 to 37 percent of employer premiums in "employers' liability" were paid out as benefits in some form by the insurance companies (56, pp. 286-290). With the addition of reasonable presumptions concerning occupational disease liability, the labor/Socialist proposals of 60 years ago would make a fine platform for a radical restructuring of workers' compensation today.

As labor and the Socialists had feared, almost all their demands were lost. In no state were benefits close to 100 percent of lost wages. In New York State, organized labor's program banning private insurance companies was sacrificed for fairly high initial benefits, and a state-owned company was allowed to, coexist with private companies (7, Ch. 2). In Missouri the institution of workers' compensation was held up by a strong labor movement until 1926 over the issue of a state fund, but the battle was lost (57). Only Ohio, of the big industrial states, totally excluded private insurance companies, and today Ohio pays out 96 percent of its premium income to victims and doctors (58, p. 272), as opposed to 53 percent for private insurance companies nationally (47). Today, workers' compensation benefits could be nearly doubled at no new cost to employers by eliminating the role of the private insurance companies. A good way to start would be to investigate why it costs Ohio 4 cents and the private insurance companies 89 cents to return a dollar of benefits to work accident victims.

The Depression sapped interest in worker health and safety. People were desperate for work before anything else. Even the mass slaughter of workers during the building of a hydroelectric tunnel near Gauley Bridge, West Virginia, to bring power to a Union-Carbide subsidiary, failed to awaken the public interest, although Congressional hearings were held on the disaster.

The work force at Gauley Bridge was made up of poor people, mostly blacks, who flocked to the jobs at 50 cents (later 30 cents) per hour. Workers and their families were herded into shacks no larger than chicken-coops, with 25 to 30 people per room. The water tunnel was being cut through almost pure silica, and the dust was so thick that workers sometimes could see barely 10 feet in the train headlights. Instead of waiting 30 minutes after blasting, as required by state law, workers were herded back into the tunnel immediately, often beaten by foremen with pick handles.

> Increasing numbers of workers became progressively shorter of breath and then dropped dead. Rhinehart-Dennis contracted with a local undertaker to bury the blacks in a field at fifty-five dollars per corpse. Three hours was the standard elapsed time between death in the tunnel and burial. In this way, the company avoided the formalities of an autopsy and death certificate. It was estimated that 169 blacks ended up in the field, 2 or 3 to a hole. . . .

Toward the end of the project, some workers bought their own respirators for $2.50. The purchasing agent for Rhinehart-Dennis was overheard to say to a respirator salesman, "I wouldn't give $2.50 for all the niggers on the job." The paymaster was also heard to say, "I knew they was going to kill those niggers within five years, but I didn't know they was going to kill them so quick" (42, pp. 59-63).

Altogether over 470 men died and 1,500 were disabled. Years later, when survivors sued Rhinehart-Dennis for negligence under common law (silicosis wasn't compensable), "rumors of jury-tampering abounded," and a group of 167 suits were settled out of court for $130,000, with one-half going to the workers' attorneys. Blacks received from $80 to 250, and whites from $250 to 1,000 each. Later it was discovered that one of the workers' law firms had accepted a $20,000 side payment from the companies (42, pp. 59-63).

Yet even this monstrous episode failed to catalyze reformist energy in the area of health and safety. Shortly after the adjournment of the Gauley Bridge hearings in 1936, a group of large industrialists and scientists met under the auspicies of the Mellon Institute in Pittsburgh to discuss the problem. Out of these meetings the Air Hygiene Foundation was formed, whose name was later changed to the Industrial Health Foundation. Its publicly announced purpose was to promote "better dust conditions in the industries." But the real purpose of the work of the Foundation was to forestall massive claims. The confidential report of the proceedings noted (59, pp. 176-196):

Because of recent misleading publicity about silicosis and the appointment of a Congressional committee to hold public hearings, the attention of much of the entire country has been focused on silicosis. It is more than probable that this publicity will result in a flood of claims, whether justified or unjustified, and will tend toward improperly considered proposals for legislation.

One of the first programs of the Air Hygiene Foundation, a public relations campaign to "give everyone concerned an undistorted picture of the subject," was almost wholly successful. Occupational disease claims hardly rose at all, and the Foundation, under its different names, became a permanent and important part of the "compensation-safety establishment," specializing in debunking the seriousness of occupational health problems. By 1940 there were 225 member companies, including many corporate giants. At the Foundation's fifth annual meeting, the chairman of the membership committee made a pitch in the following terms (59, p. 179):

A survey report from an outside, independent agency carries more weight in court or before a compensation commission than does a report prepared by your own people. One of the brilliant features of AHF is this; it is a *voluntary* undertaking by industry to protect industrial health. And where industry attacks a great social-economic problem voluntarily, there is no necessity for government to step in and regulate.

The Foundation later branched into other areas of occupational health, successfully providing medical cover for many other industries, until its credibility came under question by the new activists in the last decade.

Despite the lack of a national movement around health and safety after 1920, working conditions were sometimes prime issues in rank-and-file unrest. In 1935, 108 black steelworkers in Northern Indiana sued subsidiaries of U.S. Steel for negligence, in failing to provide healthy working conditions. The worker-plaintiffs were mostly furnace-cleaners and coke oven workers who had been given the dirtiest jobs in the mills, like immigrants before them. They charged that their jobs had caused tuberculosis, silicosis, and other lung diseases. The suit was settled out of court for an undisclosed amount in 1938 (60, pp. 215-219).

Union organizer Stella Nowicki tells of one incident in the '30s in Chicago where safety triggered a union organizing drive. She was canning meat (and cockroaches) in an atmosphere so "hot and steamy" that women used to pass out repeatedly.

> The thing that precipitated it is that on the floor below they used to make hotdogs and one of the women, in putting meat into the chopper, got her fingers caught. There were no safety guards. Her fingers got into the hotdogs and they were chopped off. It was just horrible.
>
> Three of us "colonizers" had a meeting during our break and decided that this was the time to have a stoppage and we did. (Colonizers were people sent by the [Young Communist League] or [Communist Party] into points of industrial concentration that the CP had designated.... The colonizers were like red missionaries. They were expected to do everything possible to keep jobs and organize for many years.) All six floors went on strike. We said, "Sit, stop." And we had a sit-down. We just stopped working right inside the building, protesting the speed and the unsafe conditions. We thought that people's fingers shouldn't go into the machine.... The women got interested in the union.
>
> We got the company to put in safety devices. Soon after the work stoppage the supervisors were looking for the leaders because people were talking up the action. They found out who was involved and we were all fired. I was blacklisted (61, pp. 71, 72).

The Second World War's labor shortage, with its huge influx of workers into new jobs, led to much higher accident rates. For management it "forcibly brought to light the importance of conserving manpower in order that production . . . be maintained" (62). For the first time federal support was granted to state occupational safety and health programs. Some of these grants were maintained as late as 1950 (62). Senator Hubert H. Humphrey introduced a bill in 1951 which proposed that the federal government write and enforce safety standards, and other bills were introduced that year and in 1962 to procure aid for the states to promote job accident prevention, but these were unsuccessful (42, p. 64) and never attracted much attention.

In 1952 a seven-month strike over a sand-like dust which produced a lung disease similar to silicosis at a mine and mill in Lompoc County, California failed to incite national interest in worker health on the job, though it received much publicity in the California press and was successful in attaining many of its objectives (63). While the problems with diatomaceous earth at Lompoc have been mostly resolved, new investigation has revealed that Johns-Manville has been exposing workers there to large amounts of asbestos dust for years, without informing them. As a result many have been killed (64).

In the 1950s the Ladish Blacksmiths and Boilermakers Local 1509 made a major effort to secure routine compensation for severe occupational hearing loss in Wisconsin. They were unsuccessful, and were so disappointed with the lack of support on the noise issue that they quit the Wisconsin AFL-CIO in protest (65). Carl Carlson of United Auto Workers Local 6 at International Harvester near Chicago began investigating the problem of noise in 1959 as head of the union's safety committee, but in the absence of a wider movement active in such problems, progress was slow. Fifty years of domination of occupational safety and health by large corporations had made it almost impossible for workers to find sympathetic specialists or a suitable climate of opinion for action.

THE NEW MOVEMENT IN HEALTH AND SAFETY

Only since the late 1960s has the "compensation-safety establishment" come under serious attack. It began in the coal mines over the issues of black lung and safety, and was taken up by workers and unions and their allies in industries throughout the United States.

In the mid-1960s coal miners began to fight for state laws granting them workers' compensation benefits for disability caused by black lung. Actively opposed by the leadership of the United Mine Workers, they founded their own organizations—the Black Lung Association and the Association of Disabled Miners and Widows—aided by sympathetic physicians, lawyers, and other specialists. In February 1969, 42,000 of West Virginia's 44,000 coal miners carried out a wildcat strike for three weeks, and marched on the state capital to get a black lung compensation bill passed. The miners' organizing and agitation led to passage by Congress of the Coal Mine Health and Safety Act of 1969 and the Black Lung Benefits Act of 1972. The nucleus of people who worked on the health and safety issues eventually combined with the leadership of Miners for Democracy, a rank-and-file group which took control of the leadership of the United Mine Workers from the corrupt and murderous Tony Boyle clique (66-68).

The working conditions issue was first brought up in a new forum in 1964 at a "President's Conference on Occupational Safety" without specific legislative proposals in mind. In 1965 the Department of Health, Education, and Welfare published a report recommending vastly increased expenditures to deal with the multitudinous new health hazards, but there was as yet little interest in the issue from the unions, natural allies of such a proposal. Finally in 1968 a bill was introduced from President Lyndon B. Johnson's office, fashioned by reformers within and outside the government as a way to call attention to the issue. Management testimony opposed the bill, and initial union reaction was favorable, if desultory. But interest generated by the 1968 hearings, the environmental movement, and the high attention paid to coal mine conditions (renewed, typically, by an explosion which killed 78 miners) kept the issue alive until 1969, when Richard M. Nixon became President (42, Ch. 7).

The most lucid support for a strong law came from the Oil, Chemical, and Atomic Workers; Nader and his supporters; the Steel Workers; the AFL-CIO; the United Auto Workers; and a few Senators and members of Congress. The hearings show that groups from the "compensation-safety establishment" (including the National Safety Council and the organized representatives of company medicine, safety engineering, and industrial hygiene) followed the line of the National Association of Manufacturers and the U.S. Chamber of Commerce in backing weak bills proposed by the Nixon

Administration. Given the lukewarm support from the top leadership of the unions, the wonder is that any legislation passed at all. The authors of *Bitter Wages* (Ralph Nader's Study Group Report on Disease and Injury on the Job) recount that (42, p. 144):

> the most surprising source of apparent support came from the Nixon Administration's attempt to grab hold of the safety and health issue. The Republicans were making a loud pitch for blue-collar support and had unleashed a torrent of rhetoric concerning the "silent majority" and the "forgotten Americans."

The Occupational Safety and Health Act of 1970 was finally signed into law by President Nixon on December 29, 1970.

The OSHA law promises much more than it has delivered. Employers are boldly required to provide a workplace "free from recognized hazards that are causing or are likely to cause death or serious physical harm to employees" and to meet the specific standards promulgated by the Labor Department's Occupational Safety and Health Administration (OSHA). To guarantee compliance, the law gives OSHA the power to inspect workplaces, make citations for violations, and propose penalties. In situations of "imminent danger," the Secretary of Labor is authorized to seek an injunction in federal court to shut down the offending operation.

The law makes explicit provision for workers to call in inspectors without giving employers advance warning. Workers have the right to a "walk-around" with OSHA compliance officers and to point out suspected violations. Anonymity is guaranteed (if requested) to the worker making a complaint, and workers are supposed to be protected against employer reprisals.

Standards are set by the OSHA administration with the advice of the National Institute for Occupational Safety and Health (NIOSH). All of the early standards for safety and health were adopted directly from private standards created by industry-supported organizations such as the American National Standards Institute, and the setting of new standards has proceeded extremely slowly because of deliberate OSHA obstructionism. A memo from OSHA's chief administrator to Nixon's 1972 election staff recommended that the promulgation of "highly controversial standards" (i.e. cotton dust, etc) be avoided, and that "four more years of properly managed OSHA" should be used "as a sales point for fund raising and general support by employers" (69).

Five years of OSHA have led to few improvements in working conditions—only a small proportion of work sites are inspected every year, and inspections are fairly common only in workplaces of at least 500 workers (37, p. 260). Penalties for violation of the standards are rather small: "From its inception on April 28, 1971, through January 1975, OSHA made a total of 206,163 inspections resulting in 140,467 citations alleging 724,582 violations with proposed penalties totaling $18,186,627 ..." an average of about $25 per violation (37, p. 258). In the first eleven months of fiscal 1975 OSHA inspections of some type were carried out in workplaces employing only 11.5 million workers out of a national total of over 80 million (37, p. 259). Appeal of penalties and work orders written by inspectors has become routine, especially for large companies, further slowing down the "enforcement" process. Only one union, the Oil, Chemical, and Atomic Workers Union, routinely contests appeals by employers, and successfully contesting employer appeals has become bewilderingly complex for workers without a lawyer (70). Workers' "rights" under the OSHA law are often so hedged with restrictions or so little known that they are impossible to exercise without support from a knowledgeable union staff, making them almost meaningless for most workers, particularly in the 25 states where enforcement has been returned to state governments (71).

Thus since the passage of the OSHA law in 1970, the "compensation-safety establishment," backed by the large corporations and a compliant administration, has been able to absorb and neutralize most threats to its dominance of the new federal regulatory apparatus. The "teeth" of OSHA have been pulled through low enforcement budgets, restrictive regulations, appeals favoring employers, low fines, and the partially successful effort to return rule making and inspection to the states. Away from the coal mines, health and safety has rarely escaped the bureaucracy to become a mass issue, except at isolated factories and mines. Workers fearful for their jobs in a period of pemanent high unemployment have been reluctant to push very hard for improved conditions on the job. Even the victory of passing a stringent new standard for exposure to vinyl chloride was an ambiguous one. The battle for a strong standard, fought mostly within OSHA's labyrinthine bureaucracy and the mass media, successfully tied up a good share of the reformers' scientific and legal talent for months, and the outcome only affected a few thousand production workers. The slightly increased production costs of polyvinyl chloride plastic will be paid for by the public, since vinyl chloride is in high demand and its monopoly sector producers are able to "coordinate" their prices upward as their need arises (72, 73). Comparable new restrictions on the use of asbestos by small firms in the competitive sector have been largely ignored where union pressure couldn't be exercised (74).

Given such policies of lax enforcement and delay, the most important consequence of the OSHA law has been to place the issue of the work environment on the agenda for workers, unions, the health specialists, and the general public. Unions are forming health and safety departments and teaching their members to identify and correct hazards, often under pressure from their memberships. Workers and progressive scientists, lawyers, and health specialists are organizing and working together through grassroots health and safety coalitions, such as the Chicago Area Committee for Occupational Safety and Health; Urban Planning Aid (Massachusetts); and the Philadelphia Area Project on Occupational Safety and Health. Medical researchers, led by Doctors Selikoff and Epstein, have formed the Society for Occupational and Environmental Health, admitting nonprofessionals as members; and the general public's awareness of working conditions has increased through a few books and mass media programs. Within this context it is possible to point to specific advances for working people: the general acceptance of higher and more realistic estimates of the size of the problem; the new questioning of the traditional role of the company doctor; the new interest in occupational disease; the increased number of collective bargaining and research initiatives in health and safety; and coal field gains regarding black lung compensation.

However, it is doubtful that the advances of the past decade can be preserved (let alone extended) in the context of a capitalist system where real wages have been stationary or declining (75); where the proportion of unemployed and marginalized workers continually creeps upward (76); where multinational firms increase their power over U.S. and foreign production, and thus their ability to lower costs by exporting production or driving down U.S. production costs (77, 78); where social and environmental program cutbacks are the order of the day (5, 79, 80); where the proportion of the unionized work force has been declining (81); and where the posture of union leadership generally has been one of "public aggression and private coopera-tion" (82). Though some shops and industries will move against the general trend, there is no reason to believe that working conditions can improve if the overall standard of living of the working class is being pushed back; for after all the problem of job health and safety is only one issue in many that workers must contend with.

Much evidence is already available which suggests that corporate and governmental expenditures on working conditions have already peaked and begun to drop (83). Employers and their associations have come closer and closer to gutting the OSHA law in Congress (84), and have already forced the weakening of 1973 Williams-Javits workers' compensation bill. Even the revised bill can expect to meet severe resistance in Congress this year (85). Unions for the most part have not dedicated substantial resources to the problems of health and safety, and hiring of staff has leveled off (86). Neither are the grassroots groups very healthy in most cases. Finally, fundamental questions concerning the role of the private insurance industry in workers' compensa-tion, or the right of workers on their own initiative to shut down dangerous jobs, have hardly advanced beyond the threshold of concern, though they are crucial to the ability to make progress for workers. In a general atmosphere of political conservatism, a holding action seems to be the order of the day. What happens in the workplace cannot be separated from what happens in the rest of society.

REFERENCES

1. Rubsamen, D. B. *Professional Liability Newsletter*. Berkeley, November 1973.
2. Selikoff, I. J. Letter to author, June 7, 1976.
3. Vela, M. Interviews with author in person, June 1975, and by telephone February 1976.
4. Berman, D. M. Death on the Job. Ph.D. dissertation, Washington University, St. Louis, 1974.
5. O'Connor, J. *The Fiscal Crisis of the State*. St. Martin's Press, New York, 1973.
6. Kolko, G. *Triumph of Conservatism*. Free Press, New York, 1963.
7. Weinstein, J. *The Corporate Ideal in the Liberal State*. Beacon Press, Boston, 1968.
8. Foner, P. S. *History of the Labor Movement in the United States*, Vol. 2. International Publishers, New York, 1955.
9. Foner, P. S. *History of the Labor Movement in the United States*, Vol. 3, International Publishers, New York, 1964.
10. Radosh, R. The corporate ideology of American labor leaders from Gompers to Hillman. *Studies on the Left*, pp. 66-96, November-December 1966.
11. Hofstadter, R. *The Age of Reform*. Vintage Press, New York, 1955.
12. Woodward, C. V. *The Strange Career of Jim Crow*, 1954.
13. Du Bois, W. E. B. *The Souls of Black Folk*. Crest Books, Fawcett Publications, New York, 1961 (originally published in 1903).
14. Rosengarten, T. *All God's Dangers, The Life of Nate Shaw*. Avon Books, New York, 1975.
15. Weinstein, J. The IWW and American Socialism. *Socialist Revolution*, pp. 3-42, September-October 1970.
16. Boyer, R. O., and Moraes, H. W. *Labor's Untold Story*. Cameron Press, New York, 1955.

17. Stone, K. The origins of job structures in the steel industry. *Review of Radical Political Economics,* pp. 61-97, summer 1974.
18. Sinclair, U. *The Jungle.* Harcourt, Brass, Jovanovich, New York, 1906.
19. Hoffman, F. L. Industrial accidents. *Bulletin of the Bureau of Labor,* September 1908.
20. Berman, D. M. *Death on the Job.* Monthly Review Press, New York, in press.
21. Sennett, M. *King of Comedy.* Doubleday, New York, 1954.
22. Sparge, J. *The Bitter Cry of the Children.* Quoted in Hofstadter, R. *The Progressive Movement in the United States 1900-1915,* pp. 39-44. Prentice-Hall, Englewood Cliffs, N.J., 1963.
23. Foster, W. Z. *American Trade Unionism.* International Publishers, New York, 1947.
24. Fitch, J. A. *The Steel Workers.* Arno Press, New York, 1969 (originally published in 1911).
25. Brecher, J. *Strike!* Straight Arrow Books, San Francisco, 1972.
26. Brody, D. *Steelworkers in America: The Nonunion Era.* Quoted in Page, J. A. and O'Brien, M.-W. *Bitter Wages,* p. 53. Grossman Publishers, New York, 1973.
27. Foner, P. S. Comment. *Studies on the Left,* pp. 91-96, November-December 1966.
28. Oliver, T. *Dangerous Trades.* Quoted in Fitch, J. A. *The Steel Workers,* Ch. 7. Arno Press, New York, 1969.
29. Brody, D. *Steelworkers in America: The Nonunion Era.* Harvard University Press, Cambridge, Mass., 1960.
30. Gary, E. H. *Addresses and Statements.* Quoted in Stone, K. The origins of job structures in the steel industry, *Review of Radical Political Economics,* p. 78, summer 1974.
31. Hard, W. Making steel and killing men. *Everybody's Magazine,* pp. 579-591, November 1907.
32. Palmer, L. History of the safety movement. *The Annals,* pp. 9-19, January 1926.
33. Close, C. L. Safety in the steel industry. *The Annals,* January 1926.
34. Cowee, G. A. *Practical Safety Methods and Devices.* Van Nostrand, New York, 1916.
35. Chaney, L., and Hanna, H. S. The Safety Movement in the Iron and Steel Industry, 1907-1917. Bulletin No. 234, Department of Labor Statistics, Washington, D.C., 1918.
36. Jensen, G. M. The National Civic Federation. Ph.D. dissertation, Princeton University, Princeton, 1956.
37. Ashford, N. *Crisis in the Workplace.* MIT Press, Cambridge, Mass., 1976.
38. Destler, C. M. The opposition of American businessmen to social control during the Guilded Age. *The Mississippi Valley Historical Review,* March 1953.
39. Domhoff, W. *The Higher Circles.* Random House, New York, 1970.
40. Hamilton, A. *Exploring the Dangerous Trades.* Little, Brown and Company, Boston, 1943.
41. *Spotlight on Health and Safety.* Industrial Union Department, AFL-CIO, Washington, D. C., 1976.
42. Page, J. A., and O'Brien, M.-W. *Bitter Wages.* Grossman Publishers, New York, 1973.
43. Hofstadter, R. *The American Political Tradition.* Vintage Press, New York, 1948.
44. Edelman, M. *The Symbolic Uses of Politics.* University of Illinois Press, Urbana, Ill., 1967.
45. Lubove, R. Workmen's compensation and the prerogatives of voluntarism. *Labor History,* pp. 254-279, fall 1967.
46. Marcus, B. Defending the rights of the injured. In *Occupational Disability and Public Policy,* edited by E. F. Cheit and M. S. Gordon, pp. 77-90. John Wiley & Sons, New York, 1963.
47. Price, D. N. Workers' compensation: Coverage, payments, and costs, 1974. *Social Security Bulletin,* pp. 38-42, January 1976.
48. Selby, C. D. Studies of the medical and surgical care of industrial workers. Quoted in H. B. Selleck, *Occupational Health in America,* pp. 103, 106. Wayne State University Press, Detroit, 1962.
49. *The Annals,* January 1926.
50. Cox, C. B. Putting safety across to the worker. *The Annals,* pp. 191-196, January 1926.
51. Powles, W. E., and Ross, W. D. Industrial and occupational psychiatry. In *American Handbook of Psychiatry,* edited by S. Arieti, pp. 588-601. Basic Books, Inc., New York, 1966.
52. Ryan, W. *Blaming the Victim.* Vintage Press, New York, 1971.
53. Braverman, H. *Labor and Monopoly Capital: The Degradation of Work in the Twentieth Century.* Monthly Review Press, New York, 1975.
54. Cameron, W. H. Organizing for safety nationally. *The Annals,* pp. 27-32, January 1926.
55. Orth, S. P. *The Armies of Labor.* Yale University Press, New Haven, Conn., 1919.
56. Eastman, C. *Work-Accidents and the Law.* Russell Sage Foundation, New York, 1910.
57. Kerstein, R., and Goldenhersch, E. Workmen's Compensation in Missouri. Missouri Public Interest Research Group, St. Louis, 1972 (processed).

58. *Compendium on Workmen's Compensation,* edited by M. Rosenblum. National Commission on State Workmen's Compensation Laws, Washington, D. C., 1973.
59. Scott, R. *Muscle and Blood.* E. P. Dutton and Company, New York, 1974.
60. Balanoff, E. A History of the Black Community of Gary, Indiana, 1906-1940. Ph.D. dissertation, University of Chicago.
61. Nowicki, S. Back of the yards. In *Rank and File,* edited by A. Lynd and S. Lynd, pp. 67-88. Beacon Press, Boston, 1973.
62. Trasko, V. M. Status of occupational health programs in state and local governments, January 1969. In *Occupational Safety and Health Act, 1970,* pp. 103-109. Hearings before the Subcommittee on Labor, Committee on Labor and Public Welfare, United States Senate.
63. Abrams, H. K. Diatomaceous earth pneumoconiosis, *Am. J. Public Health,* pp. 592-599, May 1954.
64. Tulledo, S. *Lompoc Record,* p. 1, December 3, 1975.
65. Ginnold, R. Workmen's compensation for hearing loss in Wisconsin. *Labor Law Journal,* pp. 682-697, November 1974.
66. Lynd, A., and Lynd S., editors. *Rank and File,* pp. 285-297. Beacon Press, Boston, 1973.
67. Benson, H. W. Labor leaders, intellectuals and freedom in the unions. *Dissent,* pp. 206-216, spring 1973.
68. Diehl, R. UMWA reform insurgency—A recent history. *People's Appalachia,* pp. 4, 5, winter 1972-73.
69. Guenther, G. C. Letter. Republished in *Facts and Analysis,* Industrial Union Department, AFL-CIO, July 22, 1974.
70. Cottine, B., with L. Birrel and R. Jennings. *Winning at the Occupational Safety and Health Review Commission.* Health Research Group, Washington, D. C., 1975.
71. Hyatt, J. G. U.S. inspection unit finds itself in critical crossfire. *Wall Street Journal,* August 20, 1974.
72. Brody, J. E. *New York Times,* February 16, 1974.
73. Cottine, B., and Pancake, R. R. In the matter of the economic impact study on the proposed permanent standard on occupational exposure to vinyl chloride. Health Research Group, *Comments,* Docket No. OSH-36 before the Occupational Safety and Health Administration, U.S. Department of Labor, September 6, 1974.
74. Schoenberg, J. B., and Mitchell, C. A. Implementation of the federal asbestos standard in Connecticut. *J. Occup. Med.,* pp. 781-784, December 1974.
75. Faltenmeyer, E. Ever increasing affluence is less of a sure thing. *Fortune,* p. 92, April 1975.
76. Beman, L. The slow road back to full employment. *Fortune,* June 1975.
77. Barnet, R. J., and Müller, R. E. *Global Reach.* Simon and Schuster, New York, 1974.
78. Magdoff, H. *The Age of Imperialism.* Monthly Review Press, New York, 1969.
79. Notes and comments. *The New Yorker,* pp. 31-33, October 27, 1975.
80. Notice in Boston Edison Company electric bill explaining why the utility was switching to high-sulphur coal for power generation, February 1976.
81. Raskin, A. H. Nonunion workers are an expanding majority. *New York Times,* section 3, November 2, 1975.
82. Raskin, A. H. Labor: Public aggression, private cooperation. *New York Times,* section 3, August 31, 1975.
83. *First Annual McGraw-Hill Survey of Investment in Employee Safety and Health,* May 25, 1973, McGraw-Hill, New York.
84. Labor Letter, p. 1. *Wall Street Journal,* October 12, 1976.
85. Kalis, D. B. Workmen's comp: Will Uncle Sam deal himself in? *Occupational Hazards,* pp. 35-38, December 1975.
86. Personal knowledge of author.

CHAPTER 11

Work, Disease, and Occupational Medicine in the Federal Republic of Germany

Hans-Ulrich Deppe

ON THE DUAL NATURE OF WORK AND DISEASE

The relationship between disease and work is generally considered to be part of the professional realm of occupational medicine. Occupational medicine originated as a branch of physiology, and even today tends to avoid the social aspects of occupational disease. Occupational medicine in the Federal Republic of Germany has concentrated almost exclusively on the physical, chemical, and biological threats to health and has largely ignored the psychosocial impact of the structure and organization of work under capitalism. Certainly it is hard to quarrel with the conventional orientation, as the noxious effects of adverse physical, chemical, and biological agents have been amply proven. But it is necessary to go beyond the presumption that occupational diseases, injuries, and accidents can be prevented by the simple removal of harmful agents from the workplace, as if the worker were an inert object outside of society and incapable of acting in his own self-interest. In fact, the so-called "scientific" causes of occupational disease are largely determined by the ensemble of social conditions.

The dominant conception of working people held by traditional occupational medicine abstracts them from family, management, society, and their own history, as if work itself could be reduced to its physical-mechanical dimensions. Work, however, is a social activity in which people organize their relationships to nature and each other in order to ensure their survival. The nature of work, its character in different historical epochs, and the particular modes by which it is executed, are basic to all other aspects of social life.

193

In order to explain the relationship between work and health (or work and disease), it is necessary to set forth some basic definitions:

1. The precondition for human existence is work, which is the planned exploitation of nature. Of all the creatures in the world, only humans work and produce in a conscious manner. Through work, people broaden both their needs and the possibility for fulfilling their needs. As a part of this process, they improve their health.

2. Work is a technical struggle of people against nature. People give up their labor power—both physical and mental—as they act upon the object of labor with their tools—the means of labor. In the process, they change themselves as well as the external environment. To the degree that people "outsmart" the mechanical, physical, and chemical properties of things, they gain power over them.

3. But work, as human production, is more than a technical relationship between workers and the objects of their labor. Work always creates a set of social relations between people, both through the division of labor and through the buying and selling of the products of work. The real history of human labor is the story of how people learn to cooperate and communicate with each other, because production is impossible without cooperation. The most important characteristic of work is its collective character.

4. Human work has the unique ability to produce more than it needs for its own reproduction, that is to say, it creates surplus value.

5. The distribution of this surplus value is determined by society and in each society is oriented according to the essential nature of that society. The socially created surplus value can be used for the general satisfaction of social needs (including health), or can be employed to amass huge private fortunes, depending on the historically determined organization of society. In bourgeois society, the vast majority of workers do not own the means of production and therefore must sell their labor power in order to live. Their work thus becomes wage labor. Decisions about what is to be produced and how the surplus product is to be divided between the owners of capital and the workers are largely made by the capitalists, though these decisions are constantly opposed by the organized working class.

6. Good health is both a prerequisite and a product of work. A person must be healthy in order to work, and one of the principle benefits of work is to increase the chances of leading a healthy life. Though closely linked, good health and work also contradict each other. Since ancient times, and more recently since the time of Paracelsus and Ramazzini (1), we have known that work can ruin people's health and actually make them sick.

7. The close relationship between health (or sickness) and work means that the causes and incidence of disease are strongly determined by social relations and the class interests of the dominant groups in society. These relationships reveal themselves rather strikingly in the health care system, particularly as relates to working conditions and the institutions designed to deal with problems of occupational safety and health. To the degree in which the state participates in health care, the general character and specific functions of the state must be analyzed (2, pp. 61-84).

8. A discussion of the role of medicine should not be limited to the treatment of disease, but must also include efforts aimed at the prevention of disease. In order to

go beyond mere symptomatic relief, medicine must attack the technological and social roots of the problem. At this point, medicine inevitably becomes involved in politics.

Occupational medicine and industrial sociology in the Federal Republic of Germany tend to abstract people from their social context. These disciplines conceive of work as a mechanical series of actions and reactions by individual human beings. Mechanization and automation are treated as "natural" phenomena rather than as processes controlled by the owners of capital. It is forgotten that the purpose of automation is to increase profits and capital turnover rather than to better the workers' welfare. It is also conveniently forgotten that labor, in a system organized to maximize private accumulation, is inevitably alienated labor, since the owners of capital rather than the workers decide what is to be produced and how production is to be organized. The practical consequences of such a narrow theoretical point of view will be illustrated in the rest of this paper.

WORK-RELATED DISEASE

The main focus of occupational medicine is the officially recognized occupational diseases. There is no formally accepted general definition of occupational diseases, only lists of particular diseases and administrative procedures by which to investigate individual cases. So the registration of an occupational disease can best be described as an insurance-related event rather than the result of systematic medical investigation. At the present time, there are 55 officially registered occupational diseases caused by physical, chemical, or biological agents, or the effects of cumulative trauma. Diseases which can be caused by the alienated social organization of work, especially psychosocial health disorders, are not officially recognized. In 1978, 45,484 new claims for occupational disease compensation were reported, and over 7,248 received compensation for the first time (see Table 1).

The change in recorded occupational disease rates has been caused by the constantly increasing mechanization of industry, which has exposed workers to new and different hazards. In general, the new changes tend to polarize workers between those who do jobs requiring ever-increasing technical expertise and those for whom the work content sinks to a semiskilled level. The proportion of complex operations which require intermediate skill levels declines constantly, and the skills required tend to shift from manual to mental (3). At the same time, we should not exaggerate the speed with which such changes occur. In 1969, for example, the proportion of employees in the iron and steel industries engaged in hard physical labor was estimated at 25 to 30 percent (4, p. 201). For the economy as a whole in 1971 it was estimated that 1.5 to 2 million workers did hard physical work (5, p. 171), and in 1975 a sample survey indicated that over 40 percent of skilled laborers and 20 percent of workers as a whole felt that they were being physically overworked. The same study showed that one seventh of all workers have to deal with heavy loads on the job and that one worker in thirteen in the Federal Republic works with heavy tools.

With the change in working conditions, the types of stresses and strains which workers must handle tend to change in the following ways (6, pp. 54-144):

1. Acceleration of the pace of work has become possible by two different types of

Table 1

The main occupational diseases, FRG, 1949-1978[a]

| Year | Hearing Loss, Noise-Induced Deafness | | Silicosis | | Infections | | Injuries to the Meniscus | |
	No. Claims Reported	No. Claims Compensated	No. Claims Reported	No. Claims Compensated	No. Claims Reported	No. Claims Compensated	No. Claims Reported	No. Claims Compensated
1949	26	7	23,698	5,184	3,243	909	–	–
1950	67	18	21,038	6,619	3,149	904	–	–
1951	83	12	19,281	5,263	2,755	987	–	–
1952	147	15	25,374	5,018	2,543	1,085	637	2
1953	140	32	28,041	10,385	2,211	970	1,385	227
1954	126	24	29,558	6,422	2,310	776	1,191	357
1955	109	13	22,560	4,947	1,894	677	1,226	417
1956	105	23	16,866	4,244	1,818	660	1,237	466
1957	135	22	8,822	4,323	1,732	542	1,272	632
1958	103	23	7,797	4,483	1,486	608	1,722	804
1959	129	16	6,599	3,976	1,622	520	1,978	1,147
1960	149	25	6,691	3,802	1,647	552	2,191	1,379
1961	274	22	6,229	3,238	1,595	619	2,284	1,299
1962	382	43	6,221	3,269	1,470	609	2,249	1,324
1963	444	78	5,618	2,817	1,558	491	2,136	1,266
1964	526	100	5,343	2,450	1,744	514	2,308	1,361
1965	722	124	5,285	2,415	1,725	561	2,442	1,369
1966	903	165	5,399	2,070	1,672	601	2,214	1,541
1967	1,123	173	5,206	1,870	2,270	781	1,964	1,379
1968	1,192	324	4,996	1,525	2,272	802	2,070	1,050
1969	1,833	524	5,814	1,396	2,161	878	2,279	1,093
1970	2,007	622	5,244	1,300	2,728	874	1,774	866
1971	3,163	715	4,964	1,314	2,908	996	1,675	829
1972	4,607	979	5,482	1,272	2,887	1,014	1,584	731
1973	6,337	1,145	5,241	1,337	3,251	1,077	1,731	619
1974	9,890	1,589	3,726	1,208	3,437	1,072	1,712	746
1975	12,418	2,028	6,324	1,092	3,291	1,077	1,636	624
1976	13,789	2,452	4,901	976	3,468	1,244	1,598	672
1977	20,592	3,514	4,418	1,054	3,463	1,282	1,552	546
1978	18,121	3,268	4,071	1,002	3,542	1,060	1,325	684

[a] Source, reference 2, S.262f.

Table 1 (Cont'd.)

Diseases of Tendon Sheath		Skin Diseases		Occupational Diseases (Total)		Occ. Diseases per 1,000 Full-Time Workers	
No. Claims Reported	No. Claims Compen- sated	No. Claims Reported	No. Claims Compen- sated	No. Claims Reported	No. Claims Compen- sated	No. Claims Reported	No. Claims Compen- sated
–	–	1,784	104	34,414	8,394	2.07	0.47
–	–	3,336	173	37,551	10,289	1.96	0.54
–	–	3,698	267	34,624	9,306	1.73	0.47
802	–	4,727	339	43,321	8,769	2.14	0.43
3,858	56	4,966	359	53,456	14,521	2.50	0.68
3,628	74	5,593	377	55,916	10,478	2.56	0.48
3,926	74	6,123	416	51,348	8,952	2.27	0.40
4,135	55	5,648	333	43,819	7,960	1.89	0.34
4,206	37	5,047	410	33,759	7,960	1.45	0.34
4,572	15	5,929	501	33,710	8,339	1.43	0.35
4,514	6	6,197	462	32,851	7,942	1.36	0.32
4,547	14	6,387	539	33,727	8,048	1.36	0.32
4,189	4	6,420	519	33,184	7,306	1.36	0.30
3,417	9	5,902	549	29,261	7,445	1.19	0.30
3,503	7	7,068	494	27,947	6,779	1.14	0.28
3,263	5	7,618	456	28,042	6,284	1.12	0.25
2,948	5	7,719	492	27,467	6,464	1.10	0.26
2,578	3	6,965	500	26,061	6,152	1.04	0.25
2,474	3	6,647	460	26,280	5,836	1.09	0.24
2,137	2	6,910	435	25,793	5,316	1.06	0.22
1,830	3	6,997	518	27,427	5,449	1.07	0.21
1,647	3	6,642	543	25,951	5,173	1.03	0.20
1,525	4	6,852	500	27,201	5,374	1.10	0.22
1,591	3	7,597	513	30,273	5,488	1.23	0.22
1,334	5	8,327	476	32,827	5,580	1.31	0.22
1,274	6	7,756	501	36,124	6,072	1.49	0.25
1,088	4	7,778	390	38,296	6,104	1.64	0.26
1,232	1	8,820	361	43,197	6,474	1.64	0.27
1,762	5	10,001	378	48,189	7,581	1.98	0.31
1,506	3	10,259	399	45,484	7,248	1.84	0.29

measures: (a) simplifying the operations and increasing the speed of the machinery, and (b) closer supervision and piece-work wage systems. Such speed-up leads to a greater number of accidents, heightens the burden on the heart and circulatory system, and leads to increased mental stress.

2. Both night and shift work are increasing in prevalence. They have been shown to cause digestive disorders, and most workers on such schedules find that they sleep less and work less efficiently.

3. The new technological developments have given some workers responsibility for extremely expensive machinery which requires extreme manual precision and split-second timing to operate correctly (7, p. 166). Such workers suffer a great deal from a fear of making mistakes.

4. Cooperation and communication at work become more and more difficult as people work farther apart or find themselves separated from others by a curtain of sound. Such isolation makes people tired and bored and more reluctant to cooperate when the opportunity presents itself. Isolation also makes it more difficult to pay attention to the demands of work.

5. The social atmosphere at work, especially relationships with the boss, is very often a factor in creating stress (8).

6. And finally, in a privately dominated economy, the fear of unemployment and layoffs must be seen as a constant source of insecurity and stress. With every cut in pay, every job transfer, every plant relocation, workers and their families are forced to drastically change their way of life. These events leave workers with a profound sense of inadequacy and inability to control their own fate. Research on the long-term unemployed shows how damaging such stress can be (9, p. 194).

A feeling of stress is usually the result of a combination of all these types of factors (10, p. 103). For that reason, it is conceptually difficult to make a clear distinction between sources of physical and psychological stress. Clearly the two types of stress are interdependent. In addition to the specific sources of stress we have discussed here, it is clear that stress and strain inevitably accompany economic growth and social differentiation.

WORK INJURIES

An on-the-job injury is legally defined as a single, sudden, externally caused occurrence which causes noticeable damage to the body. Depending on the jurisdiction, the time period during which the damage is defined as occurring can be as long as an entire work shift (8 hours).

In 1977, over 1.8 million job injuries and almost 190,000 "commuter" injuries (which happened en route to or from work) were officially registered among the 24.3 million full-time workers in the Federal Republic, or one worker in thirteen. Of these, 2,970 on-the-job accidents and 1,305 commuter accidents were fatal (11, p. 103).

It must be emphasized that these totals include only those injuries officially reported, i.e. those in which there were at least three work days lost. So the less-serious injuries go unreported, even though a table saw which cut off only a fingertip might as easily have cut off a couple of fingers. The total number of work accidents causing injury is thus a great deal higher than the official statistics suggest (12, pp. 131-151). Official data from a mini-census taken in 1976 imply that the number of actual work accidents was almost a third higher than the official tally reported by the compensation system (13, pp. 125-129).

Trends in Officially Reported Work Injuries

In 1949 there were 61 reported job-related injuries per 1,000 full-time workers. In 1961 the comparable rate was 118 (up 93 percent), but in 1978 it was down to 74 (see Table 2). When discussing the reasons for the decline in registered work injuries since 1961, official commentators usually refer to the salubrious effect of increased health and safety efforts by government and industry. They rarely look for other possible causes. The improvements in occupational safety and health efforts were, in fact, largely a result of trade union pressure in the 1960s and early '70s. Unfortunately, these efforts had only limited effect. For a real explanation of the decline in reported injury rates, it makes more sense to examine structural changes in the economy.

For example, the proportion of workers in accident-prone fields (agriculture, forestry, mining, construction, and industrial production) has decreased while the proportion in safer fields (the service sector and public employment) has increased, so it is not surprising that the overall injury rate has declined in the last decade and a half. Overall, the proportion of blue-collar workers declined almost 63 percent, to around 49 percent, between 1961 and 1976, while the percentage in white-collar jobs rose from 29.5 to almost 41. At the same time, the proportion in public sector jobs rose from 8 to 10 percent (14, p. 15).

In addition, the increase in mechanization and automation in the '60s has meant that many workers have become less and less important to the production process. Difficult and dangerous work is more likely to be carried out by machine, and as a result the accident rate has declined. Nevertheless, technological change has also created its own new hazards. Sometimes the machines run faster, and sometimes the repair work is particularly dangerous. All in all, however, the number of dangerous jobs eliminated has overshadowed the number of dangerous new jobs created by the introduction of new technology.

Certainly the available figures suggest (though absolute proof is impossible) that the sharp decline in registered work injuries since 1961 can best be attributed to structural changes in the economy and reductions in total hours of work (12, p. 140).

Work Injuries and Economic Crises

Table 2 documents decreases in the rates of registered work injuries in 1963, 1966-1967, and 1974-1975, accounting for much of the overall decline since 1961. Interestingly, these decreases coincide with periods of economic recession, which reduces total employment and thus the work population subject to industrial accidents. But above and beyond the decrease in the working population, it is likely that the number

Table 2

Development of occupational accidents, FRG, 1949-1978[a]

Year	Full-Time Workers (in 1000s)	Recorded Accidents and Occupational Diseases (Total)	Subtotals Occupational Accidents	Occupational Diseases	Commuter Accidents	Occupational Accidents Per 1000 Full-Time Workers	No. Occupational Accidents Compensated	Accidents Compensated Per 1000 Full-Time Workers	No. Fatal Occupational Accidents	Fatal Accidents Per 1000 Full-Time Workers
1949	18,033	1,193,511	1,099,811	37,414	56,286	60.99	84,916	4.71	6,966	0.39
1950	19,183	1,382,353	1,258,220	37,551	86,582	65.59	98,963	5.16	6,429	0.34
1951	19,989	1,595,867	1,453,734	34,624	107,509	72.73	105,635	5.28	6,098	0.31
1952	20,209	1,836,516	1,653,107	43,321	140,088	81.80	107,411	5.32	5,890	0.29
1953	21,304	2,086,581	1,854,127	53,456	178,998	87.03	115,411	5.42	6,374	0.30
1954	21,779	2,242,156	1,992,424	55,916	193,816	91.48	106,457	4.89	6,020	0.28
1955	22,575	2,476,107	2,179,834	51,348	244,925	96.56	105,006	4.65	6,017	0.27
1956	23,133	2,605,674	2,305,144	43,819	256,711	99.65	107,538	4.65	5,844	0.25
1957	23,133	2,615,716	2,341,506	33,759	240,451	101.22	100,241	4.33	5,375	0.23
1958	23,523	2,792,753	2,491,428	33,710	267,615	105.91	100,458	4.27	5,235	0.22
1959	24,123	2,861,961	2,555,432	32,851	273,678	105.93	97,767	4.05	5,134	0.21
1960	24,883	3,028,410	2,711,078	33,727	283,605	108.95	94,881	3.81	4,893	0.20
1961	24,324	3,187,614	2,870,765	33,184	283,665	118.02	95,406	3.92	4,920	0.20
1962	24,440	3,022,884	2,722,415	29,261	271,208	111.39	99,694	4.08	5,446	0.22

1963	24,345	2,934,655	2,618,544	27,947	288,164	107.56	92,328	3.79	4,831	0.20
1964	24,859	2,990,975	2,694,962	28,042	267,971	108.41	87,345	3.51	4,941	0.20
1965	24,951	2,938,127	2,655,363	27,467	255,297	106.42	88,895	3.56	4,784	0.19
1966	25,028	2,808,302	2,542,299	26,061	239,942	101.58	86,750	3.47	4,849	0.19
1967	24,129	2,417,256	2,181,464	26,280	209,512	90.41	81,077	3.36	4,524	0.19
1968	24,327	2,513,433	2,263,841	25,793	223,799	93.06	75,701	3.11	4,290	0.18
1969	25,599	2,631,299	2,359,956	27,427	243,916	92.19	76,384	2.98	4,289	0.17
1970	25,218	2,673,197	2,391,757	25,960	255,480	94.84	77,935	3.09	4,263	0.17
1971	24,828	2,586,718	2,337,926	27,200	221,592	94.16	76,833	3.09	4,589	0.18
1972	24,668	2,481,107	2,237,366	30,273	213,468	90.70	72,030	2.92	4,082	0.17
1973	24,965	2,482,637	2,221,268	32,827	228,542	88.98	68,887	2.76	4,011	0.16
1974	24,288	2,212,266	1,989,315	36,124	186,827	81.91	67,825	2.79	3,644	0.15
1975	23,301	1,970,529	1,760,713	38,296	171,520	75.56	61,590	2.64	3,137	0.13
1976	24,458	2,056,960	1,828,743	43,197	188,179	74.77	59,278	2.42	3,154	0.13
1977	24,340	2,044,431	1,809,810	48,189	186,432	74.36	58,933	2.42	2,970	0.12
1978	24,668	2,057,285	1,817,510	45,484	194,291	73.68	56,408	2.29	2,825	0.11

[a] Source, *Unfallverhütungsbericht 1980*, Bundestagsdrucksache 8/3650 vom 8.2.1980, S. 144-146.

of *reported* (as opposed to the actual) work injuries declines during recessions simply because workers are afraid to risk their jobs by reporting minor injuries. Even the government seems to recognize this dynamic: the official 1974 report on occupational injury incidence states (15, p. 7) that since the recession of 1966-1967, "the anxiety over unemployment pressures, has tended to pressure workers against reporting minor work injuries." In 1974, for example, it is likely that 100,000 work injuries (or 5 percent of that year's total) went unreported (15, p. 7).

The Unequal Incidence of Work Injuries

As might be expected, the work injury frequency rate varies by industry (16, pp. 96-112). It is highest in those economic activities requiring heavy physical labor. The most dangerous industries are mining, quarrying, iron and steel, and lumbering. Agriculture, as well, has a high and rising injury rate.

In addition, particular social groups are especially subject to work-related injuries. The injury rate of foreign workers is 2.5 times that of native Germans. Part of this difference is no doubt explainable by language and communication difficulties, but this is only part of the story. Foreigners hold the most dangerous jobs in mining, construction, and steel, and work in an atmosphere of constant fear of unemployment, as the present economic crisis has proved again.

Doctrines About Accident Causation

Occupational medicine in the Federal Republic holds that there are two basic causes of work accidents: technical defects and human error. Technical defects are those related to the means of production and working conditions, e.g. plant layout, machine design and guarding, and the use of chemicals and other materials. Human error, on the other hand, means the conscious or unconscious neglect of safety regulations or correct operating procedure by the workers.

A textbook of occupational medicine (17, p. 379) claims that "around 70 percent of accidents are caused by human error, and the rest can be attributed to organizational and technical failures." This distinction between technical defects and human error suggests that accidents are caused either by objective factors in the production process or by the personal characteristics of the injured worker. But a serious analysis of the causes of work accidents must go far beyond this simplistic scheme, which hopelessly confuses cause and effect. The means of production, after all, are the products of human design and construction at another location. Thus, technical defects are the results of previous human error in the design and construction of the means of production, or to put it another way, economic decisions at an earlier phase of the production process which contribute indirectly to the occurrence of work accidents. As such, technical defects and human error are simply different aspects of the same thing—the human organization of labor.

It is just as problematic to try to attribute accidents to human error, as if a work injury could be "caused" by a specific individual characteristic. To blame accidents and injuries on the defective personality traits of individual workers, as is commonly done by safety researchers and engineers, can best be understood as an attempt to camouflage the objective social determinants of work accidents. Biological and psychological attributes are not, as a rule, the most important determinants of work accidents. More significant are the particular characteristics of the job itself, which generates specific forms of behavior and consciousness. There is certainly a great difference between the risks to life and limb of the underground miner hacking away at the coal face and the steel worker operating a rolling mill from a remote control panel. When faced with a dangerous production process, a rested and alert worker is much less likely to have an accident than an exhausted one. Moreover, there is a continual struggle, often on a daily basis, between supervisors and employees—or in broader terms, between appropriators and creators of surplus value—over who runs the workplace, that is, over concrete issues of wages and hours and working conditions. This struggle bears directly on the safety of the workers, and constitutes one illustration of how social relations condition occupational health. It is also necessary to look outside the factory, to a culture dominated by individual consumption and the nuclear family, to understand the roots of the safety consciousness and behavior of the worker.

These social factors and relations should not be neglected when examining human error as a cause of job accidents and injuries. On closer examination, individual or personal "errors" turn out to be social failures to the degree to which behavior and consciousness are expressions of social, economic, and political processes. For that reason, the investigation of the causes of industrial injuries, if it is to go beyond mere symptomatic description, cannot overlook such basic factors (16, pp. 112-121).

Let us consider, for example, the question of speed-up. The pace of work is, at first glance, merely a technological event which depends on a given combination of machines and labor power. But the goal by which the work tempo is set is socially determined by factors outside the realm of technology. Under a system of private ownership of the means of production, the power of decision over the rate of production lies almost entirely with the owners of capital or their agents in the enterprise. The major goal of capitalists is to maximize production and profit, which they must do in order to stay in business, faced as they are by competition from other capitalists. That part of the labor surplus which is privately appropriated—the profit rate—increases in proportion to the speed of production and the ability of the owners to beat down expenditures for labor, equipment, and raw materials. As a result, management constantly presses for a faster work pace, and the formal organization of work is geared to speed-up.

The workers themselves, who tend to be paid on a piece-work basis wherever possible, get sucked into this system of productivity worship, of working as fast and as long as possible in order to maximize earnings, which are of primary importance in a culture dominated by the consumer ethic. Even workers who are paid by the hour often have their salaries supplemented by production bonuses. The entire work situation is thus organized to give workers every personal incentive to break safety regulations which might cost them extra movements and slow down their pace of work. Workers are repeatedly seduced into bettering their income at their own risk.

How, after all, do cranes become overloaded? Is it solely the fault of the crane operator? Why do supervisors tolerate behavior which goes against safety regulations? Do supervisors get promoted on the basis of their safety records or their production quotas? Production bonuses and piece-work are proven methods of increasing the pace of work. In such cases, *the short-term interest of the workers in the highest possible income contradicts their long-term interest in maintaining their health.*

MEDICAL CARE ON THE JOB

After examining the background causes of occupational injuries and disease, we must ask a number of questions about the practice of occupational medicine in the Federal Republic: What is the legal framework of occupational medicine? What roles do occupational physicians fill? Where do they work? Who pays for their services?

The Work Safety Law (*Arbeitssicherheitsgesetz*) took effect on December 1, 1974. Under the provisions of this law, empoyers were, for the first time, obligated to hire occupational physicians and safety specialists to aid in worker protection and accident prevention. In addition, the employer is required to provide the occupational physicians with appropriate support, including an office, a staff, and the necessary equipment and whatever else they need to carry out their duties.

In examining the history of the Work Safety Law, two questions arise: Why did it take so long to pass a Work Safety Law? Why was the passage of this law so strongly opposed?

The Work Safety Law was the outcome of real political struggles. Not surprisingly, the creation and maintenance of an occupational medical service has come to mean something profoundly different for business and for labor. For a business required to maintain one, an occupational medical service represents a large capital expense, which nevertheless pays for itself in increased productivity and reduces the costs of work-related sickness and absenteeism. It should lead to an increase in profitability. For the workers, on the other hand, an occupational medical service is a means to protect their lives and health, and should be organized with those goals in mind.

After more than a decade of opposition to the Work Safety Law, business finally gave in. The convincing factor was studies carried out since the mid-sixties showing that occupational medical services could in fact be profitable for large-scale enterprises and should no longer be considered a form of "social charity." According to one analysis carried out at a large automobile firm, the cost-benefit ratio of an occupational medical service was 1:1.8 and could probably be increased to 1:3.7 with appropriate streamlining (18, p. 99). In other words, investment in such a service could return more than three times its original cost to the company. It must be noted, of course, that the profitability of such a service is greatest in giant, highly centralized enterprises. For that reason, big business was much less vehement in its opposition to the Work Safety Law than small business.

Despite the Work Safety Law, the number of active occupational physicians is still rather low. In 1975 there were 1,022 full-time and 1,380 part-time occupational physicians in the Federal Republic. Since a factory physician spends an average of only 15 minutes a year with an employee and works a 40-hour week, it can be argued that there should be 15,000 factory-based physicians in order for most workers to be covered. Moreover, most of the full-time factory physicians work for large-scale private enterprises, as well as the Federal Railroad (*Bundesbahn*) and the Federal Postal Service (*Bundespost*).

The general tasks of factory-based occupational physicians are specified in the Work Safety Law. The most important are: to support and counsel the employer on job safety; to cooperate with the Workers' Council (*Betriebsrat*) in the factory and advise it on health and safety matters; to conduct physical examinations of employees and advise them; and to assure a safe workplace. Occupational physicians are not required to treat or report cases of occupational disease.

In their daily work, factory-based occupational physicians are free of any specific formal regulations on how they should apply their medical conscience and the general requirements of medical practice. They are directly responsible to management in the hierarchy, though their job description and hiring and dismissal are subject to the advice and consent of the Workers' Council. Occupational physicians, in fact, devote up to 90 percent of their working time to routine employment and screening examinations. The purpose is to screen out the chronically ill and other high-risk categories of workers, and to remove workers from hazardous work environments (e.g. noise) as soon as clinical signs of illness begin to appear. Thus, the primary focus of the practicing occupational physician is selection of workers rather than prevention of risk.

The introduction of the Work Safety Law was basically a progressive step, because it made the employment of occupational physicians and safety specialists mandatory. As a student of the issue, I believe it is the obligation of the unions to take advantage of all the new opportunities opened up by the law. But from the workers' point of view, there are also limitations:

- The law is unclear in many ways and provides too many loopholes for the corporations.
- Physicians have no power of decision over the construction of the workplace as it relates to occupational health and safety.
- The physicians and safety specialists are not independent employees; thus they are subject to pressure from management.
- The law should regulate more closely the terms of the relationship between the occupational physicians and the Workers' Councils, which are the elected representatives of the employees, the physicians' potential patients.

CONCLUSIONS

In conclusion, I believe that there are a few important demands which should be made in regard to occupational health and safety in West Germany:

1. Industrial physicans must be cut off from their present dependence on the private employer. This area of medicine is too important to leave open to considerations of profit if medicine is to live up to its humanitarian pretensions. To escape the cross-fire of competing interests, perhaps it would be best to have industrial

physicians employed by professional insurance associations (*Berufsgenossenschaften*)[1] or similar agencies. The unions would have to assure that these agencies would be under the control of the workers. Under such circumstances, we would welcome the repeal of the present prohibition of treatment by company physicians (19, p. 17).

2. A greater stress on prevention is imperative, an emphasis which must go beyond mere early detection of disease. This is the only way to reduce the number of work-related casualties.

3. There must be a great expansion of the use of engineering techniques as the first line of defense against work-related diseases and injuries. Personal protective devices such as respirators should be used only temporarily, or as a last resort.

4. The present standards for the training and selection of occupational physicians and safety specialists should be raised and made more specific. It is not enough to take doctors from some other specialty, rush them through a two- or four-week course in occupational medicine, and expect them to perform adequately. The specialty of occupational medicine must develop in new directions, and this will be possible only if salaries are raised to competitive levels.

5. The range of officially recognized compensable diseases must be broadened to include psychosocial diseases such as stress.

6. All occupational injuries and diseases must be recorded in the official statistics, not just those which cause over three days absence from work.

In order to understand the relationship between work and health in a capitalist society, it is not enough to limit the area to a consideration of physiological problems and individual psychological characteristics. There must also be a careful examination of the concrete influences of the structural relations of property and surplus value appropriation in society. And it is hardly sufficient to limit medicine to a curative role. Medicine should be required to broaden its concern with prevention in order to ensure the health of working people. For this to occur, prevention must go beyond the superficial relief of particular symptoms to an attack on the technological and social roots of disease. Without such a fundamental strategy, occupational medicine in the Federal Republic of Germany will continue to find itself trapped on a sometimes fascinating and always dizzying merry-go-round of activities which has little to do with the humanization of the conditions of work and life.

REFERENCES

1. Deppe, H.-U., and Regus, M. Seminar—Medizin, Gesellschaft, Geschichte. Frankfurt a.M., 1975.
2. Deppe, H.-U. *Vernachlässigte Gesundheit, Zum Verhältnis von Gesundheit, Staat, Gesellschaft in der Bundesrepublik Deutschland.* Köln, 1980.

---

[1]Professional associations (*Berufsgenossenschaften*) are the financial backers of workers' compensation insurance programs in the Federal Republic. Legally, they consist of publicly organized corporations which manage themselves. Premiums are paid by employers only. Compensation hearings boards are half composed of management representatives and half of labor. The professional associations have the authority, in the Federal Republic, to issue legally binding occupational health and safety regulations aimed at the prevention of work-related injuries and disease.

3. Kern, H., and Schumann, M. *Industriearbeit und Arbeiterbewußtsein*, 2 volumes. Frankfurt a.M., 1970.
4. Hettinger, T. *Die physische Belastung an Arbeitsplätzen der Eisen- und Stahlindustrie*. Arbeit und Leistung, 1969.
5. Hettinger, T. *Stärker belastet als ein Fußballstar*. Der Gewerkschafter, 1971.
6. Mergner, U. *et al. Arbeitsbedingungen im Wandel*. Göttingen, 1975.
7. Volkholz, V. *Belastungsschwerpunkte und Praxis der Arbeitssicherheit*. Bonn, 1977.
8. Friedeburg, L.v. *Soziologie des Betriebsklimas*. Frankfurt a.M., 1963.
9. Thomann, K.-D. Die gesundheitlichen Auswirkungen der Arbeitslosigkeit. In *Vom Schock zum Fatalismus? Soziale und psychische Auswirkungen der Arbeitslosigkeit*, edited by A. Wacker. Frankfurt a.M., 1978.
10. Meyer, S. *et al. Gesundheitsversorgung, Daten des Gesundheitssystems in der BRD*. Hamburg, 1978.
11. *Unfallverhütungsbericht 1978*. Bundestagsdrucksache 8/2328, November 1978.
12. Priester, K. *Zur Entwicklung der Arbeitsunfälle in der BRD. Das Argument, Jahrbuch für kritische Medizin*, vol. 3. Westberlin, 1978.
13. *Wirtschaft und Statistik, 1978*.
14. Bundesminister für Wirtschaft (ed.). *Leistungen in Zahlen 1976*. Bonn-Bad Godesberg, 1977.
15. *Unfallverhütungsbericht 1976*. Bundestagsdrucksache 8/2328, 1976.
16. Deppe, H.-U. *Industriearbeit und Medizin*. Frankfurt a.M., 1973.
17. Valentin, H. *et al. Arbeitsmedizin*. Stuttgart, 1971.
18. Deppe, H.-U. *Medizinische Soziologie*. Frankfurt a.M., 1978.
19. Hauptvorstand der Gewerkschaft Öffentliche Dienste, Transport und Verkehr. *Perspektiven der Gewerkschaft ÖTV zur Gesundheitspolitik*. Stuttgart, 1977.

PART 4

Occupational Health in Underdeveloped Capitalist Countries

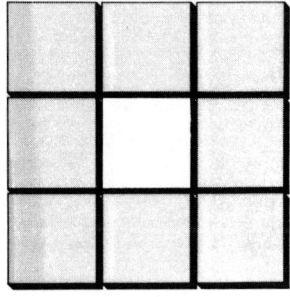

CHAPTER 12

Work and Health in Mexico

Asa Cristina Laurell

Lately there has been in a number of countries a rediscovery of the importance of the study of the relationship of health to work. What was for many years the realm of experts on productivity (1) is now becoming the preoccupation of people who are trying to make the interests of workers prevail.

I will argue that to hold a working-class point of view in the study of the relationship between health and work implies the exploration of two dimensions of the problem: the technical one, traditionally developed by occupational health experts, and the conceptual one, which is necessary to the formulation of a working-class understanding of the problem of health.

Part of the difficulty in developing new ideas and modes of action in occupational health is derived from the way work is conceived. Although work is the central category of the problem under study, it seems that it is treated in a very spontaneous way; there is almost no attempt to transform work from an empirical category into a scientific one.

In the classical occupational health approach, work is understood as an environmental problem since it puts people in contact with chemical, physical, biological, and psychological agents that make them have accidents or get sick. Obviously this conception reproduces the view traditionally held by medicine under capitalism of illness as an individually occurring biological phenomenon.

211

The great merit of radical occupational health analysis is that it has demonstrated that health risks for workers are indissolubly linked to the functioning of capitalist industry, and that, therefore, the implementation of solutions depends more on power and struggle than on technical modifications (2).

Work in the capitalist view is usually ignored when the causes of disease are considered. The most common way of considering work in this context is to transplant it from the realm of production to the realm of consumption, viewing work as the generator of resources that determine a particular pattern of satisfaction of needs. The great number of studies on income and other socioeconomic factors and health differentials testifies to the prevalence of this view (3). It is hardly coincidental that this ideological displacement from production to consumption occurs in societies that are organized according to the principle of exploitation of alienated labor. A total resolution of the problem must conceptualize work so as to include it as a central analytical category in the understanding of health and disease as social and collective situations embedded in the structure of society.

The materialist epidemiological current of thought has addressed the problem in a different way, however. The central category of Eyer and Sterling's (4) important work, for example, is stress, and social phenomena are analyzed in relation to this factor. Such a procedure minimizes the importance of a careful analysis of social categories (among them work), and tends to group them as an undifferentiated, stressful complex under the rubric of advanced capitalism.

Stark (5), on the other hand, makes a very suggestive analysis of work; he emphasizes, and rightly so, the social and collective nature of work in advanced capitalism, proposing that the analysis of work be valid insofar as it places the understanding of the work process at the level of society as a whole. This level of abstraction, however, does not offer the necessary tools to explore how the parts relate to each other as a whole.

Some Latin American groups have approached the problem in a different way, although their propositions are relatively unknown outside their home countries. Fassler (6), for example, underlines the necessity of developing an understanding of health which departs from the analysis of the work process in order to explain "individual pathology as the concrete expression of social antagonisms and contradictions." She also stresses that different kinds of work processes find their point of expression in different moments of the life cycle.

TOWARD A DIFFERENT CONCEPTUALIZATION OF WORK AND HEALTH

The first point to make concerning the study of work and health is that work is a *social* category and consequently should be treated as such at an analytical level, and not just as one more environmental risk factor. Because of the central place that work occupies in any society, it seems inevitable that it must be the keystone of any structured attempt to explain the social origin of disease.

What, then, is work? According to Marx (7, 8), work is a conscious process by means of which man appropriates nature in order to transform it into elements that are necessary to his life. The production of material life, always developed by means of a particular form of society, occurs in the work process. Work, then, is basic to all social life, since the reproduction of life is impossible without it. This, however, is the most abstract level of understanding of work and the work process, since it does not specify the social relations under which they occur. The essential determination of the work process under capitalism is that it is organized so as to maximize the creation of surplus value and therefore profit, a fact that, as we will see, transforms it profoundly.

The particular mode of production in a given society also generates a particular mode of consumption (8, p. 247). An important element in the social determination of what are the necessities in a social formation is thus derived from the work process, and to a much lesser extent from biological elements. As a matter of fact, biology determines only the very basic physiological needs (7, p. 279), and even then there are some very serious disagreements as to what is "normal" to the reproduction of human life. This highlights why it is inconvenient in the analysis of health to dissociate the sphere of consumption from the sphere of production, and why it is incorrect to reduce work into a simple generator of goods.

At least in capitalist society, where the productive part of the productive-reproductive process of social life predominates (9), it seems possible to argue that the requirements of the work process organize all social life. In certain situations this becomes quite clear, and the ideologically imposed separation between the world of work and the world of consumption disappears. For example, the working-class neighborhood built around the factory in some places shows how the social space is organized based on the needs of the workplace: at the school, named after the boss, children are educated to become workers; on the playground children learn what kind of leisure is good leisure; and the shrill whistle which signals the start of each work shift imposes the rhythm of the factory on the surroundings.[1] The central organizing role of work is also very clear in the life of agricultural workers who are forced to move from place to place depending on the needs of the commercial agricultural cycle. Their homes, then, are the barracks of each farm where they work; their access to medical care depends on their being active workers; their children have no possibility of going to school; and even the prices of basic goods move with them—when they arrive, prices go up, and when they leave, prices go down.

As a matter of fact, the coercive organizing power of work on individual and social life becomes clear when we consider that no worker can plan any "life project" that does not consider as a starting point the time and energy that is to be spent at work. Even so, as Córdova (10) has pointed out, certain kinds of work organization, e.g. shift work, prohibit the regular development of any activity that is not work. Today, for sure, as work loses its specificity and becomes more easily interchangeable, this organizing power over life outside the workplace becomes less visible, though by no means less real.

The relation between production and consumption, however, does not explain exhaustively the relation between work and health, and it is therefore necessary to

---

[1] These kinds of working-class neighborhoods can be found in Mexico surrounding the factories that were started around the turn of the century. They are prevalent, for example, in Tizapan and Plalpan.

develop some basic notions for the study of work. An adequate concept seems to be that of work process, which on the one hand specifies the relation between work, the means of work (instruments), and the work object (7, p. 216), and on the other hand opens the possibility of studying the historical character of work.[2] The concept of work process furthermore epitomizes two fundamental characteristics of any production: that of having an essentially technical side—the labor process—and a social one. In capitalist society this means that at the same time as the work process is a technical process by means of which goods are being produced, it is also a process of valorization of capital, i.e. a process in which workers create surplus value that eventually becomes nothing but the capitalist's profit and accumulative capital (7, Vol. I, Ch. 5). This double nature of the work process has some important consequences that are relevant to the problem under study.

Under capitalism, the whole productive process is organized so as to render a maximum of surplus value, value that is created by the workers but whose amount also depends on the competitive situation of the capitalist. This means that the labor process occurs in the midst of class struggle, obliging the owners of capital to develop forms of control over the workers—control that is essentially exercised by means of the organization of the work process in the factory and the kind of technology utilized. The basic principle of this control is to separate the execution of the labor process from its conceptualization (11). The first element to take into account, then, in the analysis of any particular work process is the concrete expressions of class struggle and the capacity of the workers to attain their goals.

Analyzing the three elements of the work process—work, instruments, and object—from this twofold perspective will permit a technical and social understanding of any particular work process. The study of the work object should take into account its physical, chemical, and biological properties, since these might constitute serious health risks, as is well known concerning both natural objects, such as ore, or artificial ones, such as the thousands of chemical substances used in industry. The transformation of an object into a work object, on the other hand, is socially determined.

The instruments, or the means, of work can be analyzed either in terms of their technical sophistication or as an expression of specific social relations. The first aspect informs us about the physical effort needed in the execution of the work, the risks implied in the interaction between the worker, the instrument, and the object, and the degree of control that can be exercised over the instrument by the worker. This last aspect is directly related to the analysis of the instruments of work as the expression of the social relations that have created them. For example, the instruments of work created under capitalism will have as a distinctive characteristic their imposition on the worker of a specific manner of working. This means, among other things, that the machine dictates the rhythm of work and limits the relative decision-making power of the worker. The first fact is related to what seems to be the major work risk under advanced capitalism—stress—and the second increases in certain conditions the accident proneness not of the worker but of the instrument.

---

[2] Work process is a concept that permits analysis at different levels of abstraction: as a general process, as a process of a particular mode of production, as a process of a particular social formation, and as a concrete process.

The most important analytical element of the work process for the understanding of health, however, is work itself. It is possible to distinguish different forms of consumption of labor power in work, which in turn imply different forms of wearing out of the worker. These forms of consumption are linked to the extraction of absolute and relative surplus value. The extraction of absolute surplus is the most primitive form of exploitation of the worker, since it consists simply in the increase of work hours without any change in the instruments or organization of the work process (7, Ch. 8). The extraction of relative surplus value, on the other hand, can be obtained in two ways: increasing the productivity of work by means of technological change, or by intensifying work. The extraction of relative surplus value is thus the predominant form under advanced capitalism (7, Ch. 10).[3]

The extraction of absolute surplus value that occurs typically in the work processes with little development of technology would mean a combination of different elements: high caloric cost, heavy physical effort, and insufficient time for rest. On the other hand, since the wage is the most important element in the determination of the absolute amount of profit at a low level of technology, the extraction of absolute surplus value tends to be combined with a low wage level which establishes a limit on the adequate reproduction of labor power and accelerates even more the wearing out of the worker.[4] The effects of this kind of work process find their expression not only in the worker but also in his family. This has been very clearly demonstrated by Gross and Underwood (12), who showed that the combination of high caloric cost and low wages in the production of sisal caused malnutrition not in the workers but in their sons.

The work process in which the extraction of relative surplus value is dominant (4) is characterized by a different form of consumption of labor power determined by the effects of the increase in productivity (which implies working with machines) and in work intensity. The introduction of a more complex technology implies, at least up to a certain limit, exposure to more risks from accidents and chemicals. Both intensification and productivity increases provoke stress reactions and fatigue that cause physiological changes in the body, giving rise to disease proneness in both the short and long term. The wearing out of the worker in this case is a more common phenomenon than the "overwork-underconsumption" pattern of the producer of absolute surplus value. In underdeveloped countries like Mexico, an important part of the population does not participate directly in the capitalist productive process but rather in petty commodity production in agriculture. The linkage of this form of production to the dominant capitalist mode of production obliges the peasant or artisan to invest more and more labor power trying to maintain a minimum level of consumption in a situation of increasingly unequal exchange between his products

---

[3] It is clear that in any work process (under capitalism) both kinds of surplus value are produced, but as there occurs a reorganization of the work process and the development of the instruments of work, the production of relative surplus value becomes dominant since it is possible to increase the extraction of surplus value without prolonging the workday.

[4] If wages represent a higher percentage of the costs of production, as is the case when there is a low level of technology, the possibility of limiting wages means that the capitalist increases his profit if he sells the product at a fixed price or guarantees his profit by lowering prices to a more competitive level.

and the industrial ones. The peasant work process, then, is similar to the one of extraction of absolute surplus value given that, with the low technological level, there occurs a rapid physical erosion from long hours of work and inadequate nutrition.

Thus far, it seems possible to postulate the formation of different collective patterns of consumption-reproduction that would be determined by the following four elements: predominant type of surplus value extracted; development of the productive forces; degree of relative control over the labor process by the worker; and class struggle situation.

The analysis of these elements and of the work process could be done both at the level of the social formation as a whole and at the level of the particular work process in, for instance, a factory. It seems necessary to stress once more that the social determination is as real at the level of the concrete workplace as it is at the level of society as a whole; the failure to understand this can mire the occupational health worker in technical questions of production and prevent a broader understanding of the problem.

MEXICAN ECONOMIC AND POLITICAL STRUCTURE

During the period from 1940 to 1970, the economic and class structure of Mexico was profoundly transformed. In 1940, Mexico was predominantly an agricultural and raw material producer with a mostly rural population. By 1970, it had developed an economy whose central and dynamic sector undoubtedly was manufacturing and a population in which the industrial working class played an important role. But the year 1970 also marks a turning point in Mexican society since by then the results of 30 years of a particular kind of development crystalized in an economic and social crisis. This process of development could be studied from many angles, but I will try to focus only on the elements of special importance for the understanding of work and health.

Economic Structure

As can be seen from Table 1, the share of the gross national product represented by agriculture and extractive industry decreased in relative importance between 1940 and 1970, while the rest of industry and commerce increased their proportions. This process of industrialization has been sustained essentially by four elements: the maintenance of low wages, transference of resources from agriculture to industry, massive foreign investment, and a State economic policy favoring industrial capital (14).

This means that the rate of exploitation of labor has been extremely high, around 100 to 150 percent, while in Europe and the United States it is uncommon to find rates exceeding 50 percent (15). The decapitalization of agriculture, on the other hand, led to a crisis of production. During the period 1965-1970 there was a yearly decrease in the value of production of 0.2 percent (without any considerable recovery until 1976), although the annual population increase was 3.5 percent (16). One of the results of this economic policy was a growing fiscal crisis, with a 700 percent increase of the public debt from 1970 to 1975 and a 400 percent increase in the deficit of the balance of payments—two important elements that contributed to the

Table 1

Percent distribution of the gross national product by economic sector,
Mexico, 1940-1970

Economic Sector	1940[a]	1950[a]	1960[a]	1970[b]
Agriculture	22.6	22.5	18.9	11.5
Industry	29.7	30.4	33.1	33.9
Mining	(7.9)	(5.8)	(5.4)	(5.2)
Manufacture	(18.6)	(20.5)	(23.0)	(22.4)
Electricity/construction	(3.1)	(4.0)	(4.7)	(6.3)
Commerce	25.9	26.2	25.8	31.5
Services	21.9	20.9	22.2	23.1

[a]Source, Banco de México in reference 13.
[b]Source, Dirección Gral de Estadística, SIC, Mexico.

devaluations of 1976 (17). Massive foreign investment finally led to a situation in which foreign capital controls 27 percent of the 938 major Mexican industries, 50 percent of the 10 largest ones, and 53 percent of the capital goods producing industry (18).

The central role of industry in the economic structure makes it necessary to get some indication of its development in terms of the analytical tools that were proposed earlier, i.e. the type of surplus value extracted and the development of the productive forces. Given the practical difficulties of obtaining numerical expressions of these two concepts, I will use some indirect measures that permit an approximation.

As can be observed in Table 2, the value of production per person occupied in industry rose steadily from 1940 to 1970. Since this trend could not have been obtained just by making each person work more time, it means that the productivity of work has increased and also indicates a shift from absolute to relative surplus value. The data concerning productivity per hour calculated for the period of 1971 to 1975 express the same tendency, since there was an increase of 39 percent during these five years (20).

Table 2

Invested capital and value of production per person occupied
in manufacturing industry, Mexico, 1940-1970[a]

Year	Invested Capital per Person Occupied (pesos)	Value of Production per Person Occupied (pesos)
1940	8,503	8,271
1950	25,317	30,062
1960	85,148	67,239
1970	120,133	130,696

[a]Source, reference 19, pp. 113-126.

A shift from extraction of predominantly absolute to relative surplus value by means of the increase of productivity implies technological innovation. The increase in invested capital per person could also be observed in the period from 1940 to 1970. Table 2 indicates that the instruments of work are more and more expensive, probably because more complex technology is required.

Table 3 shows the reorientation of the investments in industry, with a steady decrease in nondurable and intermediate consumption goods and a sixfold increase in the relative importance of the investment in the production of capital goods and consumer durables. It is well known that the latter industry is the most sophisticated one in terms of technology. This fact, then, together with the data of Table 2, indicate that there has been a fairly rapid process of development of the productive forces in the periods under study.

Table 4 demonstrates that there exists a clear differentiation in the wage levels of the industrial working class according to the size of the employing enterprise. But it is also clear that there is an inverse relationship between the rate of exploitation and the importance of the factory in terms of production. This exemplifies the tendency to combine the extraction of predominantly absolute surplus value with low wages, given the limited possibilities of increasing exploitation of the worker through the intensification of work and increases in productivity as a result of technological innovation. In this manner, Table 4 also indicates that different sectors of the Mexican working class wear out in different ways, which in turn should be reflected in the disease pattern of these groups.

Class Structure

The transformation in the economic structure that took place between 1940 and 1970 implied a profound change in the existing class structure. There was an important shift of the work force from agriculture to manufacturing and other urban occupations, accompanied by a rapid process of proletarianization.

As can be seen in Table 5, 67 percent of the population worked in agriculture in 1940 compared to 42 percent in 1970. Industry and services experienced a steady increase in this same period, from 13 to 24 percent and 10 to 24 percent, respectively. Commerce and finance are the only activities that did not experience a considerable change. The fact that there was an important increase in the population occupied in services while this sector did not greatly increase its relative share of the gross national

Table 3

Percent distribution of invested capital by industrial group, Mexico, 1940-1970[a]

Industrial Group	1940	1950	1960	1970
Nondurable consumer goods	54.4	54.7	47.8	39.3
Intermediate goods	41.4	34.9	38.4	37.7
Capital and durable consumer goods	3.8	9.8	12.3	21.5

[a]Source, reference 19, p. 207.

Table 4

Persons occupied, annual income, and rate of exploitation by industrial group, Mexico, 1970[a]

Industrial Group by Value of Total Production (thousands of pesos)	Persons Occupied		Value Added per Person Occupied (pesos)	Average Annual Income per Person Occupied (pesos)	Approximate rate of exploitation
	Number	Percent			
Up to 1,500	390,223	24.7	15,279	6,740	126
1,501-5,000	178,799	11.3	31,611	15,828	100
5,001-20,000	302,223	19.1	43,698	20,200	116
20,001-50,000	243,591	15.4	55,012	23,772	131
50,001-100,000	166,520	10.5	67,652	28,010	141
100,001 and over	299,897	19.0	109,692	36,590	200
Total/Average	1,581,253	100.0	52,100	20,865	149

[a] Source, IX Censo Industrial, SIC, Mexico.

Table 5

Distribution of the economically active population by economic sector, Mexico, 1940-1970[a]

Economic sector	1940		1950		1960		1970	
	Number (thousands)	Percent	Number (thousands)	Percent	Number (thousands)	Percent	Number (thousands)	Percent
Agriculture	3,831	66.8	4,824	60.9	6,144	55.3	5,104	41.8
Industry	747	13.1	1,319	16.7	2,008	18.1	2,974	24.4
Commerce and finance	552	9.6	684	8.7	1,075	9.7	1,197	9.8
Services	599	10.5	1,090	13.7	1,884	16.9	2,934	24.0
Total	5,729	100.0	7,917	100.0	11,111	100.0	12,209	100.0

[a]Source, Census Grals de Población, SIC, México. Includes only population with specified occupation.

product (see Table 1) reflects the agglomeration of underemployed rural migrants in the urban areas as the result of the process of development and proletarianization in the countryside.

There is some difficulty in quantifying the degree of proletarianization because of the peculiar characteristics of petty commodity production, especially in agriculture, in which the same person employs workers at some periods of the productive cycle and becomes employed as a worker during other parts of the year. This explains why there are such large fluctuations in the employer group in Table 6. Even so, there is a clear tendency toward the separation between the direct producers and their instruments of work, as can be seen in the increase in salaried workers from 54 percent in 1940 to 62 percent in 1970. As has been noted above, the "half-proletarianized" peasantry works in conditions that have many similarities to the process of extraction of absolute surplus value.

As was noted in Table 4, there is a relatively wide range of wages among industrial workers, although the majority (55.1 percent) get close to the legally established minimum. The rapid rate of inflation has also had an important impact on the real wage level, since prices have increased faster than wages.

Another direct effect of the economic crisis, which began in 1971 and continues today with shorter periods of recovery, is an important increase in unemployment and an intensification of work in the factories. It was calculated that 3 million were unemployed in 1977, half of whom had lost their jobs as a direct effect of the economic crisis in industry (21). The intensification of work is shown by the 39 percent increase in productivity per worker hour occurring between 1971 and 1976, which could hardly be attributed to rapid technological innovation since it took place in a period during which there was a very low rate of investment (20).

The State, the Trade Unions, and Legislation

The basic defense organization of the working class at the workplace is the trade union. In Mexico, it was not until after the Revolution of 1910-1917 that this basic form of worker organization was legalized. The history of trade unionism since then is the history of the struggle between the State, which tries to subordinate the unions, and groups of workers who try to pry the unions loose from the State apparatus.

The right of workers to organize themselves in trade unions and to strike was included in the Constitution in 1917, and in 1931 the relations between labor and capital were formally regulated by the Federal Labor Law (22). In 1934, Nationalist President Cardenas came to power, and it was during the six years of his presidency that today's most important labor confederation was founded. Simultaneously, however, Mexican trade unions became a part of the State apparatus of control. In 1938, the Mexican Confederation of Labor (CTM) was converted into one of the basic sectors of the official government party, the Party of the Mexican Revolution (PMR). In 1948, Vicente Lombardo Toledano, a progressive trade-union leader, was expelled from the CTM, which remained under the control of the conservative state bureaucracy. In 1965, the CTM, together with the other major trade unions, formed the Congress of Labor, representing around 95 percent of the organized working class. Today, it has become the "sector of labor" in the official government party—the Institutional Revolutionary Party (PRI).

Table 6

Distribution of the economically active population by position in the system of production, Mexico, 1940-1970[a]

Economic Position	1940		1950		1960		1970	
	Number (thousands)	Percent	Number (thousands)	Percent	Number (thousands)	Percent	Number (thousands)	Percent
Salaried workers	3,069	53.7	3,831	46.4	7,268	64.1	8,055	62.2
Petty producers and family workers	1,417[b]	24.9	4,373	52.8	3,976	35.1	4,103	31.7
Employers, entrepreneurs, and managers	1,220[c]	21.4	68	0.8	88	0.8	797[d]	6.1
Total	5,706	100.0	8,272	100.0	11,332	100.0	12,955	100.0

[a] Source, Censos Generales de Población, SIC, Mexico.
[b] Of these, 700.5 (12.3 percent of total) were in agriculture.
[c] Of these, 1,218 (21.4 percent of total) were in agriculture, and most should be included in the petty producers category.
[d] There was a change in classification criteria; the majority in fact belongs in the petty producers category.

222

Control by the official trade unions is exercised over the workers by means of a highly bureaucratic structure, corruption, threats, violence, and State support (23, p. 45). This situation has limited considerably the possibilities of even the most basic bread-and-butter struggles. Nevertheless, there have been constant organized attempts to break this control—by railroad workers in 1958-1959, by State employees in 1965-1966, and on a broad scale from 1970 to 1977. Though this worker insurgency has not succeeded in breaking the control of the State, it has at least gained concessions for the trade-union membership. Trade-union membership stood at 17.7 percent of the labor force in 1940, 21.3 percent in 1950, 17.9 percent in 1960, and 24.5 percent in 1970 (24). Despite this recent rise in the rate of unionization, most wage workers lack even the minimal defense provided by a union and therefore have serious problems securing the recognition of their most basic legal rights. Generally, it can be stated that Mexican labor legislation has some rather progressive characteristics that essentially are used to legitimize the government as the representative of the Mexican Revolution. Nevertheless, the Mexican law enforcement system is arbitrary, to say the least.

The relatively effective control to which the working class is subjected obviously explains why it has been possible to maintain the high rate of exploitation already mentioned; it also influences the conditions of the work process.

WORK AND DISEASE

Following the approach outlined above, we will study the effects of work on health in terms which go beyond what is legally recognized as an occupationally related disease. We will first study the trends of development of the causes of death of the population of working-age men from 15 to 65 years of age, and then the causes of death in the general population as compared to particular groups of the urban proletariat. Once we have observed the existing trends, we will proceed to study the problem of work accidents and legally recognized occupational disease, and report some of the few studies that have been carried out in specific workplaces.

Causes of Death among Men of Working Age

Tables 7, 8, and 9 show the 10 principal causes of death of men aged 15 to 24, 25 to 44, and 45 to 64 years, respectively, in 1955, 1965, 1970, and 1974. As can be observed, there have not been major qualitative changes in the causes of death during the 20 years represented, but there are important increases in some kinds of disease and decreases in others. For example, rates of mortality from infectious diseases such as malaria, tuberculosis, diarrhea, and pneumonia, and nutritionally related diseases such as anemia have declined or disappeared as principal causes of death. These are pathologies which can be identified as the result of an overwork-underconsumption situation linked with the extraction of absolute surplus value and work forms in peasant agriculture. This decline, coupled with the persistence of such pathology at a lower rate, is totally consistent with the economic data presented above. The data evidence a rapid process of development of the productive forces, absorbing a considerable sector of the population into a work situation of high productivity and intensity while leaving another part laboring in activities related to the advanced sector but with a much lower level of productivity.

Table 7

Ten principal causes of death for Mexican men aged 15-24 years, 1955, 1965, 1970, and 1974[a]

Cause of Death	1955 Rate (per 100,000)	1955 Rank	1965 Rate (per 100,000)	1965 Rank	1970 Rate (per 100,000)	1970 Rank	1974 Rate (per 100,000)	1974 Rank
Homicide, suicide	87.1	1	47.6	2	46.8	2	57.6	2
Accidents	67.0	2	67.8	1	88.4	1	90.3	1
Malaria	23.3	3	–[b]	–	–	–	–	–
Influenza, pneumonia	22.7	4	14.2	3	16.1	3	9.2	4
Tuberculosis	19.9	5	13.4	4	12.7	4	7.6	5
Gastritis, enteritis, colitis	17.7	6	3.9	9	12.5	5	6.1	6
Heart disease	17.0	7	6.9	6	9.3	6	11.9	3
Arteriosclerotic	(0.1)	–	(1.6)	–	(1.9)	–	(3.3)	–
Other	(16.9)	–	(5.3)	–	(7.4)	–	(8.6)	–
Typhoid fever	8.1	8	–	–	3.4	10	–	–
Blood vessel disease	4.5	9	–	–	–	–	–	–
Malignant tumors	3.3	10	5.4	8	5.9	8	5.6	7
Psychoneurosis and personality disorders	–	–	9.5	5	–	–	–	–
Anemias, avitaminosis	–	–	6.1	7	6.0	7	3.1	9
Vascular lesion CNS	–	–	3.0	10	–	–	–	–
Cerebrovascular disease	–	–	–	–	3.5	9	3.4	8
Cirrhosis of the liver	–	–	–	–	–	–	1.8	10
All other	92.7	–	69.1	–	60.4	–	71.3	–
Total	363.3		246.9		265.0		267.9	

[a] Source, World Health Statistics, World Health Organization, Geneva.
[b] Dashes indicate category was not among the 10 leading causes of death in that year.

Table 8

Ten principal causes of death for Mexican men aged 25-44 years, 1955, 1965, 1970, and 1974[a]

	1955		1965		1970		1974	
Cause of Death	Rate (per 100,000)	Rank	Rate (per 100,000)	Rank	Rate (per 100,000)	Rank	Rate (per 100,000)	Rank
Homicide, suicide	147.2	1	92.2	2	183.2	1	102.4	2
Accidents	83.7	2	100.8	1	122.4	2	111.4	1
Tuberculosis	62.5	3	38.1	3	34.3	4	22.9	4
Influenza, pneumonia	42.7	4	33.7	5	27.9	6	20.5	5
Heart disease	41.6	5	16.7	8	31.9	5	31.2	6
Arteriosclerotic	(3.4)	–	(8.8)	–	(10.5)	–	(9.1)	–
Other	(38.2)	–	(7.9)	–	(21.4)	–	(22.1)	–
Malaria	40.3	6	–	–	–	–	–	–
Gastritis, enteritis, colitis	29.7	7	–	–	20.1	7	13.3	7
Cirrhosis of the liver	27.2	8	34.8	4	48.3	3	40.4	3
Malignant tumors	10.2	9	13.9	10	13.1	9	12.7	8
Typhoid, paratyphoid fever	7.3	10	–	–	–	–	–	–
Anemias, avitaminosis	–[b]	–	22.2	6	–	–	9.0	–
Vascular lesion CNS	–	–	17.3	7	11.2	10	–	10
Psychoneurosis and personality disorders	–	–	13.9	9	15.2	8	–	–
Cerebrovascular disease	–	–	–	–	–	–	9.8	9
All other	172.4		164.5		54.1		151.6	
Total	664.8		548.1		561.7		525.2	

[a] Source, World Health Statistics, World Health Organization, Geneva.
[b] Dashes indicate category was not among the 10 leading causes of death in that year.

225

Table 9

Ten principal causes of death for Mexican men aged 45-64 years, 1955, 1965, 1970, and 1974[a]

Cause of Death	1955 Rate (per 100,000)	1955 Rank	1965 Rate (per 100,000)	1965 Rank	1970 Rate (per 100,000)	1970 Rank	1974 Rate (per 100,000)	1974 Rank
Heart disease	197.6	1	115.6	3	201.8	1	192.1	1
Arteriosclerotic	(31.4)	–	(77.4)	–	(88.4)	–	(95.9)	–
Other	(166.2)	–	(38.2)	–	(113.4)	–	(96.2)	–
Influenza, pneumonia	155.6	2	118.6	2	141.0	3	74.2	6
Senility	146.1	3	–b	–	–	–	–	–
Cirrhosis of the liver	112.3	4	122.7	1	154.0	2	134.1	2
Accidents	101.4	5	111.7	4	136.0	4	121.4	3
Homicide, suicide	101.1	6	64.0	8	59.2	8	80.9	5
Tuberculosis	99.5	7	79.4	6	71.8	6	54.7	8
Gastritis, enteritis, colitis	97.3	8	–	–	–	–	41.4	10
Malaria	87.9	9	–	–	–	–	–	–
Malignant tumors	70.4	10	102.0	5	105.9	5	95.8	4
Vascular lesion CNS	–	–	64.5	7	–	–	–	–
Diabetes	–	–	37.7	9	–	–	48.6	9
Psychoneurosis and personality disorders	–	–	32.6	10	–	–	–	–
Cerebrovascular disease	–	–	–	–	68.9	7	62.0	7
Bronchitis, emphysema, asthma	–	–	–	–	24.8	9	–	–
Ulcer	–	–	–	–	23.9	10	–	–
All others	477.2		645.0		574.4		432.8	
Total	1,646.4		1,493.8		1,561.7		1,338.0	

[a]Source, World Health Statistics, World Health Organization, Geneva.
[b]Dashes indicate category was not among the 10 leading causes of death in that year.

226

The causes of death that show a trend of increase are accidents, certain kinds of heart disease, cirrhosis of the liver, and malignant tumors. Between 1955 and 1974, the accident death rate rose from 67.0 to 90.3 per 100,000 for men aged 15 to 24, from 83.7 to 111.4 per 100,000 for men aged 25 to 44, and from 101.4 to 121.4 per 100,000 for those aged 45 to 64. It is easy to understand how the accident death rate increase is linked to work and the necessity of living in urban areas.

The arteriosclerotic heart disease rate also rose in all age groups between 1955 and 1974, although the trend was most marked for males between 45 and 65 years of age. For this group, the death rate per 100,000 jumped from 31.4 to 95.9. The well-known relationship between this kind of heart disease and generalized stress and stress caused by a high productivity/high intensity work process turns it into the clearest expression of the pathological results of the transformation of the work process in capitalist terms (4). The rates of malignant tumors in all the studied age groups increased between 1955 and 1965, most significantly so in the 45-64 age group. The clearer trend in the older age group has to do with the character of the disease, since it usually requires decades to develop. Nonetheless, it is very probable that the increase in malignant tumors is directly linked to the use of more and more hazardous substances in the work process.

The increase in the rates of cirrhosis of the liver that can be observed in all the age groups can be taken as an indicator of alcoholism and nutritional deficiencies. Alcohol abuse could not be said to be exclusively linked to stressful work situations, but there are some important differences between the pattern of drinking in urban and rural settings. For example, the kind of alcohol consumed is different, as is the manner of consuming it.

The changes over time that have occurred in health conditions as reflected in the principal causes of death verify the association between the work process and the different ways by which it wears out the worker, giving origin to different kinds of predominant pathology. Another indication of this causal relationship would be the comparison between groups involved in work processes representative of the predominant extraction of absolute and relative surplus value and different degrees of development of the productive forces.

Unfortunately, there do not exist mortality data which identify the relationship of workers to the work process, but one can approach the problem by comparing the population that belongs to the Mexican Institute of Social Security (IMSS) with the general population. Although legally speaking all wage laborers should be members of the IMSS, 75 percent of members work in big or medium-sized enterprises, meaning that it is essentially the urban working class that belongs to this institution (25). Tables 10 and 11 present the principal causes of death and their relative importance in the total mortality for both populations. It was not possible to compute rates since the population in each age group is unknown. Nevertheless, it could be inferred that the rates of mortality are much lower among the insured, since they do not account for more than 2.5-5.8 percent of the total deaths while, as a group, they represent around 27 percent of the total population (25). The first fact to consider is that diseases like diarrhea, pneumonia, and anemia do not appear among the 10 principal causes in the insured population but do in the general population.

In the insured 15 to 44 age group, the four principal causes of death are malignant

Table 10

Ten principal causes of death in the overall Mexican population aged 15-44 and in the population covered by Social Security

Cause of Death	Population with Social Security (1976)[a]		General Population (1974)[b]	
	Number	Percent	Number	Percent
Malignant tumors	412	18.4	3,162	3.4
Heart, hypertensive disease	249	11.1	5,227	5.6
Accidents, homicides/suicides	223	10.0	22,978	24.5
Cirrhosis of the liver	169	7.5	3,088	3.3
Maternal causes	154	6.9	2,757	2.9
Tuberculosis	140	6.3	3,266	3.5
Diabetes mellitus	90	4.0	—[c]	—
Pneumonia	77	3.4	3,252	3.5
Cerebrovascular disease	77	3.4	1,701	1.8
Nephritis, nephrosis	70	3.2	—	—
Enteritis, diarrheal disease	—	—	2,529	2.7
Anemias	—	—	1,249	1.3
All others	577	25.8	44,710	47.5
Total	2,238	100.0	93,919	100.0

[a] Source, Subdirección Gral Médica, Instituto Mexicano de Seguro Social, Mexico.
[b] Source, Dirección Gral de Estadística, SIC, Mexico.
[c] Dashes indicate category was not among the 10 leading causes of death for that population.

tumors, heart disease, accidents, and cirrhosis of the liver. With the exception of accidents, each represents a greater proportion of total mortality among the insured than among the general population. Diabetes appears among the principal causes of death in the insured group but not in the general population, a fact that should be related to the increase of this disease and prolonged stress.

In the insured 45 to 64 age group, the four principal causes of death are malignant tumors, diabetes, cirrhosis of the liver, and heart and hypertensive diseases—all of which are related to the advanced capitalist work process. With the exception of heart disease, each shows a greater percentage than in the general population. The greater weight of heart disease in the general population probably could be explained by the fact that there is no distinction between arteriosclerotic heart disease and other types. As Table 9 shows, the relative weight of other heart disease is important in this age group, at least among men.

Legally Recognized Occupational Risks

The preceding discussion shows that it is inadequate to consider as work-related disease just accidents and occupational diseases. It can be argued that behind the traditional and limited definition of work-related disease can be found a class-bound

Table 11

Ten principal causes of death in the overall Mexican population aged 45-64 and in the population covered by Social Security

Cause of Death	Population with Social Security (1976)[a]		General Population (1974)[b]	
	Number	Percent	Number	Percent
Malignant tumors	935	24.3	7,211	11.0
Diabetes mellitus	532	13.9	3,128	4.8
Cirrhosis of the liver	472	12.3	6,748	10.3
Heart, hypertensive disease	443	11.5	9,765	14.8
Cerebrovascular disease	249	6.5	3,517	5.3
Tuberculosis	181	4.7	2,185	3.3
Bronchitis, emphysema, asthma	102	2.7	773	1.1
Accidents, homicides/suicides	65	1.7	5,781	8.8
Nephritis, nephrosis	50	1.3	_c	—
Colelitiasis, colecystitis	24	0.6	—	—
Influenza, pneumonia	—	—	3,623	5.5
Enteritis, diarrheal disease	—	—	2,252	3.4
All others	789	20.5	20,834	31.7
Total	3,842	100.0	65,817	100.0

[a] Source, Subdirección Gral Médica, Instituto Mexicano de Seguro Social, Mexico.
[b] Source, Dirección Gral de Estadística, SIC, Mexico.
[c] Dashes indicate category was not among the 10 leading causes of death for that population.

conceptualization of disease and a particular situation of class struggle. If disease is conceptualized as a biological and individually occurring phenomenon, the only work-related diseases would be those that could be traced directly to biological, physical, and chemical agents involved in the technical work process. Once this point of view is accepted, the struggle between labor and capital, the results of which get their expression in labor legislation, is over whether or not a particular agent causes disease. To adopt a different point of view implies questioning not just the technical side of the work process but also its social determinants.

There are some very serious problems in assessing the true number of occupational diseases and accidents that occur in Mexico, precisely because a significant sector of the working class cannot count on labor unions to impose even the most minimal respect for the existing laws. The only relatively correct estimates are from the Mexican Institute of Social Security, which, as we have seen before, includes only a minority of workers. All the data that we will analyze, then, refer to workers in medium-sized and large enterprises.

The development of work accidents and their results in terms of disability and death can be observed in Table 12. The first relevant fact is the big increase that has occurred in absolute terms. The number of accidents and cases of disability increased

Table 12

Work-related accidents, disability, and deaths, Mexico, 1960-1976[a]

	Accidents		Disability			Deaths		
Year	Number	Rate (per 1,000 workers)	Number	Rate (per 100,000 workers)	Rate (per 1,000 accidents)	Number	Rate (per 100,000 workers)	Rate (per 1,000 accidents)
1960	100,762	79.0	2,148	168.4	21.3	138	10.8	1.4
1970	245,723	89.1	4,381	158.8	17.8	471	17.1	1.9
1975	361,154	98.9	7,785	213.0	21.5	936	25.6	2.6
1976	401,303	107.8	8,940	241.1	22.3	1,077	28.9	2.7

[a] Source, Jefatura de Medicina del Trabajo, Servicios de Análisis e Información Estadística, Instituto Mexicano de Seguro Social.

fourfold between 1960 and 1976; deaths increased more than sevenfold. In relative terms there also was a considerable increase: the accident rate went up from 79.0 to 107.8 per 1,000 workers, the disability rate from 168.4 to 241.1 per 100,000 workers, and the death rate from 10.8 to 28.9 per 100,000 workers. The indices of frequency and seriousness also increased between 1972 and 1976, from 43.9 to 49.6 and 0.899 to 1.296, respectively.

These data speak volumes about the costs that workers are paying in terms of health and life for the innovation in the work process that is dictated by the social determinants of capitalist production: profit and capital accumulation.

From the data on occupational disease (Table 13), it becomes clear that serious underregistration must exist. The Federal Labor Law registers 161 diseases as occupa-

Table 13

Registered occupational diseases, disability, and deaths, Mexico, 1960-1976[a]

	Occupational Diseases		Disability			Deaths		
Year	Number	Rate (per 100,000 workers)	Number	Rate (per 100,000 workers)	Rate (per 1,000 accidents)	Number	Rate (per 100,000 workers)	Rate (per 1,000 accidents)
1960	240	18.1	48	3.8	200.0	8	0.6	33.3
1970	620	22.4	141	5.1	227.4	8	0.3	12.9
1975	1,010	27.6	623	17.0	616.8	18	0.5	17.8
1976	1,781	47.8	1,241	33.3	696.8	24	0.6	13.5
Percent Increase 1960-1976	642	164	2,485	776	248	200	0	−59

[a] Source, Jefatura de Medicina del Trabajo, Servicios de Análisis e Información Estadística, Instituto Mexicano de Seguro Social.

tional (26). It seems improbable, for example, that only 1,781 workers would have suffered serious hearing loss; or that 44,000 miners, 70,000 smelter workers, and 12,000 pottery workers would not have suffered more than 24 cases of mortal silicosis.

Despite the poor quality of the data, one can assume that the increase that occurred from 1960 to 1976 reflects real trends, because there was a considerably higher disability rate in 1976 than in 1960 (696.8 compared with 200.0), despite the existence of even stricter legal criteria for recognition of occupational disease in 1976. This means that the increase in the rate of occupational disease from 18.1 to 47.8 per 100,000 workers is an effect not of better registration but of worsening working conditions that are also reflected in the increase in the disability rate. This increase of occupational disease reflects the use of dangerous substances in the labor process.

Finally, Table 14 presents work risks, i.e. accidents and occupational disease, suffered according to income. In studying the table, it should be considered that lower incomes could correspond to smaller industries and, more importantly, to lower-level jobs among workers. As can be seen, the probability of suffering some work injury is almost 20 times as high among workers who receive less than the legal minimum wage than among the highest income group. This reflects real working conditions, in the sense that the less-qualified workers are exposed to more risks and also that they have less ability to impose safety measures.

The Health of Workers in Electrical Power Plants, Mining, and Agriculture

There are few studies published in Mexico concerning work conditions, even in the most restricted sense of the term. The investigations which are undoubtedly carried out by the Institute of Social Security and the work inspectors are not made known publicly. Despite these limitations, there are three studies of relevance to the topic under consideration: one done by electrical workers in order to change their collective bargaining position, another conducted among coal miners, and, finally, a study on poisoning of agricultural workers.

Table 14

Work risks[a] by income level, Mexico, 1976[b]

Income Level (in pesos)	Number	Rate (per 1,000 Workers)
Up to 80	197,579	287.6
81-100[c]	107,339	118.2
101-170	104,936	82.3
171-280	24,720	46.3
281 and over	5,353	15.2
Total	439,927	117.1

[a]Includes accidents and occupational disease.
[b]Source, Jefatura de Medicina del Trabajo, Servicios de Análisis e Información Estadística, Instituto Mexicano de Seguro Social.
[c]Represents legal minimum wage.

The study of the health conditions of high-voltage electrical workers (27) has two special aspects. On the one hand, it is a specific study planned by the trade union and partially carried out by the workers themselves with the technical assistance of physcans; on the other hand, it explores widely the general effects of work on health.

One group of workers was exposed to high-voltage electricity, and another group from the same company was not. It was found that the risk of accidents was 17.8 percent in the exposed group and 2.8 percent among the controls. The most impressive results of the study, however, are those presumably related to stress. Workers exposed to high-voltage cables showed significant increases in blood pressure, both systolic and diastolic, and increases in the excretion of catecholamines, a substance which characteristically appears in the urine of people under stress. Clinical examination further showed that the exposed group suffered a much higher prevalence of all stress-related diseases than the control group, e.g. 4 times more hypertension, 6 times more arteriosclerotic heart disease, 11 times more peptic ulcer, 4 times more diabetes, and 5 times more sleep disturbance. It was finally shown that 28.2 percent of the personnel exposed to high-voltage electricity had died within 10 years after retiring, while this statistic was 6.4 percent among nonexposed workers.

The working conditions in the old coal mines seem to belong to the last century. In a study of coal miners, Córdova (28) described how the miners work with a pick 10 to 12 hours a day to bring out a minimum of 5,400 kilos of coal. In addition to the extreme physical exhaustion, the miners work with the constant threat of gas explosions. Continuous mining machines are used in the newer underground mines, and the coal is constantly falling down close to the miners, who are protected only by a steel plate. In addition to the miners, there are engineers laboring in the mines supervising the machines. One of the things that was observed is that although there were more possibilities of accidents in the old mines, miners in the modern mines suffer higher accident rates. Examination of the issue revealed that there exists less direct control over the labor process by the workers in the new, mechanized mines. This means that danger signals and warnings that could be interpreted and acted on in the old mines are harder to perceive in the new mines because of the increased noise and speed of production.

The indices of accidents in the coal mines reflect the bad conditions of work in both the old and new mines. The accident frequency rate at the big mines of Fundidora Monterrey and Industria Minera Mexico in the late 1960s and early 1970s was at least five times the 1970 rate for United States coal miners (28, 29).

Agricultural workers are one of the least-organized groups of the Mexican working class, and trade unions in the countryside have been very persecuted by the state and federal governments, if not prohibited outright. This virtual absence of defense organizations is reflected in the high rates of accidents and poisonings that have been reported in this sector. During the agricultural year of 1974 in the Laguna region, one of the most developed in Mexico, there were a reported 847 cases of insecticide poisoning, corresponding to a rate of 121.1 per 100,000 inhabitants of the region, or to a rate of 1.4 per 100 men in productive ages active in agriculture. Almost none of the victims belonged to the Institute of Social Security, highlighting their totally unprotected situation (30).

HEALTH AND SAFETY LEGISLATION

The basic legislation regarding industrial hygiene, security, and worker's compensation forms part of the Federal Labor Law (26, pp. 141-216). This legislation has its own regulations in which the safety and hygiene standards and their means of enforcement are specified. Those regulations that are legally in force at the time of writing were adopted in 1934 and 1946, and are totally outdated. At present, a new law is being prepared which will be rather advanced, but it is still predictable that the new legislation will not change to any considerable extent the working conditions in Mexican industry.

The laws in any society express the domination of one social class over the other classes. It is also true that part of the function of legislation is to create an illusion of protection for the citizens, while, in reality, law enforcement is very restricted. All evidence suggests that this is the case with the legislation regarding industrial hygiene and safety in Mexico, and that the new legislation, regardless of its progressive wording, will have very little real impact at the point of production. The only way to make the law work is for organized workers to educate themselves about the problems and demand its enforcement.

The Federal Labor Law stipulates the existence of two basic structures to guarantee compliance with the law and its enforcement: the Mixed Committees of Hygiene and Safety, and the Labor Inspectorate (26, p. 152).

The Mixed Committees are supposed to exist in all workplaces and be composed of an equal number of representatives of the workers and the boss. Their basic function is to investigate accidents, inspect the work area, and promote preventive measures (31). If their recommendations are not executed, they can call in the Labor Inspection authorities. Apart from this local organization, a National Consultative Commission of Labor Safety and Hygiene was formed in May 1978 with representatives of the State, trade unions, and bosses (32).

Whatever objections one may have to the dual structure of the Mixed Committees, given the advantages of management in such a situation, this is not their main weakness at the moment. The problem is that these local committees simply do not exist. One part of Mexican industry is under federal jurisdiction and the other under state and local jurisdiction. In terms of labor legislation, this means that in the first case the federal Ministry of Labor enforces the laws, and in the second, the local state authorities. Until April 1978, there were about 18,000 workplaces under federal jurisdiction. By 1972, there existed approximately 3,000 Mixed Committees in these industries (33), and in 1977, the Ministry of Labor announced a campaign to register 1,000 new Mixed Committees a year (31, p. 4). Even if this goal is achieved, all 18,000 workplaces would not have the basic structure of safety and hygiene until 1988. To further complicate the issue, in January 1978 the supervision and enforcement of labor legislation concerning safety and hygiene was federalized for all industry. This means that the Ministry of Labor will now have to supervise and promote the formation of Mixed Committees in 120,000 workplaces rather than 18,000. It should be noted that the change in legislation was not accompanied by any substantial increase in the budget.

The second basic structure of supervision and enforcement of labor legislation, and the only one with enforcement powers, is the Labor Inspectorate that forms part of the Ministry of Labor. The labor inspectors are supposed to supervise compliance with the whole gamut of labor legislation—wages, hours of work, child labor, and so forth—and not just the part concerned with occupational hazards. To carry out this supervision in the 18,000 industries under federal jurisdiction in 1977, there were 170 inspectors in the entire country, 60 of whom worked out of the federal district. These inspectors carried out 12,830 inspections in 1977, 4,000 of which were in new industries. This suggests that the rest of the factories would be inspected on an average of only once every 14 years.

In addition to the infrequency of inspections, there is obviously a problem of their quality, which is related to the scarce resources and lack of professional training and experience of the inspectors. To carry out all its activities, the Ministry of Labor disposed of 0.11 percent of the federal budget in 1977, or 679 million pesos (U.S. $30 million) (34). Moreover, it is likely that this activity does not escape the corruption that exists at all levels of Mexican society. One more problem that obstructs the functioning of the Labor Inspectorate is the very irregular reporting of accidents. According to the law, all work accidents should be reported to the Ministry of Labor, but in reality, it is estimated that this happens only in about 30 percent of cases. There should be more coordination in this matter between the Ministry of Labor and the Institute of Social Security, which has a great deal of information about work accidents since it manages part of the compensation system.

Finally, it should be kept in mind that the situation in industry under local jurisdiction is much worse, and the federalization of all aspects of occupational safety and hygiene will have very little practical significance in most cases. Seen in this context, it is quite clear why the new legislation will probably be ignored for the most part.

Federal Labor Law establishes (26, pp. 143-150) that workers who suffer an occupationally related disease should get free medical and surgical assistance, rehabilitation, artificial limbs where necessary, and monetary compensation. It is the employer who is supposed to pay these costs, unless it is proven that the worker was drunk, drugged, intentionally caused the accident, tried to commit suicide, or was fighting. Compliance with the law is supervised by the labor courts, which also resolve cases of conflict.

The Social Security Law requires that the Institute of Social Security assume the responsibility of the boss toward the insured population. Similar job-accident insurance schemes exist in the smaller social security institutes for state employees, electrical power plant workers, railroad workers, and the subscribers to the Mexican Institute for Social Security, who comprise about one-third of the population and between 50 to 85 percent of the industrial working class, depending on the kind of industry (25, pp. 86-87). The employer pays an insurance premium according to a system of classification of risks.

Apart from paying the costs of medical care, the Institute of Social Security pays compensation for deaths and disability. In the case of total disability, the worker receives a pension corresponding to 60-80 percent of his normal wage. For a work-related death, the widow receives one month's salary and a pension of 36 percent of total disability, plus an additional 20 percent of total disability for each child (35).

For insured workers, there does not seem to be a big problem in getting the compensation due in cases of severe accidents. The problem arises when they try to get compensation for occupational diseases, which, as we have seen, are very rarely recognized in Mexico. It is also probable that the workers who do not belong to any social security system and thus have to fight their case in the labor courts seldom get the compensation which is their legal right. For all workers, it is not only rare but also next to impossible to get compensation for diseases that are intimately linked to the conditions of work as a whole, since such diseases cannot be traced to a particular causal agent.

OCCUPATIONAL HEALTH AND THE DEMANDS OF WORKERS

It is clear that advances in occupational health are directly linked to the capacity of the working class for struggle. The character of Mexican trade unions, mostly controlled from the top, has impeded to a large extent the development of struggles for better working conditions. An exception to this rule might be some of the large trade unions in the public sector, e.g. power plants and petroleum workers, which usually negotiate some improvements under pressure from the rank-and-file in order to strengthen their political control.

The extent to which the corrupt, State-controlled trade-union leadership puts a brake on demands for better working conditions can be demonstrated by the fact that almost all trade unions with a democratic internal structure have begun to make concrete demands in this area. Such has been the case for power plant, telephone, subway, and cement workers, and for dozens of other trade unions. There are two problems related to this almost spontaneous upsurge of such demands. The first is related to their priority, as such demands are usually considered less important than demands for higher wages and for guarantees of respect to the democratic union leadership. This of course means that in a negotiating situation, working-condition demands are usually sacrificed early in the bargaining.

The second problem is intimately linked to the conceptualization of work risks and their prevention. The most common demand that trade unions put up in this regard is for monetary compensation for dangerous working conditions, not for the elimination of the risk itself. This can be explained by the miserable wage level which leads workers to seek an increase at any cost. But, on another level, it reflects an ideological problem, because it shows that the worker thinks of himself as capitalism thinks of him—as labor power that has a cost, not as a human being that has a life.

A different consciousness probably cannot result from just the creation of a wider knowledge about the technical dangers of the labor process; such education only creates an understanding of the external relation between things. Analyzing the problems of health from the point of view of the work process as a social and technical whole creates the possibility of an understanding of the true meaning of exploitation and the ways in which it wears out the worker.

REFERENCES

1. Kaplan, J. *Medicina del Trabajo*, p. 337. Editorial El Ateneo, Buenos Aires, 1976.
2. Turshen, M. Worker safety and health. *HMO Packet* 3-II, 1976; Elling, R. Industrialization and occupational health in underdeveloped countries. *Int. J. Health Serv.* 7(2): 209-235, 1977.

3. Antonovsky, A. Social class, life expectancy and overall mortality. *Milbank Mem. Fund Q.* (45)1: 37-75, 1967.
4. Eyer, J., and Sterling, P. Stress-related mortality and social organization. *Review of Radical Political Economics* (9)1: 1-44, 1977.
5. Stark, E. The cutting edge in occupational health. *HMO Packet* 3-II, 1976.
6. Fassler, C. Salud y trabajo. *Salud Problema* (1)2: 1978.
7. Marx, K. *El Capital,* Tomo I, p. 215, Siglo XXI. Mexico, 1975.
8. Marx, K. *Introducción a la Crítica de la Economia Política,* p. 241. Fondo de Cultura Popular, Mexico, 1970.
9. Echeverría, B. Discurso de la revolución, discurso crítico. *Cuadernos Políticos* 10: 47, 1976.
10. Córdova, A. La dimensión humana del accidente de trabajo. *El Gallo Ilustrado* (El Día) 814: 4-5, 1978.
11. Braverman, H. *Trabajo y Capital Monopolista,* pp. 14-58. El Nuestro Tiempo, Mexico, 1975.
12. Gross, D. R., and Underwood, B. A. Technological change and caloric cost: Sisal agriculture in northeastern Brazil. *American Anthropologist* (73)3: 725-736, 1971.
13. Solis, L. *La Realidad Económica Mexican,* pp. 91-92, Siglo XXI. Mexico, 1973.
14. Alvarez, A., and Sandoval, E. Desarrollo industrial y clase obrera en México. *Cuadernos Políticos* 4: 9, 1975.
15. Gonzalez Salazar, G. *Subocupación y Estructura de Clases en México,* p. 82. UNAM, Mexico, 1972.
16. Castell, J., and Rello, F. Las desventuras de un proyecto agrario. *Investigación Económica* (36)3: 134, 1977.
17. *Punto Crítico* (6)69: 4-9, 1977.
18. Cordero, S. *Concentración Industrial y Poder en México,* pp. 17-18. CES, El Colegio de México, Mexico, 1977.
19. Carbajal, A., and Cuellar, R. *La Estructura del Proletariado Industrial en México 1940-1970.* Ph.D. dissertation, Facultad de Económia, UNAM, Mexico, 1977.
20. Arriaga, M., Velasco, E., and Zepeda, E. Inflación y salarios en el régimen de LEA. *Investigación Económica* (36)3: 227, 1977.
21. *Punto Crítico* (6)81: 10, 1977.
22. Trejo, R. *Reseña del Movimiento Obrero,* p. 11. Facultad de Ciencias Políticas y Sociales, UNAM, Mexico, 1974.
23. Leal, J. F., and Woldenberg, J. El sindicalismo mexicano. *Cuardernos Políticos* 7: 43, 1976.
24. *Anuario Estadístico Compendiado de los EUM, Censos Gral de Población 1940-70.* SIC, Mexico.
25. Instituto Méxicano de Seguro Social. *Memoria Estacística 1975.* Mexico, 1976.
26. *Ley Federal del Trabajo.* Mexico, 1971.
27. Jáuregui, A., Fernández Osrio, J., Rodríguez, C., Lloret, A., Muñiz, R., Tamez, S., and Rodríguez, M. *Estudio Fisiológico, Médico y Psiquiatrico en Trabajadores de la Cia de Luz y Fuerza del Centro Expuestos a Riesgos Electricos.* Sindicato Mexicano de Electricitsas, Mexico, 1978.
28. Córdova, A. El mundo humano del trabajo. *Condiciones del Trabajo* (1)2: 5-22, 1976.
29. *Punto Crítico* (5)48: 28, 1976.
30. *Punto Crítico* (5)50: 14, 1976.
31. *Programa para el Fortalecimiento de las Comisiones Mixtas de Seguridad y Higiene,* pp. 12-13. STPS, Mexico, 1977.
32. *Diario Oficial* (CCCXLVV) 42: 12, 1978.
33. Secretaría de Salubridad y Asistencia. *Memorias: Primer Simposio Nacional sobre Accidentes,* Tomo 1, p. 269. Mexico, 1972.
34. *Oposición* 170: 5, 1977.
35. Lazo Cerna, H. *Higiene y Seguridad Industrial,* pp. 443-459. Instituto Méxicano de Seguro Social, Mexico, 1961.

CHAPTER 13

Mortality and Working Conditions in Agriculture in Underdeveloped Countries

Asa Cristina Laurell

Around 1.5 billion men, women, and children live in the rural areas of Asia, Africa, and Latin America. Approximately 400 million are men aged 15 years or over. Since industry is not located in these areas, and commerce and services—while of great importance from an economic and social point of view—do not occupy a significant portion of the rural population, the vast majority of them are agricultural workers. In addition, millions of women and children participate regularly in agricultural production, giving us some idea of the numerical importance of those involved in agricultural work and exposed to the wide range of risks and indirect effects of the work conditions characterizing this sector.

Contrary to what is generally believed, the work and lives of agricultural workers and their families cannot be explained or analyzed in terms of simple backwardness, but rather should be seen within the context of the contradictions that the process of transformation occurring in these parts of the world is generating. Generally, the rural population has to confront this process of change in very difficult conditions for economic, political, and social reasons. Unorganized, poor, and with little knowledge useful to the manipulation of externally imposed conditions, the rural workers—wage laborers and peasants—pay a high price for "modernization."

This paper was presented at a seminar on Biological and Social Aspects of Mortality and the Length of Life organized by the International Union for the Scientific Study of Population and held in Fiuggi Terme, Italy, May 13-16, 1980.

Despite the large numbers involved in agricultural work and their unfavorable insertion in the process of change, there exists virtually no information concerning the general working conditions of this group nor basic morbidity and mortality data. It does not seem an exaggeration to state that, outside a fairly empirical knowledge held by those involved in practical health work with this population, there is little systematic scientific work being done on the problems of agricultural workers in underdeveloped countries.[1]

An important obstacle to a more specific knowledge concerning this sector is the poor quality of demographic data, which are incomplete for most countries of Africa, Asia, and Latin America, with the exception of those like Cuba that have a health service covering the whole population.[2] Furthermore, given the acute shortage of medical personnel and rudimentary systems of registration of vital statistics, data from the rural areas of these countries are even less reliable. Besides these problems, information regarding occupation is inexact or altogether lacking in the death certificates. This means that the possibilities for implementing studies using secondary data are very restricted. Most research, then, has to be done through direct studies, with all that this implies in terms of time and money.

Given these restrictions, the present paper necessarily will suffer from some serious shortcomings with respect to the empirical demonstration that should properly support some of the hypotheses presented. The method that will be used is to try to describe and specify the general characteristics of the distinct types of basic processes taking place today in the rural areas of the underdeveloped countries, analyzing them in relation to their possible impact on health conditions. In so doing, we will draw on different kinds of empirical evidence, combining clinical, epidemiological, statistical, sociological, and economic knowledge. The result will be what in painting is known as a collage, and even though it might not supply any final evidence, it seems to be a valid method for the formation of hypotheses and the definition of areas for further research.

URBAN-RURAL MORTALITY DIFFERENCES

There is quite a body of historical evidence showing that the process of industrialization in Europe was associated with clear urban-rural mortality differences (1). The urban centers, especially the industrial ones, exhibited higher mortality rates than the rural areas, particularly in the lower age groups. This was the case, for example, in England during the 1830s when the ratio of urban-rural mortality ranged from 1.65 to 1.55. The same situation was still observed about 1900 in that country, with a crude mortality rate for the cities of 24.2 per 1000 and for the rural areas of 19.5;

---

[1] This situation was confirmed by the fact that use of the N.L.M.'s National Interactive Retrieval Service for a bibliographic search using the key words "agricultural workers" and "rural health in underdeveloped countries" produced a very restricted number of articles for the last 15 years on rural-urban mortality differences and not a single paper concerned with mortality of agricultural workers in underdeveloped countries.

[2] For more information on the reliability of the demographic data of each country, consult the WHO publication *World Health Statistics Annual*.

the corresponding data for Prussia were 30.4 and 28.0, and for Italy, 32.7 and 28.7 per 1000 (2, pp. 20-21).

During the 20th century, however, the decline in mortality that took place in the industrialized countries was more rapid in the urban than the rural areas. This created a tendency toward the disappearance of the clear urban-rural difference in overall mortality. In fact, today mortality is consistently higher only for men in urban areas of industrialized countries (1, pp. 249-283).

Contrary to what has historically been the dominant pattern of urban-rural mortality differentials, data from most countries of Africa, Asia, and Latin America show a higher mortality in the rural than urban areas, and in many cases there is even a clear trend for mortality to decline with increasing urbanization (3). These two characteristics can be seen in the data presented by Seklani (4) in his study on mortality in the Arab countries (Table 1).

The same trend is shown with more detail by Vallin (5) for Algeria, where the crude mortality rate was 9.0 per 1000 in the capital, 14.1 in other towns, 16.6 in villages, and 19.8 in rural areas. Analyzing mortality by age group, however, he found that the association with urbanization decreased with age. A similar situation is reported by Gaisie (6) in his work on tropical Africa, as he found that studies on urban-rural mortality in Ethiopia, Ghana, Sierra Leone, Kenya, and Sudan all show higher death rates for rural areas than for the cities. It was further demonstrated that in Sudan, as in Algeria, there is a negative relationship between mortality and the size of the urban center. The above observations are also verified by Cantrelle (7) for Senegal, where general mortality is three times higher in the countryside than in the capital, Dakar. The Turkish Demographic Survey (8) reaches similar conclusions, registering crude death rates in the urban areas of 10 to 13 per 1000 and in the rural zones from 15 to 21 per 1000.

The situation in Latin America is not quite as clear-cut as in Africa and Asia, since it seems possible to distinguish countries that show a higher rural mortality from

Table 1

Urban and rural mortality[a] in selected Arab countries, 1960-1970[b]

Country and year(s)	Overall Mortality Rate	Mortality Rate in Capital	Urban Mortality Rate	Rural Mortality Rate
Algeria (1960-1969)	16.5	9.0	11.7	18.6
Tunisia (1968)	14.6	7.5	—[c]	—
Egypt (1969-1970)	15.5	12.0	13.4	16.0
Lebanon (1970)	9.0	8.0	—[c]	—
Morocco (1962)	19.0	13.0	15.0	20.0
Syria (1970)	14.0	9.0	11.0	17.0

[a] Per 1000 population.
[b] Source, modified from reference 4.
[c] Data not available.

Table 2

Urban and rural mortality,[a] Honduras, 1971-1972[b]

Age Group	Urban Mortality	Rural Mortality	Ratio Rural-Urban Mortality
Under 1[c]	85.6	127.1	1.8
1 to 4	10.5	22.6	2.2
5 to 14	2.7	4.5	1.7
15 to 44	2.2	4.8	2.2
46 to 64	12.2	16.6	1.4
65 and more	39.6	58.2	1.5
Crude mortality rate	9.0	16.5	1.8

[a] Per 1000 population.
[b] Source, reference 9.
[c] Per 1000 live births.

others that exhibit essentially no rural-urban difference and at least one in which a higher urban mortality is observed.

Using data from the national demographic survey of Honduras, Behm (9) demonstrated a rural-urban mortality differential that holds for all age groups (Table 2). On the other hand, mortality data from Mexico (Table 3) do not clearly show the same trend, since there is hardly any difference between the urban and rural mortality and even one year in which urban mortality was higher than the rural one. (It should be taken into account that there is a known underregistration of mortality in Mexico that is as high as 15 percent for infant mortality (10). Nevertheless, even when

Table 3

Rural and urban mortality,[a] Mexico, 1950-1970[b]

Year	Overall Mortality Rate	Rural Mortality Rate	Urban Mortality Rate	Ratio Rural-Urban Mortality
1950	16.2	16.4	15.9	1.03
1955	15.3	11.6	16.5	0.70
1960	11.5	11.8	11.3	1.04
1965	9.5	9.5	9.5	1.00
1970	10.1	10.2	9.9	1.03

[a] Per 1000 population.
[b] Source, Annuario Estadístico de los Estados Unidos Mexicanos, Dirección General de Estadística, México.

an underregistration factor of about 10 percent in the rural areas compared to the urban centers is calculated in, the rural-urban differential does not get as high as in the rest of the countries we have considered.) A situation similar to the Mexican one was also found in Panama, where the rural-urban differential was even reversed in middle and old age, especially among men (3).

Finally, reliable data on Cuba show an inversion of the rural-urban mortality differential that holds over time, as can be seen in Table 4. The situation in Cuba is obviously quite dissimilar from that in the rest of the Latin American countries, because, among other things, health facilities are universally available (12) and the nutritional status of children good (13, p. 282).

The review of the urban-rural mortality differentials highlights two problems that seem to be important for the understanding of what determines the differences that are registered. First, it is necessary to explain the discrepancies between the industrialized and the underdeveloped countries both regarding their historical experience and their current situation. A second problem that should be explored is the possible transition that may be taking place in Latin America today and that is expressed in the non-uniform patterns of urban-rural mortality.

These two issues show that the urban-rural differentials of mortality cannot be analyzed just in terms of crowding-dispersion, poverty-wealth, and so on, but have to be understood in relation to the concrete historical processes taking place at a given moment and that combine specific socioeconomic, environmental, and medical elements. After a short presentation of the mortality suffered by agricultural workers,

Table 4

Ten principal causes of urban and rural mortality,[a] Cuba, 1973 and 1978[b]

Cause	1973		1978	
	Urban Mortality	Rural Mortality	Urban Mortality	Rural Mortality
Heart disease	151.2	99.1	168.1	124.2
Cancer	93.9	77.3	76.4	67.7
Cerebrovascular disease	60.4	40.6	46.0	40.7
Influenza and pneumonia	56.8	27.8	47.1	36.1
Disease of arteries, arterioles, capillaries	28.5	27.7	13.9	15.1
Accidents	19.1	20.0	25.6	20.8
Bronchitis, emphysema, asthma	14.7	8.7	7.5	5.9
Suicide	14.6	10.6	7.3	10.7
Diabetes mellitus	13.3	5.6	13.6	6.2
Hypertension	11.1	14.5	8.2	5.6

[a] Per 100,000 population.
[b] Source, reference 11.

we will outline some considerations concerning how to go about including these elements in the analysis.

SOME CHARACTERISTICS OF THE MORTALITY OF AGRICULTURAL WORKERS

As we have pointed out, information concerning the mortality of agricultural workers in the underdeveloped countries is extremely scarce; therefore, it will be necessary to rely on data that are not, strictly speaking, related to this group but do have some indicative value.

Vallin (5, p. 1044) compares the probability of dying by occupation and by age in Algeria, showing that the risk is almost twice as high for 10 to 35 year olds working in agriculture as for those occupied in industry, commerce, and services, a difference that goes down slightly between ages 36 and 60. Assuming that the rural population is essentially active in agriculture, the data on Honduras in Table 2 show a very similar pattern in the 15-44 and 45-64 age groups.

Analyzing the Cuban data (11), we find a different pattern, since the ratio of male rural-urban mortality between 15 and 34 years varies from 1.35 to 1.18, i.e. the rural population suffers from a higher mortality than the urban population. Nevertheless, from age 35 on, the ratio of rural-urban mortality goes from 0.94 to 0.59, showing a clear trend of rural mortality advantage with increasing age.

On the other hand, it is interesting to note that the higher mortality among men characteristic of the industrialized countries is not consistently present in the productive age groupings in the underdeveloped world. For example, the Algerian study (5, p. 1039) found an overmortality among women 15-35 years of age that changes into an overmortality among men aged 36 or above. A similar situation was observed in a study of the rural population of Punjab (14), where the male death rate in the 15-44 age group was 2.2 compared to the female rate of 5.8, a difference that persisted in the 45-64 age group with rates of 14.3 and 17.1 per 1000, respectively. This female overmortality was not only due to risks related to childbirth, but also to higher rates of infectious and neoplastic diseases.

As for the causes of death, the Punjab study reported a clear predominance of infectious disease that contributes 52 percent of the adult mortality, the single most important cause of death being tuberculosis, while heart disease and cancer together account for 20 percent. An even higher death rate from infectious disease was reported in another Indian study (15, p. 54). Although we do not have data relating specifically to agricultural workers, the general information on causes of death in Africa indicates a similar pattern, with a clear predominance of infectious causes ranging from diarrheal disease and pneumonia to diseases subject to specific prevention such as tuberculosis, smallpox, tetanus, yellow fever, and malaria (6, pp. 6-7). The epidemiological and clinical data reviewed by Hughes and Hunter (16) also confirm the extremely high prevalence of infectious and parasitic diseases among the African population (16).

The only systematic data on mortality among men 15 years of age and over living in rural areas that could be found for Latin America are the Cuban statistics (11). The principal causes of death for rural men between 15 and 49 years of age are accidents, cancer, and heart disease; for men age 50 and above, heart disease, cancer, cerebrovascular disease, and pneumonia are the main causes. This coincides with the causes of death in the urban zones. It seems evident that these data are not representative of the rest of the Latin American countries, where the pattern would most likely be similar to that in Africa and Asia but with lower rates or absence of the diseases with known measures of specific prevention.

SOCIOECONOMIC PROCESSES AND HEALTH CONDITIONS

The incompleteness of knowledge regarding the patterns of mortality among agricultural workers poses several questions to be resolved in order to advance toward a more thorough understanding of this problem. Obviously there is a woeful lack of information that needs to be remedied, but, in our opinion, there are also some theoretical and methodological aspects that should be developed. Since the object of our study is a group defined by a social characteristic—its occupation in agricultural work—it seems necessary to take into account its social character and not just reduce the problem to a biologically determined one. Our suggestion, therefore, is that one of the main analytical tools in the understanding of health conditions of the collectivity should be a body of social scientific knowledge that allows us to approach health as a socio-biological phenomenon.

The health conditions of socially defined groups can be described by certain typical patterns which have been termed epidemiological profiles (17) and hold a causal relationship to the social characteristics of the group. The empirical form of the epidemiological profile is the type of pathology and its frequency in a given population. This expresses one aspect of the specific biological existence of that population. It is necessary to stress that the epidemiological profile is a characteristic of the group and is meaningful only if the criterion used to constitute the group rests on some systematic interpretation of that conglomeration of individuals and is not just derived from an arbitrary grouping of unconnected persons.

The social characteristics of a group determining the causal relationship to the epidemiological profile are those which define the group in relation to other social groups and, therefore, in terms of its role in man's appropriation of nature by means of the social forms of production. This means that each social group participates in a concrete work process which implies precise forms of work and also of consumption (18). Our interest in specifying these characteristics is derived from the fact that what in economic and social terms are work and consumption are in biological terms forms of wearing down and reproduction.[3] That is, they correspond to specific forms of socially determined biological life that are at the basis of disease and that eventually determine the mortality of a population or social group (19).

We will give some concrete examples of why and how work and consumption are related to health and disease in a given social group, but at this point it seems necessary to outline some basic premises. Traditionally, work has been considered

---

[3] The biological process of wearing down occurs as a person works and is a part of aging; its complement is the process of reproducing that which is lost in the process of wearing down.

important in relation to disease only because of the so-called professional risks, i.e. accidents on the job and occupationally linked disease. It seems increasingly clear, however, that what is legally recognized as occupational disease conceives the causal relationship between work and health only in limited form. This can be seen, for example, in the fact that certain forms of work organization create stress which in turn has a wide range of morbid expressions (20), or that there is a clear overmortality from different types of cancer in specific occupational groups (21, pp. 26-30). Moreover, there is a less specific but perhaps more important relationship between work and health reflected in the forms of wearing down and aging of workers, phenomena that have been very little explored even though they are often quite visible in the particular biological constitution of the members of different occupations.

The influence of work on health conditions, however, reaches far beyond the concrete work process in a particular workplace. Work in modern society organizes all social life (22), so the effects of work are not just a problem of the laborer but also reach his family. Work determines the forms of consumption by different roads that are related to the historical forms of production. For example, in peasant subsistence agriculture consumption is linked to production, since what is produced is directly consumed. But work also determines consumption by means of the wage, which marks the limits of consumption within socially determined patterns.

If we wish to analyze the wearing down and reproduction of a specific socially defined group as a social and biological process, the basic elements are related to the understanding of how the wearing down, or consumption, of the worker occurs in the work process and identification of the forms of reproduction that occur with the socially given means at a specific moment. The linkage between the wearing down of workers and social reproduction can be expressed as different types of adaptation with clear biological characteristics. It seems possible to distinguish two forms of socio-biological adaptation: one in which the social process provokes a process of genetic selection with long-term effects, and another in which the social process expresses itself in different biological forms without genetic mediation.

Using the case of an agricultural social process, the first type of adaptation could be exemplified by a study on the sickle-cell trait and agricultural development done by Wiesenfeld (23), in which he shows how different forms of agriculture giving rise to specific ecological systems imply different frequencies of malaria, which in turn provoke a differential selection of individuals with the sickle-cell trait. The process of selection obviously does not express itself in the biological group character immediately, but only after a period of time. The second type of adaptation expresses itself without the necessity of a long time lag, since it acts not through a process of selection but through variations in the human biological process. This can be exemplified by the historical variation of disease (19) and also by the differences in disease rates between social classes (24, 25).

Even though we consider that the analysis of the social and economic determinants of the process of health and disease of a given group should be carried out in terms of work and consumption, it is also necessary to consider the general socioeconomic dynamic of a given society, because it makes possible the understanding of these two elements.

SOME CHARACTERISTICS OF AGRICULTURE
IN UNDERDEVELOPED COUNTRIES

The study object—agricultural workers in underdeveloped countries—needs to be specified so as to define what is in reality a very heterogeneous group. That is, it is necessary to point out some basic characteristics common to members of this group as a whole, but also to define some traits that mark delineations between some clearly distinguishable subgroups. Since both the characteristics that unify the group and separate the subgroups are derived from the agricultural structure and process of the underdeveloped countries, we will start by outlining some of its elements. The exposition will be limited to the underdeveloped capitalist countries, since the agricultural process is quite different in the socialist ones.

It should be kept in mind from the beginning that agriculture can be understood only in relation to the economy as a whole at a national level and as a part of international capitalism (26). The role of agriculture in the process of capital accumulation, then, is related to the industrial sector, and as a pool of accumulation in itself. The relationship between agriculture and industry takes place at many different levels. First, agriculture provides the industrial sector with raw materials, ranging from fibers to foodstuffs. Second, modern agriculture is an important market for a wide variety of industrial goods, e.g. machinery, fertilizers, and pesticides. Third, the agricultural sector has a decisive influence on the wage level, at least in the underdeveloped countries. Because food is the basic element of consumption in these countries, food prices to a large extent determine the wage level. On the other hand, the agricultural sector provides industry with large contingents of laborers looking for periodic work, which tends to keep the industrial trade unions weak and generates a downward pressure on wages.

Nevertheless, agriculture is not just a sector that supports industry. It is frequently the principal sector of capital accumulation, especially in countries with little industrial development. According to some authors (27), the agribusiness sector also plays the role of absorbing profitable investment during periods of economic crisis.

Even though the overall logic of agriculture is that of capitalist development (i.e. it obeys the laws of profit and accumulation), the concrete form that the process of transformation assumes in a given moment has to be understood in relation to the particular historical stage of each country or region. The basic elements of the agricultural structure, however, are the same, even if they assume distinct forms. These elements can be summarized as follows: (a) property relations determining the degree of proletarianization and the relationship between the capitalist and peasant sectors; (b) extent of control over production, determined by the types of crops, mechanisms of commercialization, and credit; (c) the degree of technological development; and (d) characteristics of the rural labor force: the relations between the peasants and the agricultural wage laborers on the one hand, and between the urban and rural labor forces on the other. The particular form of these elements and their combinations generate different types of work processes and patterns of social reproduction that determine the epidemiological profile of the groups.

Although each country has its own particular form of agricultural development, it is possible to outline some general trends characterizing the overall dynamics of agriculture in the capitalist world from the middle 1960s to the present. These trends mark a changing relationship between the underdeveloped countries and the metropoly (26, 28) and imply a rapid process of transformation of the agricultural structure in the former (29).

The basic trend is the increasing penetration of the agribusiness complex in the countryside of the underdeveloped countries, and this has provoked a series of changes in crops, property relations, and the labor force. Regarding the type of production, there has been a shift from basic subsistence crops to export products. For example, the per capita production of subsistence crops in Latin America decreased by 10 percent between 1964 and 1974, while export crops increased by 27 percent in the same period (30). The result of this process is an increasing dependence of the underdeveloped countries on the grain-exporting countries, i.e. United States, Australia, and New Zealand (29, p. 70). This situation was aggravated by the "food crisis" which started with a scarcity of cereals in 1972 and provoked a fourfold price increase of wheat and rice and a tripling of the price of corn by 1974 (29, pp. 64-65). The destruction of subsistence agriculture should be analyzed together with the levels of undernutrition in the underdeveloped capitalist countries. The United Nations estimates that 30 percent of the population of the Far East suffers from malnutrition, 25 percent in Africa, 18 percent in the Middle East, and 13 percent in Latin America (31). This chronic undernutrition has reached levels of outright starvation, and it has been calculated that 750,000 persons died from hunger between 1972 and 1974 (29, p. 66).

The penetration of capital into the agricultural zones of the underdeveloped countries also has meant the displacement of peasants from the most fertile soils and an increasing concentration of land in a few hands. To the peasants, this process means either increasing proletarianization or subordinate incorporation to cash cropping controlled by the agricultural capitalist sector (26, pp. 76-77; 28, pp. 12-15).

THE EPIDEMIOLOGICAL PROFILE OF SUBSISTENCE AGRICULTURE

From the point of view of the concrete conditions of work and life, it is possible to distinguish two large groupings of agricultural workers: one formed by those who are occupied essentially in subsistence agriculture or small-scale cash cropping and constitute what is generally called the peasantry, and another composed of workers of the plainly capitalist sector of agriculture, i.e. the rural proletariat. It is not possible to completely separate the two groups in reality, since they are actually interrelated, sometimes to the point that the same people perform both types of activities in different parts of their life cycle. Nevertheless, it is possible for analytical purposes to establish some basic characteristics of each work process and pattern of consumption which are related to the epidemiological profile and, therefore, to patterns of mortality.

The peasantry involved in subsistence agriculture and petty commodity production undoubtedly make up the majority of the agricultural workers of the underdeveloped countries. Their basic characteristics are given by their direct access to small plots of land that they work with very simple implements in a process that absorbs a comparatively large amount of labor. The relations that the peasants establish with the capitalist agricultural sector are basically twofold: the historical relation, linked to the overall development of capitalism in the countryside, and another of day-to-day exploitation.

The gradual and sometimes violent displacement of the peasantry to the least fertile land, the mechanisms that oblige it to abandon subsistence agriculture for cash cropping, and the subsequent monetization of its economy and the continuous process of proletarianization form part of the historically given relations. The day-to-day relations of exploitation occur in the unequal interchange between the peasants' products and those of industry and in the different forms of credit and commercialization.

The increasing monetization of the peasant economy and the scarce and overexploited resources frequently oblige the poor peasant to perform wage labor during some part of the year, activity that very frequently implies migration. On one hand, this might be a part of the process toward complete proletarianization, but on the other hand, subsistence agriculture can also be seen as a capitalist alternative to outright proletarianization, since it provides large contingents of periodic workers who need not be paid wages during the whole agricultural cycle but only for the few months of intensive labor.

Furthermore, the concrete work process in which this population participates has a distinctive feature: a very low level of control over nature. This means that the susceptibility to natural disasters is great, and the peasantry cannot profit from the overall social development of productive forces because of the unequal distribution of technology and wealth in society. Some authors have shown that the particular articulation of subsistence and petty commodity production agriculture in the overall capitalist development increases the vulnerability of the former to natural disaster. Ball (32), for example, analyzes the drought of 1968-1973 in Sahel from this perspective, pointing out that the natural phenomenon of drought was potentiated by the ecological degradation due to the process of overcultivation and overgrazing that had occurred in the area.

The characteristics of the wearing down and reproduction of the peasantry, understood as the specific forms of biological life derived from their concrete work process, are little known, but we will try to identify some elements. In bio-social terms, the work process of the peasant agricultural worker is characterized by hard physical work with a high caloric cost (because of the nature of agriculture and the rudimentary instruments used) and periods of intensive labor with long work days alternating with periods of inactivity. The sphere of consumption, on the other hand, is usually characterized by precarious life conditions, and correspondingly, an irregular nutritional situation.

One of the fundamental expressions of the distinct forms of human biological life is the life span, reflected in statistics on life expectancy or mortality. Using the data from Honduras (see Table 2) and Punjab, India (14, p. 911) as exponents of underdeveloped capitalist countries and Cuba (33, pp. 102-103) as a comparison given its similarity in terms of technological and industrial development but with socialist

Table 5

Death rates[a] by age, Honduras, Punjab, and Cuba[b]

Age group	Rural death rate[c]	Rural death rate[d]	General death rate[e]
15-44	2.2	2.2	1.4
45-64	12.2	14.3	4.7
65 or more	39.6	77.4	51.5

[a] Per 100,000 population.
[b] Source, modified from references 9, 14, and 33.
[c] Men and women, 1971-1972.
[d] Men, 1957-1959.
[e] Men, 1972.

relations of production, we find very high mortality rates in the former countries (Table 5). This expresses the relatively short life span of peasant workers, a fact that also has been observed in capitalist developed countries such as the United States (34, p. 522), where the life expectancy of agricultural workers is less than that of the average person. Furthermore, it is possible to observe a close relationship between the concrete conditions in which agriculture is developed and the mortality. Cantrelle (7, p. 159), for example, found a direct relationship between mortality rates and rainfall, population density, extension of farmland per person, and the type of crops.

While mortality undoubtedly has been declining in the countries under study, it is necessary to analyze it in relation to other expressions of health conditions. In this sense, the findings of Teller and collaborators (35) are very important, since they show that the mortality reduction has been combined with an increase in the prevalence of malnutrition. This fact should be closely analyzed, since it indicates some important changes in the relationship between morbidity and mortality.

The epidemiological profile of the peasant worker, in general terms, is dominated by the infectious and nutritional diseases. Hughes and Hunter (16), for example, point out that in different studies of tropical Africa it has been shown that there are, on an average, two infections per person, with prevalences of bilharziasis of 15 to 66 percent, filariasis of 20 to 65 percent, yaws of 27 to 50 percent, leprosy of 13 to 53 percent, malaria of 26 to 80 percent, and so on. General information seems to indicate a similar situation in Asia (14) and a similar but more favorable situation in Latin America (36). Another element that should be kept in mind in the analysis of the epidemiological profile is the fact that professional medicine does not intervene systematically among the rural population, which means that the prevalence and course of disease is different than in populations covered by medical services.

As we have pointed out, one of the characteristics of the peasant work process is its relatively low level of control over nature, which is reflected in the epidemiological profile. This has been clearly demonstrated by Cantrelle (7, p. 161) in his analysis of the mortality rate over time in relation to natural phenomena and the agricultural cycle. He finds a close relationship between the increases in mortality and abnormal climatological situations, e.g. rainfall and drought, that provoke a dialectical process between nutrition and infectious disease. He also points out the important seasonal variation of disease and death, which has been described by Gordon (14, p. 914) and Malina and Himes (37).

The great vulnerability to natural disaster expresses this same dependence on nature, since the overall development of the productive forces could, in principle, to a large extent reduce this type of mortality (32, pp. 273-274). Nevertheless, tens of thousands of persons die each year as a result of earthquakes, drought, cyclones, and floods. For example, the East Bengal cyclone of 1970 had a mortality rate among the adult population of at least 6 percent (38), and the drought of 1973-1974 killed approximately 750,000 persons (29, p. 66). As was pointed out before, the low level of control over nature should be analyzed together with the ecological effects of the type of agricultural development in these countries, since the latter frequently increases the vulnerability to natural events.

As most of the peasant workers are living in a phase of transition from subsistence agriculture to cash cropping and wage labor, we would like to point out some problems related to this transition which need to be taken into account in the analysis of the mortality of agricultural workers. The crucial issues relate to the changes in landholding and use of land, a changing relation to the monetary market, and the corresponding changes in the social composition of the population.

In a study on morbidity in two Mexican villages (39), it was shown that there existed a morbidity differential between subsistence agricultural workers, cash croppers, and waged agricultural workers in the sense of a gradual increase from the former to the latter. Analyzing the mortality in the Philippines during the last century, Smith (40) found that the increase of mortality observed was closely related to the change from subsistence to commercial agriculture.

Some studies point to the concrete dynamics of this process that can explain the interrelation between socioeconomic events and health conditions. Hernandez and collaborators (41) evaluated the health effects of a development project in Mexico which consisted of an irrigation plan and the introduction of commercial exportation crops. Thirteen years after its initiation, there had been a substantial decrease in mortality as a result of water and malaria control. Nevertheless, the benefits of economic growth were concentrated in the hands of a small group of immigrants, and the original population had experienced virtually no positive change. It had actually suffered some deterioration in its diet, and malnutrition was as common among them as before the transition.

Gross and Underwood (42) analyzed the effects of the introduction of sisal as the dominant crop in what had been areas of subsistence agriculture in northeastern Brazil. Although in economic and technological terms the sisal fiber meant an advance, the social changes that it provoked left the great majority of the population in worse conditions. Control over concrete life conditions shifted from the local level to the international market where the price of the fiber is decided; a large majority of the peasants were dispossessed of their land and turned into wage laborers with an extremely low wage level; all subsistence articles had to be acquired in the market. Analysis of the caloric cost in the work process of sisal as compared to the wage received showed that the latter was hardly enough to replace the calories spent by the worker and totally insufficient for the satisfaction even of the nutritional requirements of his family. This was reflected in the fact that 45 percent of the children of sisal workers were undernourished. Hughes and Hunter (16) show extensively that "development" is not inert from the point of view of ecology, since it changes patterns of water flow and use, man-habitat relationships, increases population movement and mixing, and changes the vegetation cover and the micro-environmental conditions, all of which have potentially far-reaching consequences for health.

The migrations that in some regions of the world are part of the life cycle of subsistence agricultural workers have important implications for their health and will be analyzed in relation to the agricultural proletariat.

THE EPIDEMIOLOGICAL PROFILE OF THE RURAL PROLETARIAT

The expansion of capitalist agriculture in the countryside of the underdeveloped countries is an inevitable historical trend that also has been accelerated by the economic crisis of the 70s (28). As a product of this process, the agricultural proletariat is formed and constitutes a rapidly growing social class in all underdeveloped countries. Capitalist agriculture is characterized by comparatively capital-intensive methods and the use of technology and industrial products to increase productivity. Usually the entrepreneurs of this sector control large extensions of land and grow commercial crops destined for the international market. This kind of agriculture consumes comparatively little labor, with the exception of some social points of the cycle such as the harvest.

One of the outstanding problems faced by rural wage laborers is the long periods of unemployment; it is common for them to find work just 3 to 6 months a year (28, pp. 29-31). The scarcity of work also provokes migrations, sometimes over long distances. The relative overpopulation of the rural areas, which is a result of the continuous process of proletarianization of peasants and the population growth, together with the periodic character of employment, pose great obstacles to the union organization of these workers, with consequences for their wage level and working conditions.

The concrete work process in which the waged agricultural workers participate has some features in common with that of the peasantry, so we will emphasize the elements that are unique or especially important. The productive moment incorporates new risks incurred in the handling of machinery and a wide range of toxic chemical substances (34, pp. 523-524). Some of the commercial crops, like cotton, are in themselves health risks or could carry significant residuals of pesticides (43, p. 172). Most studies on the working conditions of agricultural laborers note days of 10 to 13 hours of hard physical labor (44).

The patterns of consumption of this group increasingly are dictated by the market, since the subsistence agricultural strategies for survival disappear when there is no direct relation of control over production. The agricultural laborer depends for survival on the wage and on what he can acquire in the market with it. This means, among other things, the disarticulation of the extended family, changes in food patterns, and frequently, migration.

There is almost no information that allows us to specify the concrete aspects of the wearing down of agricultural workers, but there is some evidence pointing to the types of problems that should be studied. For example, different studies from Central America show that the rural workers are young, e.g. approximately 75 percent under age 35 (44, p. 16), and that their active working life is about 12 years (28, p. 32). Furthermore, the data related by Gross and Underwood (42) indicate that the new generations of landless workers are to a large proportion undernourished. In addition, studies of agricultural workers from other parts of the world have noted that they suffer from high rates of disability (45), a situation that most likely also holds true for corresponding groups in the underdeveloped countries.

The epidemiological profile of the wage laborers, like that of the peasantry, is dominated by infectious disease and problems of nutrition. Nevertheless, it seems important to emphasize that the causes of this pathology in social terms are partially different than in the case of subsistence agriculture. For example, the nutritional problems are less dependent on a deficient control over nature than on the low wage level and the rupture of cultural food patterns. Regarding infectious disease, one of the problems that should be taken into consideration is the previously noted migration of these workers.

Migration is important not just in terms of infectious disease, but is also directly related to accidents, alcoholism, stress-related disease, and venereal disease (46). Agricultural migrant workers in Africa have been found to be especially at risk of contracting tuberculosis or trypanosomiasis (16, pp. 166-183). Although most studies on the health risks of migration refer to rural-urban migration (47, 48), some of the phenomena observed could also apply to rural-rural migration, since the problems have more to do with the rupture of subsistence agriculture than with city life as such. For example, the rate of sickness found among non-migrant adult males in Senegal was 18.9 percent and among migrants 21.1 percent.

A second set of problems specific to workers in the capitalist agricultural sector relates to the risks derived from its level of technological development. The accident rate among agricultural workers, where it is being registered, is very high. In a Central American study on occupational health among banana workers, the index of frequency of accidents was found to be 216.9 and the index of seriousness 1618.3, both extremely high (44, p. 521). These data coincide with statistics from the United States. While agricultural workers make up only 4.4 percent of the U.S. labor force, they suffer 16 percent of the fatal accidents and 9 percent of the disabling diseases (34, p. 521). Apart from the handling of machinery, the most important risk of agricultural work is derived from the use of pesticides. Those substances, as is well known, are dangerous because of their immediate toxic effects, but also since some of them are suspected carcinogens. Moreover, the risks related to pesticides are greater in the underdeveloped countries, since some of the substances banned in other countries are freely used, without even minimum precautions (49). A study from a cotton-producing area in Mexico showed that in the agricultural cycle of 1974, the rate of intoxications from pesticides was 121.1 per 100,000 population, or 1.4 per 100 men in productive ages (50). In Ceylon, it was found that 30 percent of the accidental poisoning was provoked by agricultural chemicals, especially by insecticides, and that the great majority of the victims were between 15 and 50 years of age (51).

CONCLUSIONS

It seems to me that the methodological elements presented in this paper open the possibility of analyzing health conditions as part of the social process. The rupture with the clinically and biologically oriented approach permits a more profound understanding of how and why disease and death occur in society. For a period of time, national and international public health agencies seemed to believe that the improvement of health conditions was a matter simply of technology, methods of specific control, and good planning. The events of the last twenty years, however, show that these elements are not enough and oblige the search for a different approach to the dramatic health situation found in the underdeveloped countries.

REFERENCES

1. Federici, N., De Sarno Prignano, A., Pasquali, P., Cariani, G., and Natale, M. Urban/rural differences in mortality, 1950-1970. *World Health Statistics Report* 29(5): 254, 1976.
2. Berlinguer, G. *Malaria Urbana.* Ed. Villalar, Barcelona, 1978.
3. Johnson, G. Z. Health conditions in rural and urban areas of developing countries. *Population Studies* 17: 293-309, 1963.
4. Seklani, M. L'Evolution de la Mortalité dans les Pays Arab Depuis le Milieu du 20e Siecle. Paper presented at the Conference on Socioeconomic Determinants and Consequences of Mortality, Mexico City, 1979.
5. Vallin, J. La mortalité en Algerie. *Population* 30(6): 1041, 1975.
6. Gaisie, S. K. Some Aspects of Socio-economic Determinants of Mortality in Tropical Africa. Paper presented at the Conference on Socioeconomic Determinants and Consequences of Mortality, Mexico City, 1979.
7. Cantrelle, P. Niveaux, typeo el tendance de la mortalité. In *Croissance Demographique et Evolution Socio-économique en Afrique de l'Ouest,* edited by J. C. Caldwell. Population Council, New York, 1973.
8. Rumford, J. C., Heperkan, Y., and Fincancioglu, N. The principals and preliminary results of the Turkish demographic survey. *Public Health Rep.* 83(7): 578, 1968.
9. Behm, H. Socioeconomic Determinants of Mortality in Latin America. Paper presented at the Conference on Socioeconomic Determinants and Consequences of Mortality, Mexico City, 1979.
10. Cordero, E. La subestimación de la mortalidad infantil en Mexico. *Demografía y Economía* 2(1): 56-58, 1968.
11. Matos, C. Differenciales de la Mortalidad Urbana y Rural en Cuba, 1973-1978. Thesis, Instituto de Desarrollo de la Salud, MINSAP, Havana, 1979.
12. Guttmacher, S., and Danielson, R. Changes in the Cuban health care. *Int. J. Health Serv.* 7(3): 383-400, 1977.
13. Jordan, J., et al. *Desarrollo Humano en Cuba.* Ed. Científico Técnico, Havana, 1979.
14. Gordon, J. E., Singh, S., and Wyon, J. B. Causes of death at different ages, by sex, and by season, in rural population of Punjab. *Indian J. Med. Res.* 53(9): 911, 1965.
15. Djurfelt, G., and Lindberg, S. *Pills Against Poverty.* Studentlitteratur-Curzon Press, Sweden, 1975.
16. Hughes, C., and Hunter, J. Disease and development in Africa. In *The Social Organization of Health,* edited by H. P. Dreitzel, pp. 150-214. Macmillan, New York, 1971.
17. Breilh, J. *Epidemiología: Economía, Medicina y Política.* Universidad Central, Quito, 1979.
18. Laurell, A. C. Work and health in Mexico. *Int. J. Health Serv.* 9(4): 543-568, 1979.
19. Laurell, A. C. *La Salud Enfermedad como Proceso Social. Memorias Seminario Salud enfermedad en México.* Instituto Politécnico Nacional, México, 1979.
20. Eyer, J., and Sterling, P. Stress-related mortality and social organization. *URPE* 9(1): 2-44, 1977.

21. Lewinson, C. *Riesgo Profesional: Agentes Químicos en el Lugar de Trabajo.* ICF, Switzerland, 1975.
22. Braverman, H. *Trabajo y Capital Monopolista.* Nuestro Tiempo, Mexico, 1976.
23. Wiesenfeld, S. L. Sickle-cell trait in human biological and cultural evolution. *Science* 157: 1134-1140, 1967.
24. Saracci, R. Epidemiological strategies and environmental factors. *Int. J. Epidemiol.* 7(2): 104-107, 1978.
25. Antonovsky, A. Social class, life expectancy and overall mortality. *Milbank Mem. Fund. Q.* 45(1): 31-73, 1967.
26. CEPAL. *El Desarrollo Social en las Areas Rurales de América Latina.* Servicios de Información No. 276, Chile, 1978.
27. Arroyo, G., and Aceituno, G. Agribusiness Ganancia contra hambre. *Le Monde Diplomatique* 1(6): 22, 1979.
28. Burbach, R., and Flynn, P. Agribusiness target in Latin America. *NACLA Reports* 12(1): 5-7, 1978.
29. Treubal, M. La crisis alimenticía y el Tercer Mundo. *Economía de Latinoamérica* 2: 61-80, 1979.
30. U.S. Department of Agriculture. *Agriculture in the Americas: Statistical Data.* U.S. Government Printing Office, Washington, D.C., 1975.
31. U.N. World Food Conference. The Assessment of the World Food Situation: Present and Future. Document E/CONF. 65/3.
32. Ball, N. Drought and dependence in the Sahel. *Int. J. Health Serv.* 8(2): 271-298, 1978.
33. World Health Organization. *World Health Statistics Annual 1972,* Volume 1. Geneva, 1975.
34. Ashford, N. A. *Crisis in the Workplace.* MIT Press, Cambridge, Mass., 1976.
35. Teller, C., Sibria, R., Bent, V., del Canto, J., and Saenz, L. Population and Nutrition: Implications of Sociodemographic Trends and Differentials for Food and Nutritional Policy in Central America and Panama. Paper presented at the IX International Nutrition Congress, Rio de Janeiro, 1978.
36. *Hechos Que Revelan Progreso en La Salud 1971.* PAHO/WHO Publición Científica No. 227, Washington, D.C., 1971.
37. Malina, R. M., and Himes, J. H. Differential age effects in seasonal variation of mortality in a Zapotec municipio. *Hum. Biol.* 49(3): 415-428, 1977.
38. Somer, A., and Mosley, W. H. East Bengal cyclone of November 1970. *Lancet,* May 13, 1972, p. 7759.
39. Laurell, A. C., and Blanco Gil, J. Disease and development. *Int. J. Health Serv.* 7(3): 401-423, 1977.
40. Smith, P. L. Crisis mortality in the 19th century Philippines. *Journal of Asian Studies* 38(1): 51-76, 1978.
41. Hernandez, M., Perez Hidalgo, C., Ramirez, J., and Madrigal, H. Effects of economic growth on nutrition in a tropical community. *Ecology of Food and Nutrition* 3(2): 283-291, 1974.
42. Gross, D. R., and Underwood, B. A. Technological change and caloric cost: Sisal agriculture in northeastern Brazil. *American Anthropologist* 73(3): 725-736, 1971.
43. Friberg, L., and Ronge, H. E. *Hygien.* Swenska Bokförlaget, Stockholm, 1967.
44. Salud occupacional en el sector bananero en Centroamerica. *Revista Centroamericana de Ciencias de la Salud* 4(9): 9-67, 1978.
45. Wan, T., and Wright, A. Occupational differentials in chronic disabilities. *J. Occup. Med.* 15(6): 494, 1973.
46. Prothero, M. Disease and mobility: A neglected factor in epidemiology. *Int. J. Epidemiol.* 6(3): 259-267, 1977.
47. Benyoussef, A., et al. Health effects of rural-urban migration in developing countries: Senegal. *Soc. Sci. Med.* 8(2): 259-267, 1974.
48. Stromberg, J., Peyman, H., and Dowd, J. E. Migration and health: Adaptation experiences of Iranian migrants to the city of Teheran. *Soc. Sci. Med.* 8(2): 309-323, 1974.
49. Elling, R. Industrialization and occupational health in underdeveloped countries. *Int. J. Health Serv.* 7(2): 209-235, 1977.
50. *Salud Pública de México* 17(5), 1975.
51. Senewiratne, B., and Thambipillai, S. Patterns of poisoning in developing countries. *Br. J. Prev. Soc. Med.* 28(1): 32-36, 1974.

CHAPTER 14

A Historical and Socioeconomic Analysis of Occupational Safety and Health in India

J. V. Vilanilam

On the morning of December 27, 1978, a terrible accident happened in a village near Sivakasi, in which 35 children were drowned when their bus was washed away by a flash flood. The poignancy of the tragedy was heightened when it became known that the victims were not school children but factory workers aged between 10 and 14 years, most of whom were girls. Sivakasi is an industrial town about 12 hours by train from Madras. It is well known for its printing, fireworks, and match industries. The children were being transported from villages around Sivakasi on a routine basis to the industrial units in the town which engaged "mostly child labour for its cheapness and availability." (1)

Twenty-year-old Anthonyswami[1] had come from an interior village of Tamil Nadu with high hopes to work as a production operative in a tire plant in Madras. One autumn day in 1962, his hand got caught in the fabric calendering machine. The unguarded machine pulled him in and he was crushed to death. After several months, his relatives were paid Rs. 2000 (roughly U.S. $250) as compensation from the company.

---

[1] The names of the victims cited in this article are not real; the accidents are.

In the summer of 1967, after the day's work in the same factory, Ramasamy Iyer was waiting in the factory bus that was about to leave the premises. Unfortunately, he felt thirsty and ran to a water cooler installed in the reception area. When he pressed the button and bent to sip the water, the young man was electrocuted. A science graduate, Iyer was a recent recruit to the supervisory cadre of the company. He was the oldest in a family of six children; his father had retired from a small government job and the family had no other income except his meager pension. That old man had to walk 10 miles almost every month for 14 months to the company headquarters to move the powers that be to sanction some compensation to Ramasamy's family. At long last, the company, which had several million dollars in assets, sanctioned at a special directors' meeting a sum of Rs. 2000 as compensatory payment to the family.

Are there not laws against child labor in India? Are there no legal requirements for higher compensation for victims' families? Has India a primitive legal system? Far from it. India has quite a modern legal system and the longest written constitution in the world.

There are laws against child labor and there are legal measures to obtain higher compensation for victims of occupational accidents. But the law is mute when the victims have no political clout. Laws are interpreted by people who have the same economic interests as the captains of industry. Moreover, the victims and their families are not aware of their rights. Nor are they aware of the legal responsibilities of the employers for the safety of workers. The media are silent on these types of accidents and deaths because the media themselves are owned or directed by people who have close ties with the industrial powers. The cross-ownership of newspapers and industrial enterprises in India is so prevalent that a former prime minister called newspapers the house organs of industrial families. It took a major accident and the loss of 35 young and innocent lives for a newspaper to report the existence of industrial child abuse. The newspapers, like the elite of India, have all along ignored this serious malady, taking shelter under the legalistic umbrella which displays tough laws against child labor. Why should children have to waste away their lives when millions of able-bodied adult workers are idle? The inherent injustice in the practice of recruiting children and paying them next to nothing for long hours of hard work is not stirring many consciences in India.

The occupational scene in India in the last quarter of the 20th century is worse than that in the United States in the last quarter of the 19th century. "Cheaper and cheaper labour! Women's labour and children's labour!" wrote Upton Sinclair. In those days nearly two million children between 10 and 15 years of age were put to hard labor in the United States. The number of working children under 12 in Alabama alone was 34 percent of the total child labor population, with those under 10 comprising 10 percent. The children worked 12 hours a day; the oldest children got 50 cents, the youngest nine cents. Boys of six to nine years worked 12 to 13 hours for 15 cents a day, with a break of 40 minutes at noon. There was no holiday for Thanksgiving or Christmas (2, pp. 112-113).

The actual conditions of work for adult men and women (and for children who are legally employed or used surreptitiously with or without the connivance of the guardians of the Factory Acts) are yet to be studied in detail in India. While there have been surveys of labor welfare sponsored by large industrial establishments, most such studies (e.g. reference 3) simply review existing laws and regulations and present the labor welfare measures adopted by government and private managements. They do not refer to occupational health, nor do they make any in-depth study of the working conditions in the major industries of the country. Studies which discuss labor welfare measures do not make any distinction between the "top-down" labor welfare approach of the employers and the legitimate human rights of labor to a healthy and safe working environment. The whole question of worker health is treated in a paternalistic manner by the Indian industrial enterprises. This is mainly because of the peculiar socioeconomic organization of the country's population.

Is an Indian worker's life worth just $250? Are the relatives of a victim of employer negligence entitled only to an outright ex-gratia payment? What about workers who are permanently disabled by occupational accidents and diseases? How cheap can a person's life be? Even if there is some insurance and government machinery to ensure a higher compensation for a victim or his or her family, can workers' safety and health be left to such machinery? Or will such a scheme or machinery absolve the employers of all responsibilities to provide a safe and healthy work environment? The experience of workers in industrially advanced societies is no better than that of workers in industrially backward societies. As Berman has noted (4), "compensation has always overshadowed prevention" in the advanced countries. In India, even compensation is considered charity and prevention is brushed aside by top management as either too costly or totally unnecessary. The political and socioeconomic conditions in India have a bearing on the perpetuation of this situation. It is therefore necessary to examine the political and economic situation in India from a historical perspective.

PRE-INDEPENDENCE INDIA

India is an ancient country with five thousand years of history behind it. In the dim, distant past, India extended from Afghanistan in the west to Burma in the east, the Himalayas in the north to Kanyakumari in the south. The extent of the geographic, cultural, and social fabric of India varied from time to time with frequent invasions from central Asia and from the Mediterranean region. A fairly uniform and consistent geographic and sociocultural concept of India took root during the period of Asoka, whose empire extended from the Himalayas to Kanyakumari, and Purushapura (modern Peshawar) to Vanga (Bengal). This was in the third century before Christ. Later on, the empire left by Asoka and his successors was divided into small kingdoms. India continued to be ruled in small kingdoms and principalities for several centuries until the Moghuls came on the scene. Throughout India's history, there have been struggles for power and extension of suzerainty among the princes and feudal lords. But the people of India who lived in small villages were largely unaffected by these power struggles because they were organized into four religiously sanctioned *varnas* (occupational and social hierarchies): the Brahmins (priestly class), the Kshatriyas (warrior class), the Vaisyas (commercial class), and the Sudras (the working class, including artisans and craftsmen). In addition to these four, there was also a non-varna class—the class of Untouchables—comprising persons who did menial jobs (such as scavenging, animal killing, and leather tanning) and the tribal and hill people. The villages had a self-sufficient economy. The agricultural workers and the craftsmen maintained the economy and the other classes reaped the fruits of their labor. The occupational health or safety of manual workers was, of course, of no concern.

It was into such a well-organized feudal system that Vasco da Gama made European commercial and religious inroads in the last decade of the 15th century. He and his fellow explorers landed in Kozhikode (Calicut) on the Malabar coast of India in 1498.[2] Other Portuguese explorers and some missionaries soon followed, and in a few years there was a sizable Portuguese and Indo-Portuguese population in the west coast of India, including Malabar (Kerala), Goa, and Bombay. Dutch traders were the next to arrive in India, but they settled on the east coast, near Madras. Then came the French, who drove out the Dutch. Finally, the English succeeded in defeating all their European rivals. The English gradually established small but firm footholds in India, especially in the harbor areas. The English East India Company established its first manufactory in Surat near Ahmedabad in 1600 during the great Moghul emperor Akbar's time. Queen Elizabeth I's envoys were gladly received by the emperor.

There were small manufactories and trading companies owned by Europeans throughout the coastal towns of India by the end of the 17th century. Under strong Moghul rulers like Akbar, Shah Jahan, and Aurangzeb, the Europeans did not assert their might, but with the weakening of the central authority toward the mid-18th century, they began to ally themselves with feudal lords in different regions and exert decisive political influence in India. The fate of India was sealed at the Battle of Plassey in 1757 in which the British, with their superior weapons and military technology, inflicted a crushing defeat on the Bengal Nabob. The East India Company made Calcutta its headquarters and, under the guise of preserving law and order in the company's territorial jurisdiction, maintained military garrisons in the major ports and towns. Traders became tax collectors and guardians of law and order. It was not difficult for them to overthrow the feudal princes who made a last organized attempt in 1857 to resist British supremacy. But by then it was too late; in 1858, Queen Victoria proclaimed herself Empress of India.

The economic influence of the first multinational company of the world—the English East India Company—on the people of India was much more devastating than its political influence. As mentioned earlier, the large majority of the people who lived in the six hundred thousand villages of India were agricultural laborers and handloom weavers. They did not see anything wrong in the traditional exploitation by the superior *varnas* since it had religious sanction from time immemorial. But they felt the pinch when their very livelihood was affected. With the establishment of British manufactures in large towns, the weavers in the villages lost their traditional source of income since all the cotton that was grown went to the large towns for ginning and from there to the textile factories of England. The cloth made in the Manchester mills was reimported into the villages of India where those who could afford it bought it at higher prices.

---

[2]Columbus's earlier attempt to reach India took him to the shores of America and he named the native population of that continent Indians, mistaking the land he had reached for India.

The role of British finance capital in the destruction of the Indian economy has been described by Levkovsky (5, p. 45) as follows:

> British capitalist enterprise did of course advance the country's productive forces (though on a restricted scale), but on the whole it was reactionary and anti-national, impeding India's independent economic and political development. In the independent European countries the new capitalist relations of production were giving definite scope to the productive forces, but in India British capital created a type of capitalism that from the very outset put a brake on their development.

The export of capital to India started with great vigor in the middle of the 19th century when England had already become the foremost industrial and military power on earth, and the British imperial "pink" had spread almost everywhere on the world map. It flowed into cotton export, textile import, mining, metallurgy, railway construction, and the steel industry. In short, almost every modern industrial activity that originated in Europe had its counterpart or subsidiary in India by the end of the 19th century. Modernization and industrialization started much earlier in India than in most countries that are called "developing" countries today. But it was an illusory industrialization, a misleading and mirage-like modernization. British capital ruined India's rural economy without replacing it with an economy that was helpful to raise the standard of living of the Indian people. Most of the productive activity was confined to the extraction of raw materials, the maintenance of a huge military force, and for railway building, which ensured not only troop movement for quelling people's uprisings against oppression but also the transportation of raw materials to the ports for export to Britain. Britain had thus become the manufacturer for India, but the manufactured articles could be purchased only by the higher classes of the Indian population. The masses were left to fend for themselves without the basic provisions of life. Some raw materials needed processing before export, and for this there were indigenous small-scale industries such as rice mills, packing houses, flour mills, cotton presses, and cotton ginning mills. But, by and large, the Indian capitalists were serving the British as agents on a commission basis. There was no real national industrial activity. The workers in those pre-export processing plants were paid the lowest possible wages by local entrepreneurs who had only one aim: to maximize their profits through service to the British masters.

The money lenders, mill owners, and merchants of Bombay, Calcutta, and Madras formed a solid comprador class for safeguarding British interests through flooding India with British goods. In serving the foreign imperialists, the local capitalists were destroying hundreds of thousands of local craftsmen, upon whose handicraft and handloom industries the rural economy depended. The modernization initiated by European feudal merchants and explorers and promoted by British industrial capitalists with the help of Indian compradors did a thorough job of destroying the Indian economy and of keeping the wages of workers extremely low. This resulted in the creation of absolute poverty and the consequent misery, malnutrition, epidemics, and fatalism characteristic of the Indian society.

As mentioned earlier, Indian capitalists started out as brokers and business agents for British companies and soon entered the coal, steel, jute, sugar, and textile manufacturing fields. There thus arose an indigenous industrial millionaire class in India in the last decade of the 19th century. This class collaborated with the imperialists in what

Worseley (6) calls the "drain" of India's wealth to Britain. The process of mechanization and industrialization initiated by the British and carried on by the local elites went against the interests of the working class of India. The industries were concentrated in the large towns of British provinces. The areas under the control of the 600-odd princes depended on rural industries and agriculture, both of which were affected by the inflow of British financial capital, technology, and communication and marketing techniques. This resulted in the outflow of wealth to Britain and the internal aggregation of wealth in the hands of the princes and the new industrial captains who cooperated with the British capitalists.

Cheap labor was available then as now from the villages. Children and women followed rural men who migrated to the cities, and laid the foundations for huge sprawling slums, absolute poverty, and organized social evils such as prostitution and begging. Whereas the modernization process transformed the lives of most working people in England and the United States, eased their drudgery to a great extent, and brought considerable improvements in their standard of living, it only aided the deterioration of the quality of life of Indian workers. The rural folk who migrated to cities lost their rural jobs, ancestral homes and land (many mortgaged their possessions to raise enough money for railway fare to distant cities), traditional social organization, and the security of an extended family. Not all of them landed jobs in the cities. Even those who did led miserable lives, and those who did not lived on the pavement, earning a pittance from carrying loads or doing odd jobs or joining the underworld of crime.

When the new industrial class recruited workers from among ruined craftsmen and illiterate peasants who had lost their land, it set wages according to rural standards and indices. This is why labor became so cheap in India. The new industrialists of post-independence India have continued the wage structure established in the 19th century. The real wage rate of factory workers remained virtually stagnant between 1939 and 1969. Even today, their wages have not gone up considerably. The share of wages in total factory output is declining (7, p. 8). This is one of the reasons for the unions considering wage increases the most important demand, even to the exclusion of demands for a healthy working environment. Another feature of the 19th-century Indian labor world was the practice of middlemen hiring labor and appropriating sizable portions of the workers' wages with managements' approval. The middlemen were responsible not only for recruiting but also paying the workers. This practice stopped later on with the formation of workers' unions, but wages did not register any substantial improvement over the years. The phenomenon of middlemen hiring workers is perhaps not prevalent in India today, but the practice of bribing recruiters and working free for some time is still widespread among certain employment areas, especially in the field of education which is very much under the control of an unholy alliance among the industrial elite (wearing the mantle of philanthropists), aristocracy, landed gentry, administrative cadres, and the religious hierarchy.

The pattern of exploitation of working men, women, and children was more or less similar in India, England, and the United States in the early days of industrialization; long hours, low wages, and a poor working and living environment. The working day ranged between 12 and 15 hours in all three countries. Weavers at the Calcutta jute mills had to work for 15½ to 16 hours a day (8, pp. 6-11). The report of the Textile Factories Labor Committee of 1907 (9) stated that the health of women was being injured by night work in over 1,000 ginning mills in India. The same report described the intolerable living conditions of the workers as follows (9, p. 7):

> The conditions can only be described as deplorable. After making allowance for the very limited space which will satisfy Indian workers and their families, the houses were distinctly overcrowded, dark, damp, and ill-ventilated. . . . the dwellings were surrounded by narrow gullies for carrying off waste water and sullage, the offensive vapour from these gullies permeating the whole of the surrounding atmosphere. . . .

The situation today is not much different, except for the fact that some of those dark, damp dungeons described in 1907 are collapsing in various parts of Bombay and Calcutta, killing tenants in the process.

Even as late as 1938, the wage of sugar factory workers was less than six cents a day (10, p. 155). Today, the average factory worker gets *a dollar a day* in some industries. This might appear a great improvement, but the price of everything—including the most basic needs such as food, clothing, housing, education, and health care—has gone sky-high. In fact, in many industries the wages are still extremely low. There are intra-industry wage differences because of the free enterprise system which allows the purchase of labor at the cheapest rate possible. Table 1 presents the wage picture as it existed in 1968. Today's wages are not substantially different. Moreover, there is

Table 1

Monthly wages for selected jobs in India, 1968[a]

Job	Monthly Wage[b]	
	Rupees	Dollars
Paper Mills[c]		
Laborers, sorters, kollar gang, rotary cutter assistant, etc.	122.40	16.32
Solvo pulper, digester, beater helper	138.32	18.44
Beater operator	190.84	25.44
Rotary cutter operator	258.37	34.44
Machine operator	188.42	25.12
Senior finisher	179.75	23.96
Textile Mills (average in 1962)	149.60	19.95
Engineering Industries		
Lowest wages[d]	87.37	11.65
Highest wages[e]	272.87	36.38

[a]Sources: Government of India, *Census of Indian Manufacturers,* New Delhi; Government of India, *Annual Survey of Industries,* New Delhi; Aziz, A., *Industrial Wage Structure in Mysore State,* Mysore University Press, Mysore, 1972.
[b]Exchange rate: $1 equals Rs. 7.50.
[c]These are the wages in a comparatively well-paying paper mill. There are mills which pay half these rates, e.g., some factories pay only $8 a month for sorters!
[d]The lowest wages are paid by a private machine manufacturer.
[e]The highest wages are paid by a government factory.

no correspondence between wages and the prices of commodities. Workers cannot afford to purchase most of the products they labor to make.

The only major improvement is the statutory limitation of working hours to eight and the payment of overtime wages for time in excess of this. In all other respects, the conditions of Indian workers of the 1900s and those of the 1970s are similar. Both groups faced starvation and poverty, ill health, harassment from merciless moneylenders, and extremely hazardous working conditions. Epidemics like tuberculosis have been widespread in both periods, despite the marvels of medical science. Unsung and unwept, thousands of workers in both periods have vanished from the occupational scene due to the toxicity of their environment and the poverty of their existence.

POST-INDEPENDENCE INDIA

The British left India in August 1947, but mere political independence has not brought any major improvements to the workers and peasants, despite several five-year plans. No basic structural changes have been made. With the attainment of political independence under the able guidance of Mahatma Gandhi and Jawaharlal Nehru, the expectations of the masses were raised. At the dawn of independence, Nehru said (11, pp. 5-6):

> The future beckons to us. Whither do we go and what shall be our endeavour? To bring freedom and opportunity to the common man, to the peasants and workers of India; to fight and end poverty and ignorance and disease; to build up a prosperous, democratic and progressive nation, and to create social, economic and political institutions which will ensure justice and fullness of life to every man and woman.

Thirty-one years have passed since Nehru gave that message to the Indian people, and India has already passed through five five-year plans and taken several gigantic steps toward economic development. In quantitative terms, and based on certain criteria for the measurement of economic growth, India has registered growth in all fields of economic activity. Compared to pre-independence days, India's national income has nearly doubled; industrial production has tripled and agriculture has improved greatly. During the 50 years preceding 1947, the annual growth rate was less than 1 percent. In post-1947 years, the growth rate went up to 3 percent, but there has been no corresponding increase in the standard of living of the workers. Conventional economic indicators do not mean much when we measure economic improvement in former colonies of imperial powers because the large majority of their populations still live substandard lives.

There is no doubt that the fruits of India's growth during the past three decades have not reached the lower strata of the Indian society. In fact, some statistics point out that the gap between the rich and the poor has become wider. The wealthiest 10 percent enjoy 34 percent of the national disposable income, while the poorest 10 percent have only 3 percent of that income. What the Mahalanobis Committee found in the 1960s is still true. There has been no significant change in the distribution of income. More than 10 percent of India's rural families (i.e. about 60 million people) are landless, and the next poorest fourth own less than half an acre. By comparison, the 437,000 families falling in the richest 0.6 percent of landholders own more than 11 percent of the total acreage (12, p. 23). The number of people below the poverty line rose from 39 percent of the total population (172 million) in 1961 to 45 percent (245 million) in 1971. The definition of poverty line as given in the draft fifth plan is a minimum standard of Rs. 40.60 (about U.S. $5.40) per capita per month at 1972-1973 prices (13). The uppermost 5 percent of the population has acquired certain material status symbols like automobiles, refrigerators, air-conditioners, and telephones; the next lower 5 percent is struggling to keep up with the Joneses. But the large majority who live in mud huts, *cheries, basties,* or slums and pavements suffer abject poverty, the dimensions of which cannot be described or compared. The workers and peasants of India are among this large majority. They are the tired millions, the deeply dejected and despondent "wretched of the earth." There is no future for them if the present economic system continues. They silently bear the brunt of the socioeconomic and political experiments conducted by half-hearted, class-ridden reformers who occupy positions of power. The tears which Mahatma Gandhi wanted to wipe off are still rolling down their sunken faces. Meanwhile, India is doing well, but not her people. Why this big paradox?

Part of the reason lies in the semifeudal economy that still persists in post-independence India. The existing economic structure is mainly responsible for the glaring contrast between India's scientific, technological, and industrial progress[3] and her enormous poverty. Feudalism is at its worst in many enterprises run by some powerful families. As Veit notes (14, p. 324):

> At the apex of India's industrial hierarchy are a few dozen family-controlled conglomerate empires which are largely the creation of businessmen from particular communities.... These industrial giants have been preserved and even expanded since 1947 despite India's desire to create a "socialist pattern of society."

This kind of economic structure and "socialism" exerts a very harmful influence on the condition of the workers. No less a personality than the current President of India has acknowledged the irony of India's economic development during the past three decades. He noted in a speech last year that every party in the country advocates socialism, but the entire economy is centered on 200 capitalist families. He drew attention to a recent convention of the Chambers of Commerce in Calcutta where it was revealed that the total capital of 45 families had grown from hundreds of crores of rupees to thousands of crores in two decades. He warned that the country's economy would be controlled by a few if proper steps were not taken (15). Despite the President's warning, the economy is already under the control of monopoly capital, both foreign and indigenous. This can be understood only when India's post-1947 development is viewed from an international perspective.

Global corporations have not only influenced India's recent economic development but created certain concepts of development and modernization among India's elite, which are ultimately detrimental to the workers. The industrial and business elite of India which rallied against the British at the height of the national movement for its

---

[3] India has advanced far in many scientific and technological fields. Indian doctors could bring about the birth of the world's second test-tube baby. Indian scientists could explode an atomic device in 1974. India ranks third in the world in the number of engineers and scientists.

own economic ends entered into technical and financial collaboration with multinational corporations without due consideration for the long-term effects on employment generation and technological dependence. The bulk of modern Indian economic activity is centered in the metropolitan cities of Bombay, Calcutta, Madras, and New Delhi and a few large cities such as Ahmedabad, Hyderabad, Jamshedpur, Bangalore, Kanpur, and Lucknow. Most of these cities were great trading centers even during the British period, and they were developed by the colonial traders and administrators in order to streamline the gathering and export of raw materials for factories in New Castle, Liverpool, and Manchester.

The indigenous business houses and industrial enterprises which came into being during the British period could not grow independently because of imperial restrictions on expansion and tariff. But once independence was achieved, these units expanded into huge conglomerate giants, without doing anything substantial for the real producers of wealth. Heavy dependence on highly sophisticated foreign technology, finance capital, and marketing and communication techniques dominates the Indian industrial scene today. Technology has been imported without due regard for the basic needs of the large majority of people. The net result of all this economic activity has been the creation of a covert foreign colonial sector and an overt, duly legitimized internal colonial sector. The ground is now clear for the import of hazardous manufacturing processes into India. Already, the process of transferring hazards from environmental health-conscious developed countries to poorly informed developing countries has started. The industrial workers in poor countries are unaware of the dangers of high technology. And even when aware, poverty forces them to take up any job that is offered. Vinyl chloride has been found to be a lethal liver carcinogen, but B. F. Goodrich has opened a plant in India, taking advantage of the non-existence of occupational health regulations against hazardous chemicals there (16). Nearly 90 percent of the patents in India are foreign-owned (17, 18). This should open the eyes of planners and development economists to the possibility that in another decade or so, more and more hazardous technology, products, and processes will be transferred to India.

The political involvement of multinational corporations in Chile, Japan, and the Netherlands has been revealed in several investigations conducted during the past five years. There have been allegations that some multinationals have bought political influence in India. A recent study (19) published by P. Ramamurti for the Center of Indian Trade Unions indicates the involvement of the West German multinational, Siemens, in the decision-making process of the Bharat Heavy Electricals Limited (BHEL), a large public-sector undertaking in India. The study points out that,

> instead of paying attention to overcoming the weaknesses . . . the top management sought the easy way of indiscriminate import of technology, rather than relying on and encouraging the creativity of their undoubtedly talented engineers and technical personnel.

This study has revealed that it is not only the private capitalist enterprises that are subject to the influence of multinationals, but also the state-capitalist heavy industries run by the central government. If the grip of the multinationals on the top management of private and public sector undertakings is of such a magnitude in India, who can prevent the technology transfer for the manufacture of dangerous products? Already there are hundreds of multinational corporations operating in India in collaboration with national enterprises. They are so powerful that they can direct the course of politics in the country and ward off the regulatory arms of health and safety authorities. Moreover, they can treat the whole subject of occupational health in a cavalier fashion because of the huge surplus labor available at short notice and extremely low wages. Unemployment is rampant not only among the rural illiterates but also among highly educated urban youth. The products which the big companies make enjoy monopolistic markets and the government comes to their rescue with price increases whenever the modern alchemy of advanced accounts manipulation indicates a loss. The government also comes forward with special incentives and subsidies for export marketing. High technology does not generate more jobs and, more often than not, produces products affordable to a minor fraction of the huge Indian population. In many cases, manpower is curtailed by the introduction of sophisticated machinery and equipment. Since the products are made for specialized markets, Indian entrepreneurs do not have to produce goods that are to be sold nationwide in order to make a profit. Even 1 percent of the Indian population is more than the population of, say, Switzerland.

Employers still consider it an act of charity to give someone a job. Workers have unions, but almost all unions concentrate—necessarily—on wage increases. They have little knowledge of occupational health problems, nor do they have the time or the means to obtain research findings. Medical institutions do not conduct epidemiological surveys in industries. Ignorance about occupational diseases is widespread not only among workers but also among the general public. Management personnel, at least those in the top echelons, are aware of the dangers of toxic substances in the industrial environment because of their frequent interaction with foreign collaborators, but this awareness is not shared down the line. Even the middle managers on the shop floor are not aware of the hazards in the working environment. It is therefore reasonable to assume that ignorance is universal outside of the highest ranks of the management hierarchy. The general public is not informed by the mass media, or by any other institution or agency, about environmental health issues.

INDUSTRIAL LEGISLATION IN INDIA

Like many other partially industrialized former colonies of imperial powers, India has a long record of industrial legislation: most legislation that was enacted during the later decades of industrialization in England had its Indian equivalents. But having laws and regulations is one thing; their implementation is another. As early as 1850, there was an Apprentices Act in India which enabled children to get training in various crafts. But today, there is very little being done for vocational education in India. An 1853 Fatal Accidents Act provided for compensation to families for loss occasioned by death of a person "caused by actionable wrong." It remains to be seen how many factories have been indicted so far for violating safety rules. Following the first International Labor Conference in Berlin in 1890, the Indian Factories (Amendment) Act was passed in 1891, according to which children up to 14 years of age were covered by the act and children under nine were not to be employed. The working hours of children were brought down to six in textile factories and seven in other factories. Later acts brought a rise in the legal working age and a decline in the legal working hours of children. Employment of children below 12 was prohibited, and persons up to the age of 15 were considered children. Night work was prohibited for women and children. But in 1948, the working of the latest act (1934) was found defective. Even today, despite the existence of laws and regulations, there is no effective monitoring machinery to detect flaws in the implementation of the various acts. Implementation of labor laws cannot succeed because of the availability of cheap labor. Employers can flout laws with impunity when workmen acquiesce to any indignity or ill-treatment for the sake of sheer survival. Legislation becomes useless in such circumstances.

There are separate acts in India for miners and plantation workers. But again, who monitors their enforcement? Who keeps statistics of how many miners get coal workers' pneumoconiosis or silicosis? The facts that statistics are sparse, that there are no complaints from unions or workers, or that there are very few compensation claims do not establish the absence of serious occupational diseases in India. The textile industry is perhaps the oldest Indian industry, but there are few studies of brown lung disease or byssinosis among textile mill workers in India.

Occupational health is equated with labor welfare and labor legislation. Reports on workers' welfare and health are prepared without any reference to occupational diseases. There has not been any comprehensive survey of major industries in India in order to gather data on occupational diseases, compensation claims, or the like. Personnel management and labor relations institutes concentrate on Factories Acts and the size of workers' bathrooms and lockers, instead of turning their attention to medical records (or the absence of such records), unsafe and unguarded machinery, lack of ventilation and lighting, high dust accumulations, unprotected handling of hazardous chemicals which leads to various skin diseases, or the ingestion or inhalation of toxic substances at the workplace.

There is a feeling among Indian managers and the Indian intelligentsia that occupational diseases can occur only in highly advanced countries like the United States and the Soviet Union. This is quite unfounded. Vinyl chloride, carbon monoxide, asbestos, benzene, petroleum products, carbon black, cotton dust, silica, talc, fiber glass, corrosive acids, mercury, beryllium, chromium, radiation, noise, rubber chemicals, chlorinated hydrocarbons, and a host of other factors in the working environment behave the same way in workers whether they be in Madras or Manchester. The speed and consequences of their action will be enhanced by workers' malnutrition and poverty. And here, the Indian workers will be affected more than their American or Soviet counterparts. Moreover, the medical community in India is by and large not aware of the diseases caused by occupational factors. Doctors do not ask patients what kind of work they do. This is not surprising when one considers the fact that, even in the United States, it is rare to find a physician who questions patients about their occupation to determine whether their illness is job-related. Medical colleges in India do not offer courses in occupational medicine or related areas on a regular basis.

ENVIRONMENTAL POLLUTION

In industrially and educationally backward nations, the awareness about environmental pollution is also very low. The connection between environmental and ecological factors and occupational health is gradually being recognized in advanced countries, but information about it in underdeveloped countries is poor. It is a misconception among the elite of the latter countries that environmental pollution means just air pollution caused by automobile exhausts. It is assumed that since poor countries do not have a plethora of automobiles, pollution is not a serious hazard. But environmental pollution can be caused by a number of factors other than automobile exhaust fumes.

In July 1976, a reactor in a trichlorophenol manufacturing plant in Seveso, Italy, exploded and its contents escaped through a safety valve directly into the atmosphere. This resulted in the fallout of a lethal chemical, TCDD, in the village of Seveso. The inhabitants had to be evacuated, and they were asked not to return to their homes for a year because the chemical had seeped through the soil and found its way into every possible object of human contact, including walls of buildings. Blood tests showed that the residents had lost their immunity and that TCDD had serious systemic toxicity, besides teratogenic effects. If this was the case with residents outside the factory, then the question is suggested: What about the workers in such factories who spend one-third of their lifetime in hazardous environments? Are not hazardous chemicals produced and handled in Indian factories? Even agricultural workers cannot escape the direct or indirect effect of hazardous pesticides, as the following incident in a region of India will indicate.

Agricultural workers (including women and children) living in Malnad, a region of Karnataka in South India, were attacked by a crippling disease in 1971. Several years later, the state health authorities began an investigation which has now revealed, though belatedly, the depth of the problem. The finding is that the victims had consumed crabs caught from paddy fields intensively sprayed with highly toxic pesticides like folidol and endrin. The Malnad tragedy is equal in intensity to the Seveso tragedy, the "Ouch-ouch" tragedy in Japan caused by cadmium in rice, or the Minamata tragedy in which hundreds of Japanese were poisoned following the ingestion of mercury-contaminated fish.

It is very rare that the news media in India report job accidents, environmental tragedies, or occupational diseases. Lack of communication is a major stumbling block in India. Barring the *Hindu* of Madras, the front-line English newspapers ignored the Malnad tragedy, or gave it a three-line report. The *Hindu* made a fairly detailed investigation of the tragedy, and portions of its report (20) are quoted below to show how far the medical profession and the public of India have to go if occupational and environmental issues are to get the attention they deserve.

> In a space of two years from 1971, a large number of landless labouring folk . . . in . . . Malnad were stricken with this mysterious disease. . . . In January 1975 some local leaders brought to the Government Hospital at Sagar four illiterate agricultural labourers of Handigodu. . . . They complained of loss of locomotion as well as excruciating pain in the limbs. Within a week, there were 30 cases in the hospital. The key symptom reported was pain in the lower part of the body, incomprehensible

and developing. . . . They came from both sexes and their ages ranged from 4 to . . . over 40. It was only when the Sagar hospital was filled with people from the villages afflicted that the State health authorities began to act. . . .

The initial studies ruled out a neurological disorder. . . . The whole question approached the stage of minimum comprehension only after the Director-General of the Indian Council of Medical Research assigned the investigation to . . . scientists working at the National Institute of Nutrition at Hyderabad. . . . Nothing can be done to the people who have been crippled by the "Handigodu Syndrome." . . . The report [by medical scientists], couched in the businesslike language of clinical and investigative medical science, cannot convey the poignancy, the dimensions, the depth, the social significance, of the suffering of the simple labouring folk in a cluster of villages surrounding the town of Sagar. . . .

These people have no control over the conditions of their work or over the natural and social environment. They get a measly one-and-half to two rupees [26¢] for a full day's agricultural work. And this work, being seasonal, is severely restricted. Nothing called land reform has so far touched their lives. . . . The "Handigodu Syndrome" has not touched those belonging to the upper sections of society . . . who live in the same villages, but in separate quarters. . . . There has been some attempt to treat the victims, although it is certainly a reflection on the state and conscience of the public health system that it took nearly four years from the time the attack began for medical science to come ploddingly to the field. . . .

"God alone knows why this misfortune befell us," the villagers keep saying, as life goes on and they struggle to make a living.

The above represents a microcosm of the village scene in many parts of India. It took nearly six years for a tragedy of this proportion to hit the headlines in one among the 800 daily newspapers of India. And when it did, it made just one of the 75 English-language newspapers read by the elite living in metropolitan areas and large cities, far removed from the villagers and their socioeconomic problems. How many workers in other parts of India have been affected this way is not known. Also unknown is the number of victims in various industries who succumb to acute and chronic poisoning by inhalation, ingestion, or percutaneous absorption of toxic chemicals in their work environment. How can the workers' consciousness and the public's conscience be touched in such a situation? This is the major problem confronting those concerned about occupational health and safety in India, however small their number.

OCCUPATIONAL HEALTH RESEARCH

There are some research organizations in India which devote their exclusive attention to occupational health and safety. Two of the more prominent ones are the National Institute of Occupational Health (NIOH) in Ahmedabad, and the Industrial Toxicology Research Center in Lucknow. In addition, the Central Labor Institute in Bombay devotes some attention to job safety as part of its supervisory training program. The Indian Association of Occupational Health has been in existence since 1936. It started as the Society for the Study of Industrial Medicine in Jamshedpur and now has its headquarters in New Delhi. Its official organ, the *Indian Journal of Industrial Medicine,* is published from Calcutta. But India has a long way to go in the field of occupational health. The workers, managements, medical professionals, unions, labor welfare and safety organizations, and the general public have yet to be made fully aware of the impact of the industrial environment on the working and general population. Working environments in underdeveloped countries are not substantially different from those in developed countries. But those in the former are more risky because of: workers' low level of education and awareness; poor nutrition; filthy working and living conditions; high unemployment, forcing workers to accept any job; a traditional resignation to fate; employers' predatory hunger for profit accumulation; 19th-century wages for 20th-century jobs; non-correspondence between wages and prices of products; multinationals' involvement in national economic, industrial, and technological problems; government's eagerness to import high technology without evaluation of the dangers involved and effects on employment generation and technology dependence; lack of proper monitoring of existing legislation; lack of political awareness of the need for further legislation; unions' preoccupation with higher wages and workers' indifference to their own health; lack of education and training for medical personnel; outdated preventive measures and absence of modern methods to evaluate risks in modern production processes; total lack of threshold limit values/maximum permissible concentration values for most industrial chemicals; general lack of research in the areas of occupational safety, health, industrial medicine, environmental pollution, and related disciplines; all-pervasive apathy and indifference of the mass media toward workers' right to a healthy and safe working and living environment; overdependence on the legalistic approach to the question of occupational health; and prevalence of a false notion among the knowledgeable that occupational health is manageable by the existing safety compensation-factory regulations-labor welfare mechanism.

Although the above factors are applicable to most developing countries, including India, a special situation in India should be noted. It is the emergence of thousands of small-scale industrial units in industrial estates that have sprung up in small towns in many parts of India. According to a 1975 NIOH survey (21):

> [A] large variety of industries are mushrooming with the direct encouragement of the Government. This is a desirable course in the interests of the economy, democratization and employment. . . . However, we suspect that in such enterprises, a risky compromise is made to ensure economic viability. This type of industry, employing a few workers in a factory shed independently owned and operated, poses the greatest problem in the organizing of occupational health services. Factors that hinder the development of suitable health care systems are: the small industries are spread over an enormous area; they frequently use a floating population of seasonal workers; they are often genuinely ignorant of the hazards to workers; and even when a group of such industries is concentrated in an area, as an industrial park or estate, their manufacturing processes and products differ so widely that no unified approach is feasible. The NIOH is taking a close look at the small-scale industries, in order to identify problem areas, assign priorities, and develop low-cost measures to protect the workers. . . .

According to another report (22), the occupational diseases identified in Indian industries are: pneumoconiosis in coal, mica, metal and other mines; carbon disulfide poisoning in rayon factories; skin ulceration from tar, dichromate, and coke; DDT and parathion poisoning; byssinosis and chronic bronchitis in textile and jute mills; lead poisoning in printing press and storage battery manufacturing companies; dye poisoning in the dye industry; visual defects in the textile and welding industries; and noise deafness in the fertilizer industry. Of these, the diseases with the highest rates of incidence are pneumoconiosis among coal miners, mica miners, and mica processors; lead poisoning among printing press workers; insecticide poisoning; byssinosis among textile workers; and dye poisoning from naphthol derivatives, azo-dyes, and benzanthrone.

The above data are based on findings from a survey of a small fraction of the working population of India. Moreover, several industries were not included in the survey, e.g. the rubber and tire industry, metal industries, plastics industry, stone quarries, cement industry, rubber chemical industry, plantation industry, and several others.

CONCLUSIONS AND RECOMMENDATIONS

Occupational health in India is still a much neglected topic. Workers and the general public are unaware of their right to a healthy and safe working and living environment. Managements cannot be expected to take the initiative, because they have inherited a socioeconomic philosophy and system rooted in industrial oligopoly and monopolistic trading and production relations. The unions have yet to recognize the gravity of the occupational health problem. They should stress both higher wages *and* better working conditions, including safe machines, ambient air monitoring, respiratory protection, pre and postemployment medical checkups, free annual medical checkups for families, and healthy living quarters. Government has to be cautious in approving or entering into further technical and financial collaboration with multinational manufacturers who are eager to transfer dangerous products and technology to poor countries. Above all, the existing occupational health research methods and industrial survey techniques have to be expanded and improved upon considerably, with a view toward arriving at a suitable, all-inclusive act which will recognize workers' right to a safe and healthy working and living environment. The machinery for implementation of existing and future laws has to be revamped to include worker representation. Workers should also be included in the day-to-day management of factories. In addition, medical colleges and general educational institutions have to start offering courses in occupational medicine, toxicology, biomechanics, occupational safety, safety engineering, human factors engineering, environmental health, ecology, and the economics of health.

Occupational health cannot be treated in isolation; it is intrinsically interwoven with the socioeconomic and political issues confronting India. Unless total structural changes occur, children will be industrially abused and millions of Anthonyswamis and Ramasamy Iyers will continue to be killed silently by machinery, lethal chemicals, and, above all, by industrial man's inhumanity to fellow beings who are forced to sell their labor at cheap prices.

REFERENCES

1. *Hindu* (Madras). December 28, 1978.
2. Sinclair, U. B. *The Industrial Republic.* Doubleday, Page & Company, New York, 1907.
3. Vaid, K. N. *Labour Welfare in India.* Shri Ram Centre for Industrial Relations, New Delhi, 1970.

4. Berman, D. M. How cheap is a life? *Int. J. Health Serv.* 8(1): 79-99, 1978.
5. Levkovsky, A. I. *Capitalism in India: Basic Trends in Its Development.* People's Publishing House, New Delhi, 1966.
6. Worseley, P. *The Third World.* University of Chicago Press, Chicago, 1964.
7. Sau, R. K. *Indian Economic Growth: Constraints and Prospects.* Orient Longmans Ltd., Calcutta, 1973.
8. Report of the Indian Factory Labour Commission, Vol. I. Her Majesty's Stationery Office, London, 1908.
9. Report of the Textile Factories Labour Committee. Her Majesty's Stationery Office, London, 1907.
10. Indian Sugar Industry Annual, 1938.
11. Nehru, J. *Independence and After.* Publications Division, Government of India, New Delhi, 1949.
12. Report of the Committee on Distribution of Income and Levels of Living, Part I. Planning Commission, Government of India, New Delhi, 1964.
13. *Times of India* (Bombay). June 21, 1977.
14. Veit, L. A. *India's Second Revolution: The Dimensions of Development.* McGraw-Hill Book Company, New York, 1976.
15. *Hindu* (Madras). July 9, 1978.
16. Elling, R. H. Industrialization and occupational health in underdeveloped countries. *Int. J. Health Serv.* 7(2): 209-235, 1977.
17. Barnet, R. J., and Muller, R. E. *Global Reach: The Power of the Multinational Corporations.* Simon and Schuster, New York, 1974.
18. Ghosh, P. K., and Minocha, V. S. *Global Giants.* Sultan Chand & Sons, New Delhi, 1977.
19. Ramamurti, P. *Stop BHEL's Truck with Siemens.* Centre of Indian Trade Unions, New Delhi, 1978.
20. The Handigodu Syndrome of Malnad: An investigative report. *Hindu* (Madras). October 2, 1977.
21. Ramanathan, N. L., and Kashyap, S. Occupational environment and health in India. *Ambio* 4(1): 60-64, 1975.
22. Ramanathan, N. L., Gupta, M. N., Chatterjee, B. B., and Rao, M. N. *Occupational Health Research in India—A Third Review 1963-1968.* Special Report Series No. 61, Indian Council of Medical Research, New Delhi, 1970.

CHAPTER 15

The Export of Hazardous Factories to Developing Nations

Barry I. Castleman

In the next decade, the export of hazards from the United States to Third World countries is likely to increase (1). Banning of unsafe consumer products, foods, drugs, and pesticides here has often led to the subsequent export of these products. Similarly, U.S. pollution control laws and occupational health standards may soon lead to wholesale exodus in major industries, as manufacturers move overseas to avoid the large costs imposed here while continuing to sell their products in the United States.

Typically, several years elapse from the time of the discovery that a high-volume chemical causes serious disease at low levels of exposure until the time that appropriate regulations are implemented to protect workers and communities. In many of our most polluting and hazardous industries, existing plants are very old and incapable of being made safe by adding on control devices. These plants need to be redesigned and rebuilt, not just fitted with exhaust fans. Faced with this reality, some manufacturers find it economically attractive to move hazardous manufacturing plants to less

Much of this text was entered in the June 29, 1978 *Congressional Record* by Representative David Obey. The research spans a five-year period, during which support was provided by the National Resources Defense Council, Environmental Defense Fund, United Steelworkers of America, and the U.S. Congress Office of Technology Assessment.

restrictive locales rather than stay where they are and meet tough regulations. Today "runaway hazardous shops" are leaving the United States, whereas in the past they only crossed state boundaries within the country.

Of course, there is not usually a one-for-one correspondence between plants closed in the U.S. and foreign sources of supply opened. Nor are all foreign plants that export to the U.S. from nonregulating countries owned by multinational firms. However, the economy of hazard export is emerging as a driving force in new plant investment in many hazardous and polluting industries.

As Table 1 shows, pollution control costs are much higher in the United States than they are elsewhere. American industrial companies are spending twice as much for air and water pollution control in the U.S. as they spend overseas, in terms of pollution control expenditures as a percent of capital spending. These figures are actually a conservative indication of the true disparity since worker protection, solid waste disposal, and land reclamation (mining) are counted in the non-pollution-control share of capital spending.

It is inescapable that, as manufacturers in industrial nations are forced to absorb the economic burdens of preventing and compensating occupational and environmental diseases caused by their operations, pressures favoring hazard export will increase. National efforts to implement environmental controls for hazardous industries may have to be complemented by measures that prevent the mere displacement of killer industries to "export platforms" in nonregulating countries. Poverty and ignorance make communities in many parts of the world quite vulnerable to the exploitation implicit in hazard export.

Asbestos Textiles and Friction Products

Occupational and environmental exposure to asbestos in this century has been the cause of a monumental tragedy whose full extent is not yet known. In the United States, the number of people now living who worked with asbestos and will someday develop cancer as a result has been conservatively estimated at 400,000 (2). In the past five years, the asbestos industry has faced increasing regulation of workplace exposure and pollution. The regulations show no sign of abating, following as they do a steadily growing body of knowledge about the effects and prevalence of "low-level exposure."

Historically, asbestos manufacturing has been done in industrial nations, and the United States has been a world leader. Now that industrial nations are applying increasingly costly controls, some of their asbestos manufacturing industries are declining. In 1975, the National Institute for Occupational Safety and Health (NIOSH) noted that the U.S. asbestos textile industry faced mounting competition from imports (3):

> Foreign facilities, which may be owned by domestic companies, typically have a competitive advantage over domestic producers since they do not have to pay for environmental controls capable of meeting the OSHA [Occupational Safety and Health Administration] standards. Consumers are already turning to foreign suppliers for dry processed asbestos products which have been discontinued by domestic producers in order to comply with OSHA standards.

Table 1

Investment by U.S. firms for air and water pollution control, 1975-1977[a]

| Industry | Overseas Pollution Control Expenditures (Millions of Dollars) | | | Pollution Control Expenditures as Percent of Capital Spending | | | | | |
| | | | | Overseas | | | United States | | |
	Actual 1975	Actual 1976	Planned 1977	Actual 1975	Actual 1976	Planned 1977	Actual 1975	Actual 1976	Planned 1977
Primary metals	43	57	45	9.8	15.0	8.5	19.7	20.4	16.0
Machinery	67	73	89	2.4	2.6	3.1	2.3	4.1	6.1
Electrical machinery	33	17	21	3.7	2.0	2.0	4.2	4.8	3.8
Autos, trucks, and parts	44	90	99	3.5	7.4	6.7	5.7	4.8	4.0
Other transportation equipment	2	2	2	4.7	4.9	4.6	4.3	4.6	4.1
Fabricated metals	18	14	14	4.9	4.4	3.0	9.0	9.3	5.8
Chemicals	138	144	113	5.3	5.5	6.1	8.9	12.3	11.8
Paper	83	46	26	11.8	7.9	5.7	21.9	25.7	25.8
Rubber	10	9	17	2.6	2.7	3.9	4.8	5.7	7.3
Stone, clay, and glass	32	15	30	8.0	4.6	5.0	17.6	9.0	7.5
Foods and beverages	18	14	40	2.6	2.1	4.6	5.3	7.3	4.7
Textile and misc. manufacturing	4	32	28	0.6	5.6	4.6	5.4	6.0	4.8
All manufacturing	492	513	524	4.4	4.8	4.6	9.8	10.7	9.0
Petroleum	500	419	478	5.1	4.5	4.7	12.8	7.5	6.4
Mining	43	56	122	3.9	6.2	12.7	8.2	7.0	5.2
All industry	1,035	988	1,124	4.7	4.7	5.0	10.3	9.8	8.4

[a] Sources, *Overseas Operations of U.S. Industrial Companies, 1976-1978 and 1977-1979*, McGraw-Hill Economics Department, New York.

The earliest runaway hazardous shops jumped state borders, as noted previously. Jones (4) reported that asbestos manufacturing firms were forced to pay very high rates for worker's compensation insurance in 1935 in New York State. Private insurers, some of whom had refused to sell life insurance to asbestos workers as long ago as 1918, were turning down the asbestos firms as unacceptable risks for worker's compensation insurance (4, 5). In 1936, Jones noted (4):

> As a consequence of these very high rates and the inability of some industries to get any kind of insurance at a price that permits continuance of operations, many establishments are laying off workmen and either closing down or sending their hazardous work out of the state.

Brodeur's book, *Expendable Americans* (6), describes an extremely hazardous asbestos insulation plant that was moved from New Jersey to Texas in 1954. Follow-up of former plant workers in New Jersey has shown that an excessive incidence of fatal lung cancer has occurred in men employed there for one month and less (7). By 1965, it was established that cancer rates among asbestos workers were extremely high; moreover, even family members of asbestos workers and neighbors of asbestos plants were dying of asbestos-related cancers (8-10).

The current U.S. workplace asbestos standard took effect on July 1, 1976. However, it was a scheduled reduction in the standard issued June 7, 1972; in other words, the Occupational Safety and Health Administration (OSHA) gave U.S. manufacturers four years to lower the asbestos dust levels in their plants from 5 million to 2 million fibers per cubic meter of air (11). Perceiving that further reductions were necessary to reduce asbestos workers' cancer risk, OSHA proposed on October 9, 1975 to lower the standard to 500,000 fibers per cubic meter (12). This was followed at the end of 1976 with a recommendation by NIOSH to lower the standard still further to the lower limit of detection by optical microscopy—100,000 fibers per cubic meter. NIOSH acknowledged that there is probably still an increased risk of cancer at that level of exposure (13).[1] OSHA will promulgate the new standard in 1980.

The asbestos industry responded to OSHA's 1975 proposal by submitting a consultant report (14) that said the asbestos textile industry and many other asbestos manufacturers would be unable to comply with the proposed 500,000 fiber limit. The report concluded that even with implementation of the best available technology, the achievement of an exposure limit of 500,000 fibers per cubic meter would not be feasible for 65 percent of the manufacturers' processing steps. The consultant forecasted that the already depressed domestic asbestos textile industry would suffer an accelerated decline, with mounting imports from countries with weaker regulations. Foreign competition is intense, and imports already supply 35 percent of U.S. demand, the report noted (14).

Penetration of the domestic asbestos friction products industry (e.g. brake linings) was also predicted if the proposed OSHA standard is implemented. The report said

---

[1] The workplace standards apply only to the largest airborne fibers, since the fibers are counted using light microscopes. Duplicate sample analyses with electron microscopy have typically shown that for every fiber seen with a light microscope, there are 100 or more submicroscopic-sized fibers present. Unfortunately, electron microscopy is very costly and few labs are equipped for it; thus it is not suitable for routine monitoring of compliance with workplace standards.

that the United States has already begun to import asbestos friction products from Korea. The U.S. friction products industry employs more workers than any other asbestos manufacturing industry (14). Raybestos-Manhattan, a leading manufacturer of asbestos textiles and friction products, declared in its 1976 Annual Report (15) that the NIOSH recommendation to OSHA was "so extreme as to be totally unrealistic and impracticable." The report went on to note (15):

> The escalating costs associated with handling this raw material and the uncertain consequences of future government asbestos regulations ... have necessitated our decision to work toward the elimination of asbestos from all our friction products and this eventuality has become an essential part of our long-term product and manufacturing plans.

Most of the company's business is in friction products.

In Cork, Ireland, Raybestos has just built a plant to produce 10 million disc brake pads a year for export primarily to countries in the European Economic Community. This plant apparently conforms to all existing (if not all pending) U.S. standards of control. As the $8 million plant was completed, the local community held a large meeting and set up an investigating committee. Early in 1977, the residents' committee issued a report declaring that the factory "constitutes a major health risk to the local population which we regard as totally unacceptable." The residents were alarmed about hazards to the community from the plant's air pollution and solid waste dumping, as well as hazards to workers. The residents now appear to be equally divided on whether to accept the 30 to 100 jobs the plant would provide if allowed to open (16). Citizens have challenged government approvals of the plant and dump sites in the courts.

Abex Corporation, a U.S. subsidiary of the British-based Imperial Chemical Industries, recently built an asbestos friction products plant in Madras, India. In 1976, the plant was covered by over $1 million in political risk insurance by the Overseas Private Investment Corporation (OPIC), an agency of the U.S. government. OPIC, whose mission is to promote needed U.S. industrial investment in developing nations, made no effort to obtain an accounting of measures that would be taken to protect workers in the design and operation of the plant. Abex replied to OPIC's perfunctory question on ecological effects by simply stating, "The company will comply with governmental regulations regarding wastage disposal" (17).

The torrent of health-related regulations for U.S. asbestos manufacturers could have been anticipated at the outset of this decade with the passage of the Occupational Safety and Health Act and the Clean Air Amendments of 1970. There is no end yet in sight: in March 1977, the Environmental Protection Agency (EPA) announced that asbestos would be one of 15 substances targeted for priority attention under the Toxic Substances Control Act of 1976. In addition to worker's compensation premiums and numerous environmental control regulations, the asbestos industry incurs the expense of high wages in the U.S., where regulations require that asbestos workers be informed of the mortal hazards of asbestos, given regular medical examinations, and monitored to assure that their exposure does not violate the standard.

U.S. imports of asbestos textiles have soared since 1970 (Fig. 1). Prior to that time over 99 percent of U.S. asbestos textile imports came from Canada, Europe, and Japan. Imports from these "regulating countries" stayed at around 3 million pounds

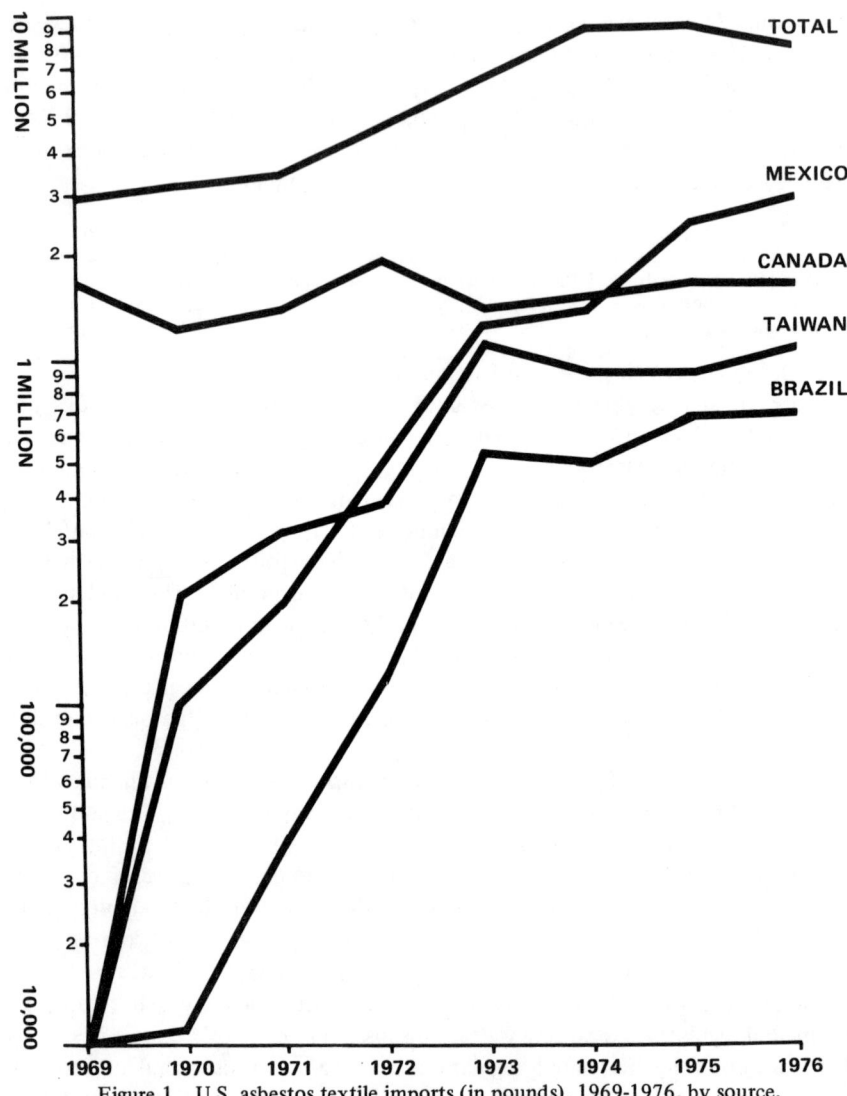

Figure 1. U.S. asbestos textile imports (in pounds), 1969-1976, by source.

per year in the years 1970-1976, while total imports from Mexico, Taiwan, and Brazil shot up to nearly 4.5 million pounds in 1976 (18).

The Asbestos Textile Institute reports that its membership included seven U.S. primary producers in 1972; currently only three U.S. primary asbestos textile producers are member companies of the organization. Fiber consumption of the U.S. asbestos textile industry fell precipitously after 1974 (Fig. 2). The depressed state of the U.S. industry is further indicated by the steep drop in U.S. imports of textile-grade

‖‖‖‖ U.S. IMPORTS OF TEXTILE GRADE ASBESTOS FIBER

■ U.S. EXPORTS OF ASBESTOS TEXTILES

(MILLIONS OF POUNDS)

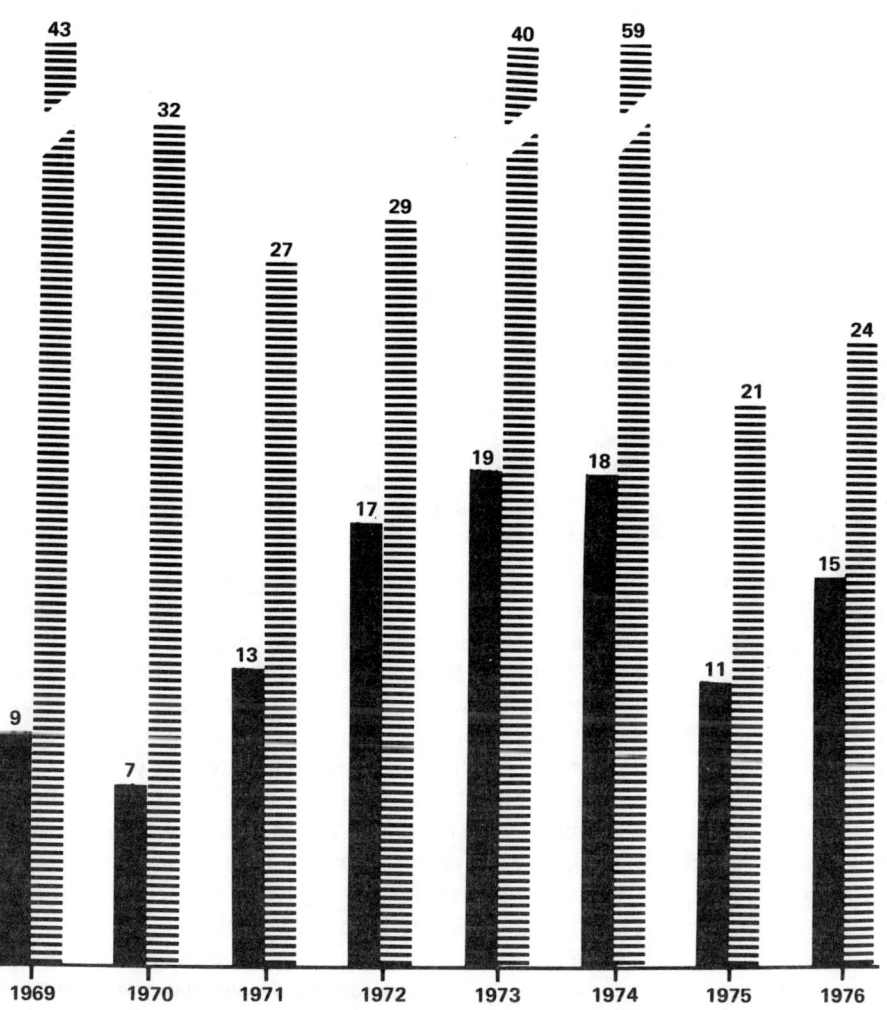

Figure 2. U.S. asbestos textiles exports, 1969-1976. This includes 4 million pounds to Mexico in 1976, most of which was processed and reimported by Amatex. Also shown are total U.S. imports of textile-grade asbestos fiber during the same period, including crudes and spinning fibers. Sources, United States Department of Commerce, Asbestos Textile Imports, TSUSA 518.2100, Asbestos Textile Exports, Sch. B 663.8120; United States Bureau of Mines.

asbestos fiber after 1974 (Fig. 2). Despite the fact that there were major strikes at the Canadian mines in 1975 and general economic conditions were poor that year, the continued depressed level of textile fiber imports in 1976 signifies that the U.S. asbestos textile industry has diminished in size. In 1976, one of the remaining U.S. manufacturers, Southern Asbestos, closed one plant and consolidated all operations at its other textile facility.

In 1972, Amatex, a firm based in Norristown, Pennsylvania, closed a new (opened in 1967) asbestos yarn mill in Milford Square, Pennsylvania (19). Since 1969, Amatex has operated an asbestos textile plant in Agua Prieta, a small town just across the Mexican border from Douglas, Arizona. The company owns another asbestos textile plant in Ciudad Juarez, across the border from El Paso, Texas (20). In December 1974, Amatex began to import asbestos textiles into the U.S. from the Juarez plant. Amatex "imported" about 2 million pounds of asbestos textiles from its Mexican border plants in 1975, about one-fourth of U.S. imports from the entire world in that year (21). The asbestos fiber used by the Amatex mills in Mexico comes from Canada; there are no asbestos mines in Mexico. Workers are paid the minimum wage.

In March 1977, a reporter from the *Arizona Daily Star* and a prominent industrial health specialist, Dr. William Johnson, visited the Agua Prieta plant. They saw part of the interior of the plant, and the reporter gave the following account of conditions (20):

> Asbestos waste clings to the fence that encloses the brick plant and is strewn across the dirt road behind the plant where children walk to school.
> Inside, machinery that weaves yarn into industrial fabric is caked with asbestos waste and the floor covered with debris. Workers in part of the factory do not wear respirators that could reduce their exposure to asbestos dust.

The *Arizona Daily Star* story was reprinted in Spanish in an Agua Prieta news-paper, and the workers in the plant called for an investigation, which was started by Sonora (state) health officials.[2] Workers must now wear uniforms to cover their street clothes and are required to leave them at the plant so their families will not be endangered. However, none of the workers have quit, and due to the scarcity of jobs, the union reportedly pressured the workers to be silent. The union, which is known for its alliance with management, has threatened workers with loss of their jobs if the complaints continue. Since publication of the first news article, the factory exterior has been cleaned regularly so there are no longer threads of asbestos clinging to the fence behind the building. However, Dr. Johnson said the company's improve-ments were "cosmetic," pointing out that clumps of asbestos fiber could still be seen on the road behind the plant and shrubs in nearby lots (22).

In September 1977, a Texas television team visited the three-year-old Amatex plant in Juarez. A worker, whose identity was concealed, said that he had not been warned that he could develop a fatal disease from breathing asbestos. He went on to describe the plant as having no dust controls in the dustiest parts, and said no

---

[2]It is unlikely that any of the Aqua Prieta workers have already developed symptoms of asbestosis. Asbestosis rarely appears until 10 or more years after the onset of exposure. Cancer rarely appears until more than 20 years have elapsed since the onset of exposure, even in cases of continuous exposure.

provisions were taken by management to provide workers with functioning respiratory protection or a change of clothes for work. Dust levels in the plant were not monitored; in its U.S. plants, Amatex has been required since 1972 to monitor fiber levels in the workplace air at least twice a year and to make the data available to workers. Despite repeated attempts, the television reporter was unable to get Amatex president and principal stockholder, John Rainey, to submit to an interview. After Juarez newspapers carried stories linking asbestos to cancer, about 25 workers quit working for Amatex out of fear for their health (23).

Mexico does not have specific regulations to protect workers from asbestos. The 1945 Regulations on Work Health have general provisions that workplaces using toxic or suffocating substances must display posters warning workers of the dangers to which they are exposed, and they must provide adequate protective means to the workers. The fine for not having warning posters and protective equipment may be no more than 1000 pesos (U.S. $45), up to 2000 pesos for a failure to take corrective action within the specified timetable. Mexico does not have specific regulations for control of asbestos air and water pollution. By contrast, the State of California began last year to implement its Occupational Carcinogens Control Act of 1976, which provides fines of $1000 for violations and $5000 for repeated violations of carcinogen standards at least as stringent as OSHA's. California also authorized $1 million for the first six months of 1977 to assure that the law would be enforced (24). OSHA has in the past assessed smaller fines, but under the law could fine employers up to $1,000 for serious violations and up to $10,000 for repeated or willful violations (25).

The Amatex plant in Meredith, New Hampshire, was until late 1977 unable to comply with the OSHA standard promulgated in 1972. This plant has just attained the degree of control required by OSHA as of July 1976. It is possible that Amatex, with its long record of repeated and serious OSHA violations, will close in New Hampshire rather than meet the further reductions of the OSHA standard recently proposed.

Raybestos-Manhattan, on the other hand, has invested $11 million in a modern wet process for making asbestos yarn in the U.S. in compliance with OSHA standards. In its 1975 report to stockholders, Raybestos acknowledged that foreign competition from nonregulating countries is a serious threat to domestic asbestos textile manufacturers. In 1974, Raybestos bought a 47 percent share of an asbestos textile plant in Venezuela. John Marsh, the company's chief of environmental affairs, claims that the Venezuelan plant operates at airborne asbestos levels lower than the peak level allowed in the U.S. by the current OSHA standard.

One of the U.S. customers of the Venezuelan plant had been Standco Industries, a Texas firm. In 1975, Standco turned to two plants in Spain for over 400,000 pounds of asbestos textiles; 1976 statistics on overall imports by country suggest that Standco is now buying most of its asbestos textiles from Mexico.

Taiwan and South Korea have been displacing Japan as a source of asbestos textiles for the United States, as this industry has come under regulation in Japan. The plant in Taiwan and one of the plants in South Korea exporting to the U.S. are owned by the Japanese firm, Nippon Asbestos. In 1976, Taiwan shipped 1 million pounds of asbestos textiles to the United States. The U.S. importer of record for asbestos textiles from Taiwan and Korea is the Japanese global trading company, Mitsui (21). These asbestos textiles may also be made largely from Canadian asbestos fiber. There are no specific health regulations for asbestos in South Korea. Taiwan's ceiling limit of 2 milligrams per cubic meter of air amounts to classifying asbestos as little more than a nuisance dust.

Brazil is the other country that supplies large quantities of asbestos textiles to the United States. There, a 1965 law established a scheme of hazard-pay increments for various industries. The law provides for three levels of wage premiums to be paid in a number of industries, determined by the official hazard class for each industry. Asbestos textile manufacture is not even listed; asbestos brake shoe and asbestos cement manufacture are rated as medium among hazardous industries. The maximum hazard-pay increment is 40 percent of the minimum wage, which might be a 20 percent increase over base pay for a typical worker. If the labor courts find that the hazard has been eliminated or controlled, the pay increases are discontinued accordingly.

By making hazardous work economically attractive and by making workers suffer pay cuts in exchange for improved working conditions, the law undermines all efforts to improve working conditions in hazardous industries. Management has the choice of taking steps to protect workers or paying them extra for losing their health, and presumably does whichever costs less. The concerned worker has little choice but to accept management's terms or look elsewhere for a job. This law is fertile soil for the growth of hazardous industries.

Mexico, Brazil, Taiwan, and South Korea are among the developing nations that recently have been declared "beneficiary countries" under the generalized preference system for tariffs on U.S. imports. Some of the asbestos textiles from these countries enter the U.S. duty-free, and the standard 4 percent duty is charged for the rest.

The Johns-Manville Corporation is the leading producer of asbestos fiber in the Western Hemisphere. Johns-Manville sales policy includes the following statement:

> We will reserve the right to refuse to sell asbestos fiber to customers who fail to meet applicable governmental regulations on asbestos exposure and thereby endanger the health of their employees, and expose Johns-Manville to unwarranted liability. In countries where there are no governmental regulations on asbestos exposure, accepted industrial hygiene practice shall apply.

The effect of this policy so far has been to assist Johns-Manville customers in complying with government standards, primarily in the United States. Johns-Manville officials do not make a point of visiting many of their far-flung customer plants around the world, however. Johns-Manville has dropped out of the asbestos textile business and is now producing only enough material to support the firm's needs for its other product lines.

The United States has long been a world leader in manufactured asbestos products, with manufacturing plants in the eastern U.S. drawing fiber from the large asbestos mines in Quebec. Little asbestos is mined in the U.S. Consumption of asbestos textiles for the U.S. economy is believed to have declined slightly in recent years, owing to the loss of some older markets to substitute materials and failure to develop new markets. However, no figures are available.

Arsenic and Refined Copper from Primary Smelters

On January 21, 1975, OSHA proposed to lower the workplace limit for airborne arsenic exposure from 500 to 4 micrograms per cubic meter of air in light of mounting reports on the carcinogenicity of inorganic arsenic (26). NIOSH recommended that OSHA adopt a standard of only 2 micrograms per cubic meter (27). In June 1976, OSHA released an Inflationary Impact Statement on its proposed standard, which would have its most severe impact on nonferrous smelters, especially copper smelters (28). Arsenic is present in copper ores, and a few copper smelters are designed to recover arsenic trioxide ("white arsenic") as a byproduct from high-arsenic ores.

The only U.S. producer of arsenic is Asarco's copper smelter in Tacoma, Washington. OSHA determined that this plant, which has supplied about half of domestic arsenic demand, would alone incur a $9.9 million annual cost to meet the standard. OSHA estimated that even if the workplace standard was set as high as 50 micrograms per cubic meter, Asarco's annual compliance cost would be $7.4 million (28). At hearings held in Washington, D.C. in September 1976, Asarco representatives said they would close the plant rather than achieve the proposed 4 microgram limit, at a cost, they said, of more than $15 million per year (29). The final standard of 10 micrograms per cubic meter was issued by OSHA on May 5, 1978.

Asarco's Tacoma smelter is also a major source of community exposure to arsenic air pollution. The application of available technology for the improved control of arsenic air pollution would put Asarco to considerable additional expense. Epidemiologists at the National Cancer Institute reported that in the period 1950 to 1969, mortality for lung cancer in U.S. counties with copper, lead, and zinc smelting and refining was significantly higher than in other counties: the researchers believed that arsenic air pollution was a contributing cause to the high rate (30).

Previous reports have demonstrated excess rates of lung cancer among smelter workers and workers exposed to arsenical pesticides (31, 32). Community exposures to inorganic arsenic near the Tacoma smelter are within an order of magnitude of the limit proposed by OSHA for the workplace, and high urinary arsenic levels have been reported in children who live near the smelter (33). Soil for miles around nonferrous smelters is ruined permanently from years of being rained on with metallic pollutants; road dust and playgrounds are likewise contaminated. It is likely that before 1980 EPA will promulgate rules requiring best available technology for the control of arsenic air pollution from smelters.

Asarco's Tacoma smelter is now in violation of sulfur oxide air pollution standards. The maximum degree of sulfur oxide control achieved by existing equipment is only 51 percent. A consultant has determined that any EPA requirements for additional sulfur oxide controls, coupled with the expected workplace arsenic standard, would make continued operation of the smelter unprofitable. EPA is trying to determine whether to approve Asarco's request for a five-year variance from complying with the sulfur oxide standards.

The smelter will probably not be allowed to operate as it does now for much longer. Already Asarco has taken steps to reduce the amount of arsenic processed at the plant. In early 1976, Asarco terminated its agreements with other companies to accept high-arsenic residues from their nonferrous smelters. As a result, Anaconda's Montana copper smelter has been stockpiling high-arsenic dusts such as those recovered by air pollution dust collectors. Anaconda has also given money to support university research on what to do to process the dusts. Asarco Tacoma still takes the Asarco Montana lead smelter's "speiss," which is 20 percent arsenic and 50 to 60 percent copper.

Two-thirds of the copper produced at Tacoma is made from ore mined in the southwestern United States and scrap. This ore is low in arsenic. Asarco could alleviate its principal problem at Tacoma if it is able to shift further in the direction of using low-arsenic raw materials. However, this would have the effect of selectively exporting the production of arsenic byproduct to copper smelters in other countries.

The remaining sources of raw materials processed at Tacoma are high-arsenic copper ore concentrates from the Philippines and Peru (34). Due to Asarco's unwillingness to renew its contract for Philippine ore, Lepanto Consolidated Mining Company has started constructing a copper smelter in the Philippines that will produce 8,800 tons per year of byproduct arsenic trioxide, beginning in 1980 (35). In 1973, over 60 percent of the arsenic trioxide produced at Tacoma came from Philippine ores (34). The high-arsenic concentrates from Peru are from a marginal mining venture owned entirely by Asarco.

Asarco might be pleased to divert some of its arsenic business to Mexico. Asarco retains a 34 percent interest in a metal and coal mining and refining company called Industrial Minera Mexico (IMM). IMM's copper smelter, formerly Asarco Mexicana, is in San Luis Potosi, about 500 miles from Laredo, Texas. This smelter has been a steady source of arsenic trioxide for the U.S. market, and is the sole source of arsenic trioxide from Mexico. In 1976, 89 percent of U.S. imports of arsenic trioxide came from the IMM smelter (36) (Table 2). This smelter is designed to handle high-arsenic raw materials, and its arsenic output could be increased without any expansion of copper capacity if the plant receives "dirtier" raw materials in the future than it has in the past. It could process residues from U.S. smelters and high-arsenic ore concentrates from Peru, to produce more arsenic for the U.S. market.

Table 2

U.S. imports of arsenic trioxide, 1973-1976 (in tons)

Country of Origin	1973	1974	1975	1976
France	1,281	480	595	462
Mexico	5,605	6,185	3,174	3,793
Republic of South Africa	409	145	—	—
South West Africa	—[a]	—	970	—
Sweden	6,144	6,889	7,172	3
Other	57	43	102	3
Total	13,496	13,742	12,013	4,261

[a] Dashes indicate zero imports.

A newer source of arsenic is Namibia (South West Africa), where a U.S. mining firm, Amax, owns 30 percent of a nonferrous mining and smelting complex. This operation, Tsumeb, supplied 8 percent of U.S. arsenic imports in 1975 (Table 2).

In Sweden, workplace and pollution controls were cited as a reason for reduced production of arsenic in 1975 compared to 1974. The Swedish government approved expansion of the Boligen smelter in 1975, so increased output of arsenic may accompany increased copper output. The expansion plan includes $40 million worth of environmental controls (37).

Thus, it appears that even if Asarco does not close the Tacoma smelter, this sole U.S. source of arsenic will have to reduce its output. High-arsenic residues from other U.S. smelters may be shipped to Mexico for refining, with reimportation of the arsenic trioxide. Imports of arsenic from the Philippines can be expected after 1980, along with increased imports from traditional suppliers (Mexico, France, Sweden), and perhaps from other new sources.

There also may be shifts in manufacturing by firms seeking to escape the new OSHA arsenic regulations. Arsenic is used to make pesticides, herbicides, wood preservatives, and soda-lime glass (28). Sources and uses of arsenic in the U.S. economy are shown in Figure 3.

Though U.S. arsenic imports have declined since 1975, domestic demand for arsenic, particularly for making pesticides used on the cotton crop, is again on the increase. In long-term forecasts by the U.S. Bureau of Mines, both U.S. and world arsenic consumption are slated to increase slightly by the year 2000, with U.S. consumption remaining at roughly half of world consumption (34).

In a 1975 report from the U.S. Secretary of Commerce to the President (38), the costs of sulfur oxide air pollution controls for copper smelters in the U.S. were compared with the corresponding costs in Canada and South America (Peru, Chile). The pollution control costs were computed as a cost increase of 6.6 cents per pound of copper in the U.S., 2.5 cents per pound of copper in Canada, and 0.5 cents per pound of copper in South America. As the price of copper then was about 65 cents per pound, the report concluded that control costs would "impair the industry's ability to finance new productive capacity and compete in an expanding world market with relatively unencumbered foreign competitors" (38). In its calculations, the Department of Commerce did not take account of additional control costs for particulate air pollutant emissions, occupational exposure to arsenic, and water pollution—which are substantial in the United States.

EPA closed a Kennecott copper smelter in Nevada in 1976 after rejecting the company's plans for meeting air emission standards. The plant was not reopened until six months later, after a preliminary injunction against the EPA ruling was granted by a federal district judge (39).

The Bureau of Mines considered the effect of air pollution regulations to be a critical factor in limiting U.S. smelter output during a period of high demand for copper (40):

> The 1972 and 1973 shortage of capacity to process available concentrates at several smelters appeared to be partly due to a curtailment of maximum operation to comply with existing pollution control regulations and to delays in expansion of facilities owing to uncertainties regarding resolution of the pollution problem.

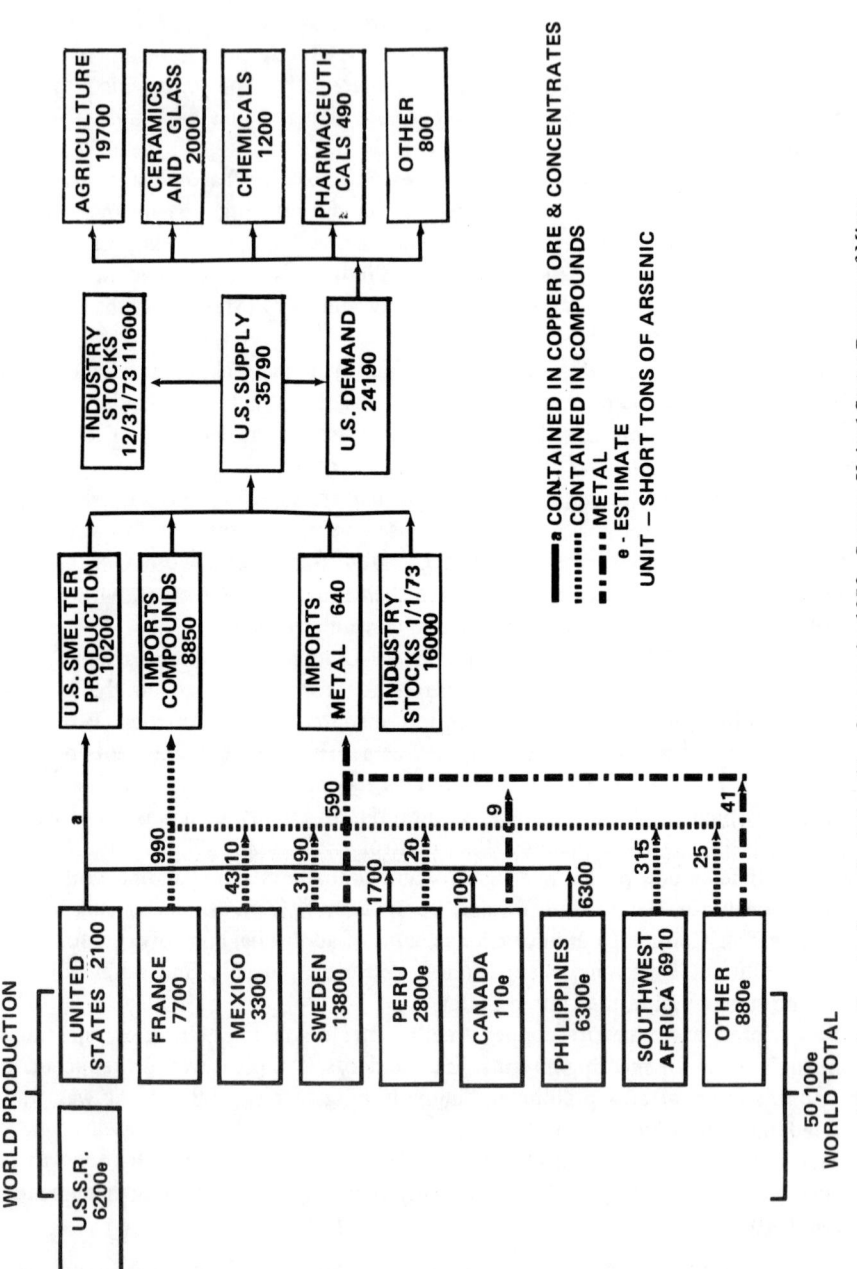

Figure 3. Supply-demand relationships for arsenic, 1973. Source, United States Bureau of Mines.

284

Smelted copper is called blister copper. It is further processed into refined copper. A small but growing amount of copper is produced directly from ores in electrolytic refineries. Some copper is also reclaimed from scrap. However, in order to assess U.S. dependence on foreign sources of copper smelted from ore, the best indicator is net imports of refined plus blister copper (Fig. 4). This indicator peaked at 392,000 tons in 1974, two to three times the volumes recorded in preceding years. Recovering from the economic downturn in 1975, net U.S. imports of refined and blister copper reached over 300,000 tons in 1976. That year, one-third of record U.S. imports of refined copper, 120,000 tons, came from Zambia (41). It is too early to say whether there is any trend toward increased U.S. dependence on foreign copper smelters, however.

One nickel-copper mining and smelting complex in Botswana, partly owned by the U.S.-based Amax, is now being expanded. Amax's 25 percent share is backed with political risk insurance from the Overseas Private Investment Corporation (42). Careless initial planning has led to costly delays in the project, extended shutdown of the sulfur recovery unit, and unanticipated heat stress among workers mining the chemically unstable ore. The Botswana government had to go to great expense to build the infrastructure (roads and a town) needed to operate this smelter at its remote location. The position of the new town relative to the smelter was designed to minimize the potential air pollution hazard to the town. Unfortunately, this planning, which was done by the World Bank and the U.S. Agency for International Development, utilized wind direction data from a place 80 miles away—where the winds were not the same as those at the smelter location. The result is that in late 1977, the town was needlessly exposed to air pollution from the smelter, whose sulfur recovery unit was still not working.

Mercury Mining

Pollution control regulations have led to a worldwide reduction in demand for mercury, increased recycling of the metal, and a steep decline in price. Between 1969 and 1976, the number of producing mercury mines in the U.S. went from 109 to 4. Domestic demand for mercury refined from ore bottomed out in 1972 and was carried down by the economic downturn of 1975 but is rising again (Fig. 5). Extremely depressed prices probably account for the shift in sources of U.S. imports since 1974 away from Canada and Mexico where large reserves exist. Most of the imports for 1975 and 1976 were from Italy, Algeria, Yugoslavia, and Spain. Industries in most, if not all, of these countries are nationalized and have accumulated stockpiles while operating at a loss. In 1976, though domestic mine output was spurred by the opening of a large new mine in Nevada, imports accounted for 69 percent of U.S. consumption (43).

Mercury was designated as a hazardous air pollutant in 1971 in the United States, and national emission standards for mercury ore-processing plants were promulgated in 1973. Small mercury producers, once numerous, are not expected to expend the capital costs necessary to control their air pollution, and barring major price increases for mercury, small U.S. producers will never again be an important factor in the market (44).

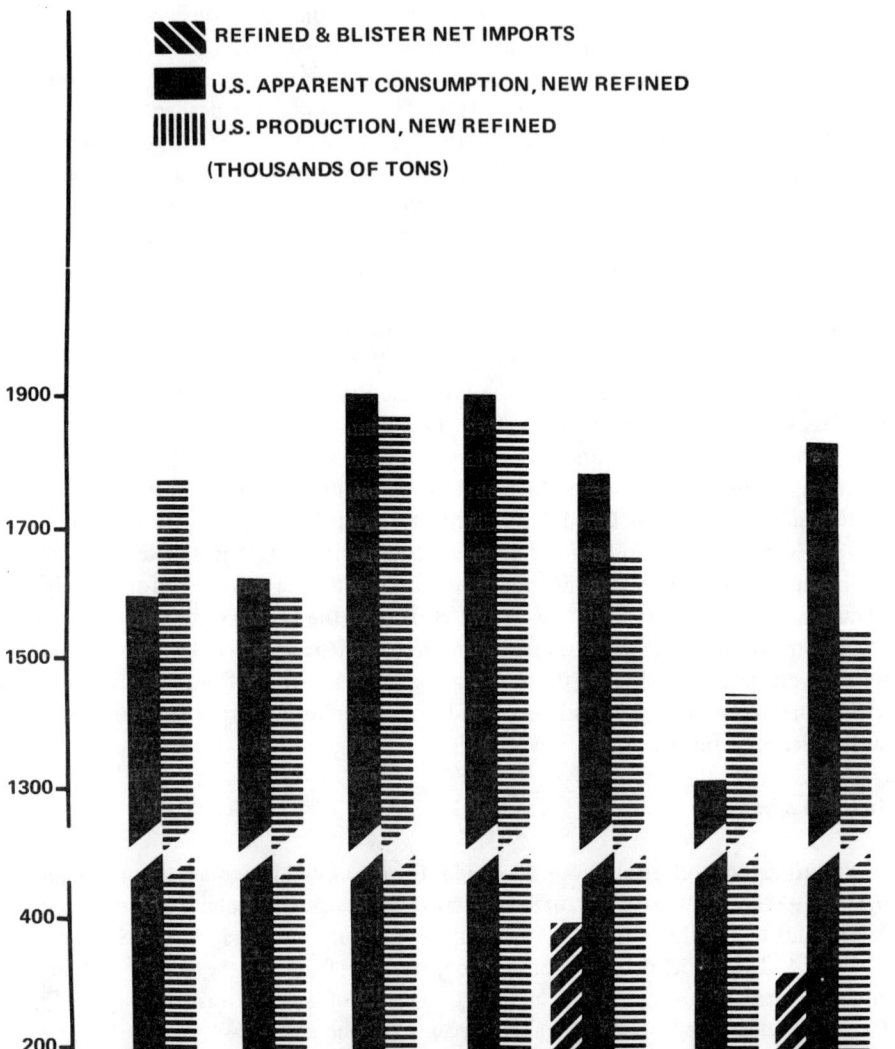

Figure 4. U.S. imports of refined and blister copper, and production and apparent consumption of new refined copper, 1970-1976. Source, United States Bureau of Mines.

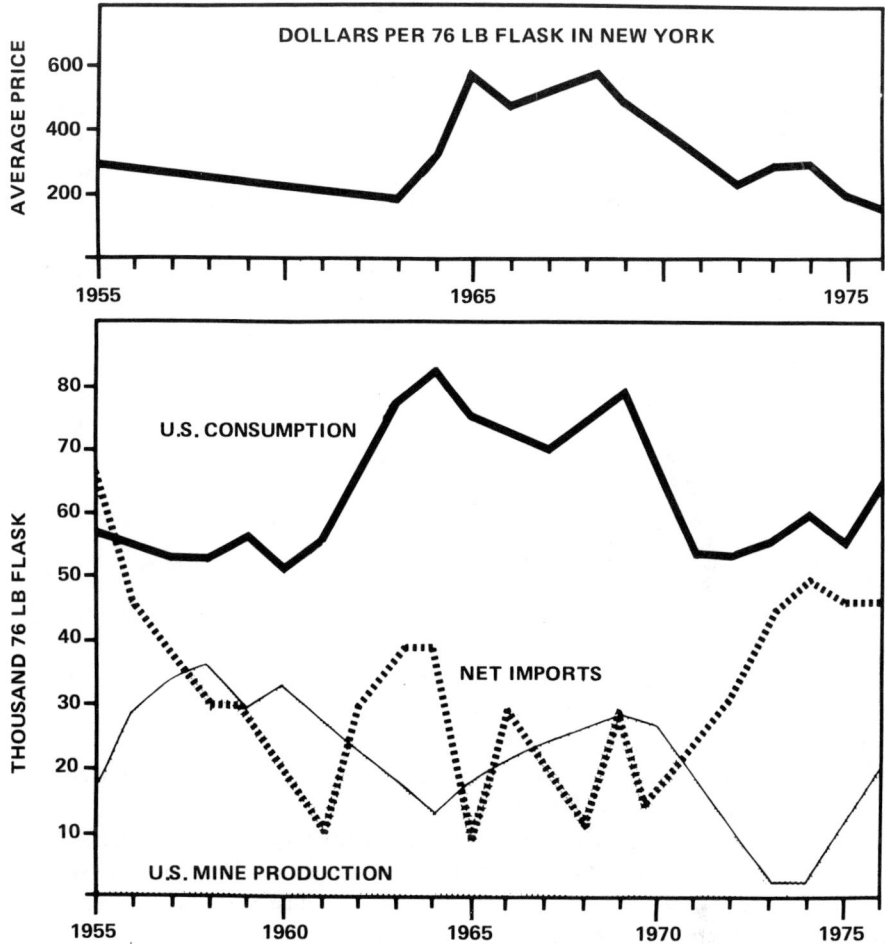

Figure 5. U.S. consumption, net imports, and average price of mercury, 1955-1976. Source, United States Bureau of Mines.

Lead Smelters and Battery Plants

The major U.S. lead industries will experience a great economic impact after OSHA enforces its new lead standard. The standard, issued November 14, 1978, was immediately tied up in court challenges by industry. Primary smelters (extraction of metal from ores), secondary smelters (scrap recycling/refining), and lead acid battery plants are mostly old, and many cannot even achieve compliance with the existing workplace standards.

NIOSH surveys in late 1975 at the Bunker Hill lead and zinc smelting complex revealed widespread violations of existing workplace standards for lead and cadmium (45). A clinical study of workers in two Indianapolis secondary lead smelters (NL Industries and RSR Quemetco) in 1976 revealed that most had a history of elevated blood lead levels and many had taken chelation drugs to be able to work at all (46). Lead poisoning has also been reported among children of lead-exposed workers, caused by household contamination by dust brought home on workers' clothes and shoes (47).

In January 1976, the State of California fined a Prestolite auto battery plant $45,000, prompting the firm's attorney to tell the *New York Times* that the company "is within half an inch" of leaving the state (48). Subsequently, the fine was reduced and the firm spent about $500,000 to achieve compliance with the state standard. Of 40 lead acid battery plants visited in 1975-1976 by southern California health authorities, 28 (including all of the large plants) exceeded state standards. In general, these plants are trying to comply with the state standards but are not so well controlled that they could meet the standard proposed by OSHA.

The California lead standard (maximum allowable lead concentration in workplace air) adopted in 1975 is 50 percent higher than the national limit proposed by OSHA in October 1975. The standards are: OSHA, 200 micrograms per cubic meter of air; California, 150; and OSHA-proposed, 100 (49). In its newly issued standard, OSHA gave some industries up to three years to get worker exposures down to 100 micrograms per cubic meter and up to 10 years to control exposures to 50 micrograms. The standard for lead in the workplace air has been 50 micrograms per cubic meter for many years in Japan and Czechoslovakia. The 1966 Soviet Union standard is 10 micrograms per cubic meter; however, it is widely doubted that the USSR actually enforces its stringent workplace standards (50).

In its January 1976 response to OSHA's lead proposal, the Lead Industries Association claimed the proposed standard was not feasible and would have an adverse effect on the U.S. economy. The trade group noted that industry members already face "enormous" financial burdens in complying with other health-related standards, and maintained that many companies would be forced out of business if the proposed OSHA standard is adopted. The standard would encourage investment by U.S. companies in lead smelters in foreign countries, contribute to general inflation, adversely affect competition, cause severe local unemployment problems, and adversely affect the U.S. balance of payments, the industry further claimed. On the other hand, United Steelworkers health representative George Becker criticized the proposed OSHA lead standard as inadequate, noting that even half the proposed limit would endanger the health of large subgroups of the work force that are especially susceptible to the toxicity of lead (51).

A survey of smelters by EPA in 1973 found that the Bunker Hill smelter complex exposed its neighbors in Kellogg, Idaho, to high levels of lead and arsenic air pollution (52). The Asarco El Paso lead smelter's air pollution has been cited by the Center for Disease Control as a cause of neuropsychological dysfunction in community children (53). Asarco was forced to spend $60 million for control and new process equipment (54). On December 14, 1977, EPA proposed an ambient air standard for lead of 1.5 μg/cm, taken as a continuous monthly average measurement. This standard, if adopted, would require stringent control for lead air pollution at lead smelters and other major sources that are not already well controlled. EPA estimated that the cost of installing the necessary controls would be $600 million nationwide.

The United States has about 35 percent of the world's known lead reserves. Net annual imports of refined lead have been declining through 1976, with imports furnishing 10 to 15 percent of domestic consumption. Major foreign sources are Canada, Mexico, and Peru. Domestic consumption has been growing, along with increasing supplies from primary and secondary U.S. smelters. Most lead is used in storage batteries. U.S. production of storage batteries has been adequate to supply domestic demand through 1976.

The cost of transporting lead ores out of the United States for refining and battery manufacture would severely limit the geographic choices of firms seeking to use U.S. lead ores and still escape U.S. regulations. However, some shift in smelting and battery manufacture to Mexico and Canada may occur in the future. Facilities in these and other countries may be able to supply refined lead and batteries to the United States from locally available ores and scrap at prices lower than some U.S. plants can offer.

Primary Refined Zinc

The Bureau of Mines notes that although U.S. demand for zinc metal has increased over the past 10 years, U.S. metal-producing capacity declined almost 50 percent from 1968 to 1975. "Plants closed because they were obsolete, could not meet environmental standards, or could not compete for concentrate feed. Consequently, metal has replaced [ore] concentrates as the major import form" (55). U.S. exports of slab zinc have not exceeded 20 thousand tons per year since 1968.

In 1976, imports of zinc metal exceeded domestic production (714,000 against 536,000 tons) (Fig. 6). Canada has been the main supplier of both ores and zinc metal imports, and Canada will be refining more of its own ores in the future. In second place to Canada's 313,000 tons of zinc metal shipments to the United States in 1976 was Mexico, at 63,000 tons. Zaire joined the traditional suppliers, West Germany, Belgium, Yugoslavia, Finland, Australia, and Italy, in the 30-50,000 ton range. Spain began to export significant amounts of zinc metal to the U.S. in 1975 and continued to do so in 1976 (30,000 tons). Japan, a major supplier as late as 1974, apparently no longer has excess capacity to refine zinc for export to the U.S. (56).

Industrial Minera Mexico negotiated loans from a consortium of U.S. banks in 1975 to construct a new electrolytic zinc refinery at San Louis Potosi (54). New Jersey Zinc is constructing a smelter near its subsidiary's zinc mine in Thailand. About half of the product will be exported. Smelters being built by the governments of Bolivia and Peru have relatively low capital cost to capacity ratios, suggesting that there may have been minimal outlays for pollution and workplace controls (56).

The Bureau of Mines expects U.S. zinc smelting capacity to increase slightly between 1974 and 1980. A new zinc refinery complex is being built in Tennessee by New Jersey Zinc, "the first totally new zinc plant to be constructed in the U.S. since 1941." United States zinc mining is expected to fall short of demand for the rest of this century. U.S. demand for new zinc metal was 1316 thousand tons in 1973 and is projected to reach 1800 thousand tons in 1985 and 2600 thousand tons in the year

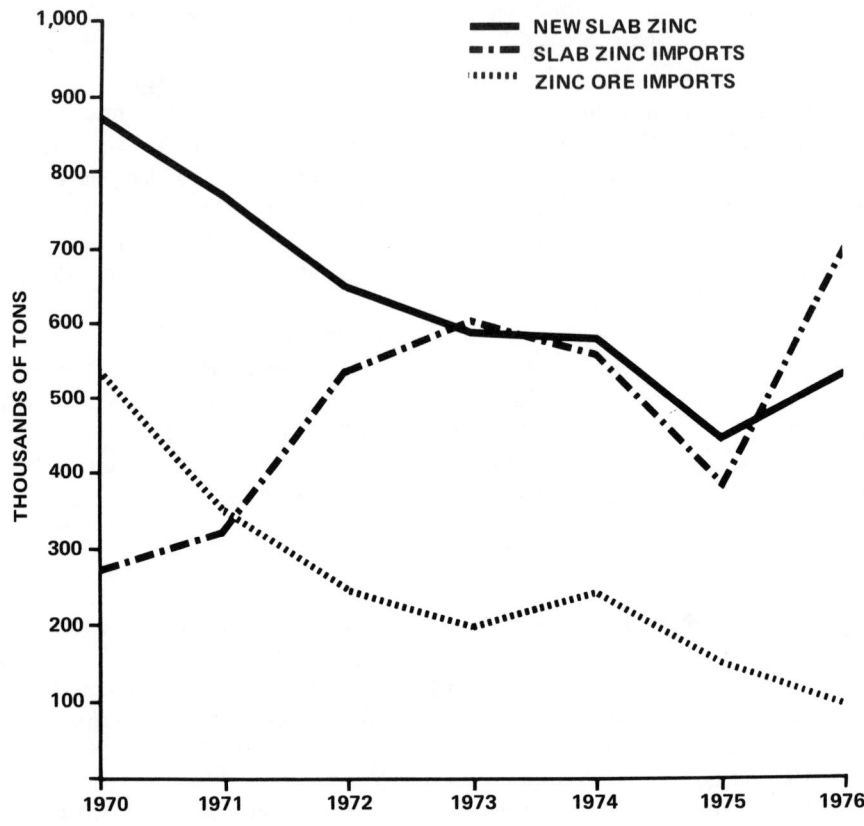

Figure 6. U.S. zinc statistics, 1970-1976. Source, United States Bureau of Mines.

2000; U.S. mine production was 479 thousand tons in 1973 and is forecasted to be 600 thousand tons in 1985 and 1100 thousand tons in 2000. However, smelting capacity is expected to increase sufficiently to process mine production between 1980 and 2000 (55, 56).

Mineral Industries in General

Mining as well as refining of ores is economically attractive in countries with lax environmental and workplace regulations. In the United States, mining is subject to standards governing air and water pollution, worker health and safety, solid waste disposal, and land reclamation. In many cases, an environmental impact analysis is required before a permit to undertake mining can be granted by the government. There is increasing pressure on the U.S. government to restrict mineral exploitation on certain public lands, e.g. the national parks. Competing demands for land use raise formidable obstacles to mining: in the western states with large coal reserves, large areas now used for raising cattle and sheep will be ruined for that purpose permanently if coal mining is allowed.

The refining of most minerals presents major additional problems for mining companies, as the preceding discussion indicates. It is illustrative to compare the sections on domestic and foreign investments in Asarco's 1975 report to stockholders. The section on U.S. smelters is densely packed with figures for pollution control and worker health expenses being forced on the company. The part on foreign investments, in contrast, mentions only the construction of two tall stacks for the expansion of a smelter in Peru.

Due to its risky nature, the mining business is dominated by global corporations that can spread their risks over many projects and raise the large sums needed to finance mineral development. Though mineral exploration has until now been concentrated mainly in developed nations, this is bound to change shortly (57).

Relatively expensive environmental controls in the United States may be crucial in discouraging global mineral companies and banks from exploiting some U.S. mineral deposits. The days of building smelters in the U.S. to refine imported ore are nearly over. There are no increased transportation costs for refining foreign ore near the mine rather than near the market. Many mineral-rich nations today have embarked on programs to develop their own refining capacities, and some accept or ignore substantial worker health hazards and pollution as the price of economic development.

Pesticides

Pesticide manufacture by U.S.-based firms has generally been done in the United States, although in some cases the manufacture of pesticides for export has caused widespread central nervous system disease among U.S. chemical workers and death among foreign users.

Until 1975, kepone was manufactured in Virginia for Allied Chemical Corporation by Life Science Products Company for sale to banana growers in Latin America, Africa, and Asia. This pesticide has caused sterility and apparently permanent nervous disorders among 75 Life Science employees, severely polluted the James River, and wreaked havoc on the local seafood industry. Allied and Life Science were indicted for over 1000 violations of federal water pollution control laws, and criminal charges were filed against Life Science owners. Employees and their families sued Allied for over $150 million. EPA and the Corps of Engineers have estimated that clean-up of the James River will cost $50-100 million. Allied was fined $13.2 million, the maximum fine allowed by law, in federal court. After Allied set up an $8 million fund to clean up the James River, the fine was reduced to $5 million, still the largest criminal penalty ever levied in a federal pollution case. In 1976, the National Cancer Institute reported that kepone caused excessive rates of liver cancer in rats and mice in lifetime feeding studies (58-64).

Another pesticide, leptophos, was manufactured until 1976 by Velsicol Chemical Company in Texas. It was granted a tolerance by EPA for residues on tomatoes and lettuce, but in May 1975 EPA announced its intention to revoke the tolerance. EPA apparently was alarmed by an article about water buffalo deaths and human injuries associated with the use of the pesticide in Egypt. When Velsicol appealed the decision, EPA appointed a panel of experts to review the matter. The panel asked Velsicol whether any of its employees manufacturing leptophos were showing signs of nerve diseases. Despite a subsequent attempt by Velsicol to drop its appeal to retain the tolerance for leptophos on crops, the investigation was followed through and serious nerve damage was discovered among Velsicol's Texas workers. One former supervisor at the plant, who quit in protest over unsafe working conditions, told of seeing a man with leptophos in his mustache eating a sandwich (65).

The revocation of leptophos tolerances in November 1976 caused consternation in Mexico, where the pesticide was used on tomatoes grown for export to the United States. Residues of leptophos were found on some shipments of Mexican tomatoes (65).

The next development in the story was the revelation that, as part of U.S. foreign assistance programs, the Agency for International Development (AID) had sent tons of leptophos to Indonesia and other countries in recent years. Other pesticides that were either banned or were being banned in the U.S. that AID had shipped to developing countries include heptachlor, chlordane, and DDT (65).

The U.S. pesticide industry is a $2.6 billion-a-year business and is growing rapidly, despite increased costs for pre-market research and declining numbers of firms that are still developing new products. The industry produces 1 billion pounds per year of pesticides for domestic use and 600 million pounds for export. The global market for these chemicals is a $7 billion-per-year business. Since 1957, AID has financed the export of over $500 million worth of pesticide chemicals (66).

In 1975 AID was sued by a coalition of environmental groups, and in early 1976 the agency announced that it would no longer sponsor the export of pesticides that are not allowed to be used in the United States for health or environmental reasons. In May 1977, AID went on to announce that its basic pesticide policies would be reversed. Less money would be given to developing countries to buy U.S. pesticides; instead, AID would help end indiscriminate use of pesticides. AID may have been influenced by a 1976 tragedy when malathion, incorrectly applied to Pakistan crops, caused five deaths and illness in 2,900 people (66).

Dibromochloropropane (DBCP) is a soil fumigant that has been produced and formulated for field applications since the mid-1950s at about 80 U.S. plants. In 1977, the Oil, Chemical and Atomic Workers Union discovered that many of the operators in Occidental Chemical Company's DBCP formulation plant had become sterile. This finding was widely publicized, and the State of California ordered a halt to DBCP production and formulation. Sterility was also found at plants producing DBCP in Alabama (Shell Chemical) and Arkansas (Dow Chemical). Federal health officials estimated that as many as 3000 DBCP workers may have become sterile or nearly sterile. Dow announced a worldwide recall of distributor's stocks. At the urging of the union, OSHA established a one part per billion emergency workplace standard for DBCP. In addition, other U.S. regulatory agencies suspended the use of DBCP on 19 food crops and banned the sale of foods containing residues of DBCP (67, 68).

Research which was done by Dow and Shell at the time they introduced DBCP and published in 1961 showed that the pesticide caused damage to sperm cells, as well as other effects, when administered to test animals. Some workers have sued these firms for damages, in light of the companies' failure to inform them of and protect them from the documented sterility hazard (69, 70).

The closing of DBCP production in the United States was followed by a surge of imports from two plants across the border in Mexicali, Mexico. Subsequent discovery of sterility among the Mexican workers led to the closing of the Mexicali plants in late 1978 (71, 72).

OSHA's emergency standard for DBCP was the first U.S. workplace standard for a pesticide. Cessation of kepone and leptophos production had obviated the need for worker protection rules for those pesticides. OSHA has announced that a general practice standard will be issued for formulators of all pesticides. The rules will cover medical monitoring, safe work practices, engineering controls, and informing workers of potential hazards. OSHA will also be writing standards for specific pesticides that will include numerical limits for worker exposure (73).

EPA has responsibility for the way new pesticides are applied. In September 1977, EPA proposed that some or all uses of 23 pesticide ingredients—most of them important to farmers and ranchers—be restricted to those users who have completed state-administered training on safe use, storage, and disposal. Pesticides containing these ingredients will continue to be freely exported, however (74).

Pesticides thus present a range of potential hazard export problems. However, the new policy of AID, coupled with OSHA's regulations and EPA's attempts to reregister pesticides, are likely to have the effect of displacing pesticide manufacture from the United States to developing nations, where incidents as bad as or worse than those discovered in the U.S. might occur. It certainly cannot be ruled out that unscrupulous firms might move some of their more questionable pesticide-for-export operations to nonregulating countries, or even manufacture pesticides for the U.S. market at plants in nonregulating countries.

Benzidine Dyes

The manufacture of dyes from benzidine has been banned in a number of countries, including Sweden, England, Italy, Japan, and Switzerland, due to the extremely high rate of cancer of the bladder observed in benzidine workers since before the turn of the century (75). A retrospective study of Allied Chemical benzidine dye workers showed that by the time of follow-up, 17 out of 76 workmen (22 percent) had developed bladder cancer (76). In Italy, 13 families of dead and sick workers recently charged a dye plant's management with multiple manslaughter, claiming that 132 workers had died from confirmed or suspected bladder cancer over the past 20 years. Three plant owners, the general manager, and the company doctor were jailed for terms of three to six years each (77).

Benzidine dyes are now made in the United States only by a small firm called Fabricolor. However, about three-fourths of the benzidine dyes made in the U.S. until recently were made by Allied Chemical, which discontinued operation in 1976. Some of Allied's former customers may have switched to substitutes for benzidine dyes; others may have turned to GAF and Fabricolor, increasing output by these domestic firms. But it is apparent that some of the textile, paper, and leather firms formerly supplied by Allied have turned to foreign sources of these dyes. United States imports of three benzidine dyes discontinued by Allied rose fivefold in 1976 (Table 3). Romania supplied half of the imported material, followed by Poland, India, and France.

Table 3

U.S. imports of benzidine dyes formerly manufactured domestically
by Allied Chemical, 1974-1976[a]

Dyes	Imports (in pounds)		
	1974	1975	1976
Direct Black 38	—[c]	—	70,753
Direct Blue 2	—	11,023	38,478
Direct Brown 2	—	2,205	24,251
Others[b]	20,353	12,520	15,906
Total	20,353	25,748	149,388

[a] Source, United States International Trade Commission.
[b] Acid Red 85, Acid Orange 45, Direct Orange 1, Direct Orange 8, Direct Red 1, Direct Red 13, Direct Red 28, Direct Red 37, Direct Blue 6, Direct Green 1, Direct Green 6, Direct Brown 31, Direct Brown 74, Direct Brown 95, Direct Brown 154, and Direct Black 4.
[c] Dashes indicate zero imports.

GAF Corporation had been second to Allied Chemical in U.S. production of benzidine dyes, but Allied's withdrawal did not leave GAF a lucrative business. GAF announced in July 1977 that, as part of a move to eliminate the company's less profitable enterprises, the firm's dye works would be put up for sale. Later that year, GAF stopped making benzidine dyes. It is now obvious that any firm that wants to make benzidine dyes in the U.S. will be expected to provide lifetime medical follow-up for every worker.

One result of a shift from domestic to foreign sources of benzidine dyes may be increased workplace and pollution dangers in U.S. dye-using industries. Allied and GAF used process controls to limit the amount of free (unconverted) benzidine remaining in their benzidine dyes to less than 20 parts per million (ppm). Benzidine dyes from other countries have been analyzed as having 500 ppm free benzidine content.

A large, new benzidine dye plant in South Korea reportedly supplies Europe with the popular Direct Black 38 dye. Attempts to identify the ownership of this plant and major markets for its products have been unsuccessful.

In 1965, Dr. R.A.M. Case noted that England had stopped making benzidine and was importing it instead. He proposed that benzidine be manufactured in extremely well-designed plants under international agreements (78). England still imports benzidine dyes, and also imports textiles colored with them, though not the deadly intermediate, benzidine.

Dr. D.B. Clayson expressed the opinion that benzidine can eventually be replaced by safer substitutes in all its applications, but he seemed to think it would be a long time before industrial use of benzidine would be abandoned worldwide. At an occupational cancer conference in March 1975, he said (79):

> Only recently has the British chemical industry been able to relinquish completely the manufacture and use of this chemical. The Italian chemical industry has introduced a range of alternatives to benzidine dyes for cotton. They are more expensive than the dyes they replace, but not excessively so. . . . I have no information on how carefully the toxicology of these alternatives has been studied.

The U.S. chemical industry has felt the pressure of imports in the general category of benzenoid dyes and pigments, of which benzidine-based colors are a subclass. Months before a fire precipitated Allied's decision to stop making benzidine dyes, a spokesman for five U.S. chemical industry trade associations asked the International Trade Commission to exempt foreign producers of benzenoid dyes and pigments from "most favored nation" tariff preference. The industry also requested a rule to deny duty-free status to any article that increases in quantity imported by 5 percent or more over the previous year, unless an affirmative decision is made to continue favored trade status for the article: "Such a rule would give the domestic industry time to adjust to increased import penetration and would stem underdeveloped countries being used as pollution havens by corporations seeking to evade the anti-pollution laws of the U.S. and other industrialized nations" (80).

About 8 million pounds of benzidine dyes were used in the U.S. in 1976. Use of these dyes has been steadily declining, and U.S. consumption was probably 50 percent more in 1972 than in 1976. Roughly half of the benzidine dye produced is Direct Black 38.

Current research by NIOSH and the National Cancer Institute suggests that pure benzidine dyes are themselves carcinogenic (81). These findings should lead to increased regulation of industries using benzidine dyes and a further drop in the market for such dyes in industrial nations. At the same time, benzidine dye production and use may even increase in other countries that make cotton goods for export to industrial nations.

Beta-naphthylamine, benzidine's notorious cousin, is another potent bladder carcinogen once widely used as a dye intermediate. Fortunately, routes of synthesis have been developed that do not involve beta-naphthylamine. The manufacture of this chemical was discontinued in Switzerland in 1938, and its use was banned in the United Kingdom in 1967. It was even abandoned in the United States in 1972. However, dyes are still made from beta-naphthylamine in India (82).

Vinyl Chloride Industries

In 1974, when B.F. Goodrich Company announced that vinyl chloride had caused liver cancer in workers exposed to the gas, it was claimed that workplace and pollution control regulations would cause the closing of plants and curtail expansion of the industry in the United States. However, despite initial industry claims that the OSHA standard promulgated in October 1974 was not feasible, compliance with the standard was achieved in virtually all plants (83).

There are three types of plants where vinyl chloride (VC) is present: a) VC manufacture, b) polymerization of VC gas to make polyvinyl chloride (PVC) resin, and c) fabrication of PVC resins into various consumer products. Production of VC would be cheaper in nonregulating countries, but added costs and difficulties in shipping VC from abroad might offset any advantage in production cost of the flammable gas. The U.S. Department of Transportation is preparing to write regulations for packaging and shipping carcinogens, and increased costs and limitations on VC are likely (84).

For PVC operations to escape U.S. regulation, the polymerization as well as the fabrication would have to be done abroad. In order to comply with the 1974 OSHA standard in polymerization plants, manufacturers employed improved stripping in polymerization reactors. This lowered the amount of residual VC that remained in the polymer leaving the reactors. Improved stripping not only reduced VC concentrations throughout polymerization plants, but also produced PVC resins with much lower residual VC content than had previously been the case. (Prior to 1975, PVC resins with as much as 1000 ppm of residual VC were common.) The U.S. customers of the PVC producers, thousands of PVC fabrication plants, also had to meet the OSHA standard of not more than one part per million of VC in workplace air. Now that these plants (which melt the PVC resins and cast them into records, garden hose, and hundreds of other products) could buy resins with 10 ppm and less of residual VC, they were able to comply with the OSHA standard without installing expensive ventilation and monomer capture equipment. Fabrication plants making PVC food packaging were especially concerned about getting the resins with the lowest possible residual VC content. As a result, domestic PVC fabricators were forced to continue to buy resins from domestic polymerization plants rather than turn to imports from nonregulating countries. Resins made in plants without improved stripping would be too high in residual VC content to be attractive to domestic PVC fabricators.

Promulgation of long-expected EPA regulations on vinyl chloride air pollution has been calmly accepted by domestic manufacturers of PVC resins; much of the cost of air pollution controls had already been incurred on improved stripping and control of fugitive emissions in PVC plants to meet the OSHA standard.

U.S. production of VC and PVC has recovered from a weak year in 1975, and the "OSHA problem" has been "solved . . . without inflating production costs to the point where PVC's growth might be stunted," in the words of *Chemical Week*. A *Chemical Week* article of September 15, 1976 tells of major new plant investment in domestic VC and PVC production. The industry looks for a 5 to 11 percent annual growth rate in the years ahead. Domestic capacity is expected to be adequate to meet demand, as it has in the past (85). The U.S. consumption of 5 billion pounds per year of VC dwarfs exports and imports, and the U.S. petrochemical industry has been a net seller of VC and PVC to other countries. In the future, as more countries develop petrochemical industries, U.S. producers will become less dominant in some export markets.

The possibility that VC and PVC manufacturing will be displaced by health-related regulations is greater elsewhere in the world than in the United States. The U.S., unlike many other industrial nations, has vast domestic petroleum resources. It is more likely that VC and PVC industries will be stunted in some petroleum-poor industrial countries, as they import increasing amounts of VC-based plastic products from nonregulating countries.

Steel Industry

Steelmaking is a highly polluting industry, and making coal into coke for blast furnaces is one of the most polluting steelmaking processes. It has been well documented that coke oven workers incur excessive rates of lung and kidney cancer (86). On October 22, 1976, OSHA issued a standard for occupational exposure to coke oven emissions. The estimated annualized cost to the steel industry to comply with the standard was $200 million to over $1 billion, and the industry immediately went to court to challenge the standard. However, implementation of the rules would only increase the price of coke 1 to 3 percent, and control costs would at most amount to only 2 to 3 percent of planned capital expenditures by the domestic steel industry over the next eight years (87).

In 1973, U.S. supply of coke was "curtailed by the inability of producers to meet environmental standards," according to the Bureau of Mines, so that it was exceeded by the enormous domestic demand in that year (88). But because of the high price and poor quality of imported coke, the fragility of coke to powdering in transit, and the fact that both the deposits of coking coal and markets for the coke are abundant in the U.S., it is unlikely that there will be any long-term trend to ship more coke in from abroad. There might be far more favorable conditions for the export of coke production to nonregulating countries from other industrial nations where coke is now made from imported coal.

In Japan, the high density of polluting industries has already led to pollution export. Several years ago, Kawasaki Steel attempted to expand production at its steel mill in the polluted city of Chiba, Japan. Faced with opposition from local citizens, Kawasaki decided to build a new blast furnace in Chiba and build a sintering plant to serve it in Mindanao, in the Philippines. The sintering plant converts iron ore dusts from Australia and Brazil to larger iron pellets in a process using coke and limestone. This product is shipped to the blast furnaces at Chiba. Pollutants from the process include trace element impurities from the ore as well as coke and iron ore dust, and gases which are predominantly oxides of sulfur and nitrogen. Particulate emissions from part of the process are controlled to some extent by dust collectors, and there are no controls for the gaseous pollutants. There are no pollution standards and the government does not monitor the pollution from the plant.

A Manila newspaper responded favorably when the agreement between Kawasaki and the Philippine government was being negotiated: "This is a case of a 'dirty' industry that can no longer be located in Japan because of pollution concerns. But the Philippine authorities have no objection to its installation in the underpolluted southern island." Reportedly, 1500 families were displaced to make way for this plant and its 6 kilometer "pollution zone." The farmers and fishermen displaced by the plant were not hired to construct it, they were considered too unskilled and uneducated. The plant employs 600 to 700 workers (89, 90).

Other Cases

On July 10, 1976, a chemical reaction went out of control and the products vented to the atmosphere included one of the most toxic and teratogenic of man-made substances–2,3,7,8-tetrachlorodibenzo-p-dioxin (TCDD). The resulting contamination in Seveso, Italy, led to the evacuation of 700 plant neighbors, many of whom may never be able to return to their homes. About 90 pregnant women who were exposed to the toxic release had abortions, despite stern opposition from the Catholic Church. The plant manufactured trichlorophenol, which was sent to Switzerland and the United States for the manufacture of the antibacterial product, hexachlorophene. The Italian, Swiss, and U.S. plants were all owned by the Swiss-based Givaudan Corporation, a subsidiary of the giant pharmaceutical firm, Hoffmann-LaRoche (91).

It was well known that TCDD was a contaminant in the process of making tri-chlorophenol, and that the amount of TCDD formed increases at high reaction temperatures. The formation of TCDD in this process was a recognized hazard in the event of a runaway reaction, an accident in which there is an excessive build-up of heat in the reactor, usually leading to an explosion. Such accidents had occurred in a number of countries since 1949, and in the United States a heat control mechanism and a holding tank back-up system are standard safety features. The Seveso plant did not have these safety devices. The workers in the plant were not even told about dioxin hazards. The Seveso incident was the first TCDD explosion to expose plant neighbors; in previous accidents the contamination had been confined to within the plants. TCDD has penetrated the soil in Seveso to a depth of 12 inches (92).

The Seveso disaster led local journalists to refer to the dense, mostly foreign-owned chemical industry in northern Italy as "the Italian Colony" (93). It is highly doubtful that this Swiss-owned plant would have been allowed to operate in Switzerland. It is certain that no one from the headquarters of Hoffmann-LaRoche will ever be sent to an Italian jail. And it is possible that a similar accident might occur again, as long as there are places where trichlorophenol plants are still designed like dioxin time bombs.

There have been street demonstrations in Tokyo against several Japanese companies charged with exporting pollution. Targets of such protests have included Toyama Chemical's closure of a mercurochrome plant in Japan and plans to move to South Korea, Nihon Kagaku's shifting of chromium refining and plating to South Korea following a long history of severe chromium air pollution and high worker lung cancer mortality in Japan, and water pollution from the Asahi Glass mercury cell chlor-alkali plant[3] in Thailand (94-96).

It is not known how much mercury cell alkali Japan imports from Thailand or other countries. However, in some industries, e.g. rayon manufacture, mercury cell alkali is preferred over alkali from the other conventional process (the diaphragm cell process). Japan has suffered the great Minamata disaster and leads the world in regulating mercury water pollution. These regulations may have displaced mercury cell alkali production that serves the Japanese economy to other nations.

Over the past three years in the United States, there have been mounting reports that foundation stones for our rubber, plastics, and other chemical industries are causes of occupational diseases. Frightening human and animal data have recently emerged on carcinogenicity of chromates, chloroform, trichloroethylene, benzene, acrylonitrile, cutting oils, 2-nitropropane, 4,4-diaminodiphenylmethane, ethylene dibromide, beryllium, and cadmium. NIOSH has urged that an emergency workplace standard be issued for chromium. On May 3, 1977, OSHA published an emergency standard for benzene, lowering the standard 10-fold to 1 ppm, in response to reports of leukemia among benzene-exposed workers. An emergency standard for acrylonitrile was issued January 17, 1978, reducing the allowable workplace limits 10-fold to 2 ppm. The emergency standards for benzene and acrylonitrile had been demanded by U.S. labor unions. More emergency standards were promised by Dr. Eula Bingham, the

---

[3] A chlor-alkali plant manufactures chlorine and sodium hydroxide from salt as the starting material. Sodium hydroxide is also called alkali, lye, and caustic soda.

new OSHA Administrator. Similarly, stringent air and water pollution control standards for newly recognized carcinogens will also be issued by EPA in the next few years.

Obvious analogies between the chemical structures of some of the newly established carcinogens and other commonly used substances cast a shadow over large segments of the chemical industry. Epidemiological and experimental reports continue to reveal the carcinogenic properties of many high-volume, industrial chemicals. In a short time, many chemicals will have to be far more carefully handled in the United States than they are today. Some export of hazardous manufacturing must be anticipated in the affected industries.

WHAT SHOULD BE DONE ABOUT HAZARD EXPORT, AND WHY?

Peter Bommarito, International President of the United Rubber Workers, has said that it is the basic right of every worker and every union to be informed about the health hazards on the job (97). Workers have the right to a full explanation of the job hazards they face and means they can use to minimize those hazards, and this warning should be issued at the time of hire. That way, a worker has the chance to reject hazardous employment before jeopardizing his health or that of his family, and before becoming economically dependent on the job. Those employed in hazardous work have the right to at least be warned from time to time about job risks and means available for their control. These warnings should be expressed in language the workers can understand.

Governments in industrial nations as well as many developing nations find it necessary to require more than just employee notification in cases where hazardous substances are handled. New plants may be held to higher standards than existing ones since process control is cheaper and more efficient in the design of a new plant than in the retrofit of an established one.

There is also increasing emphasis on environmental appraisal before permits are granted for plants to be built. The host country may be quite committed, financially and politically, to a new industrial project by the time a plant is constructed. At the stage at which a plant has opened and families depend on it for their livelihood and the workers have already incurred considerable risk of cancer or other serious diseases from working under hazardous conditions, there may be little that can be done.

Clearly, all nations need to develop expertise in toxic substances control so that they are prepared to protect their people from the time that new industrial projects are planned, as well as later, in the course of their operation. Unfortunately, few nations have so far set up regulatory agencies with sufficient resources, expertise, and authority to provide much protection to workers and communities from the dangers of operating plants. This underlines the need for careful analysis prior to construction of new plants. Requiring good process control in the design of a plant is crucial to assure that it can and will be safely operated.

There is an urgent need for ongoing and competent appraisal of the worldwide movements of hazardous industries. This hazard export information service would have to be run by a respected international organization. Its goals would be:

- To disseminate current knowledge about health risks and their controls to industrial workers everywhere, directly and through governments and unions.
- To assist interested governments and affected individuals in appraising industrial project plans and setting standards.
- To gather and distribute knowledge about the movements of hazardous industries around the world.
- To keep track of other aspects of hazard export, primarily the movements of banned foods, drugs, consumer products, and pesticides to other nations from the nation where they were banned.

Further details on how such a hazard export information service would operate are contained in the Appendix.

Trade unionists have taken stock of the high toll of occupational disease and accidents, and the prevailing view is that the abatement of job hazards is preferable to "hazard pay." The International Metalworkers' Federation has attached top priority to seeking, through both laws and collective bargaining, to ensure that workers are guaranteed the right to refuse hazardous work without reprisal. The trade unions have called for regulations to protect workers' health to the same degree everywhere, "[in order to prevent employers] from gaining competitive advantages at the cost of workers' lives" (98).

The moral and medical arguments for worldwide standards to protect humans from toxic substances are persuasive, but they pale before the bleak alternatives to hazardous work in much of the world today. The establishment of international standards is a lofty goal, but it will not be within reach until a serious, widespread effort is made to turn away from historic dependence on discredited technologies. The growing awareness of the need for clean, simple technologies, appropriate for local needs and capabilities, offers hope that models for development will arise that discriminate against polluting, hazardous industries to the extent possible.

Dr. R.A.M. Case of England, noting that his country was importing benzidine as a result of domestic plant closings in 1965, said (78):

> Now I think that most humane men will agree that it is obviously improper to expect men in other countries to face a risk which a firm considers unacceptable in its own factories; but, on the other hand, if the substances concerned are really vital to human well-being, then the solution might be to have one extremely well-designed plant which could serve the world demand, and so reduce the risk to an absolute minimum.

Benzidine dye manufacture, which is widely banned and of no military importance, might be a good candidate for the implementation of the multilateral agreement outlined by Dr. Case.

The fundamental objection to the idea of controlling hazard export is the claim that very poor people are better off with hazardous factories and goods than they would be without these things. It is of utmost importance to respect the right of people and their governments to choose what is best for them and to recognize that in some cases they will accept established mortal risks with full knowledge, and with full justification. It would seem to follow that all that needs to be done to justify hazard export is to assure from the outset that all parties involved are informed and able to understand what is at stake. Once this is done, it follows that hazard export becomes a legitimate way of distributing the world's hazards and resources to places where they are "needed."

This line of reasoning rests on the assumptions that the recipients of hazard export would be fully informed and fully able to understand the nature of the hazards, both of which are highly questionable possibilities in today's world. There are other disturbing questions raised by the notion that hazard export with informed consent is a legitimate way to do business. For example, at stake may be the destruction of the environment's capacity to continue to bring forth food that is not poisoned. A starving man might accept a polluting factory even at great peril to future generations of man and other living things. He could hardly be blamed for that, but can the same be said for those who wish to profit from his misery to the extent that they will offer him no better a bargain for putting food in his mouth? And might the hazard exporters offer the poor man more if the course of hazard export was barred?

The long-term prospects for following this line of reasoning are ominous. Industrial nations are increasingly confronted with discoveries that existing technologies are far more hazardous to workers and the environment than was ever imagined. If industry is to be expected to develop innovative solutions to these problems, and if banks are to be expected to finance a new generation of technologies, something will have to be done to make exporting the hazards of current technology less attractive. Worldwide, the pollution and worker health hazard problems posed by asbestos, benzidine, mercury, and the like are largely determined by price. As long as hazardous processes can operate without the expense of controls, their products will be cheap to manufacture and will remain competitive with other products made by safer processes. Demand for the hazardously manufactured product will remain high rather than decline in favor of safer alternatives. The resulting pollution and worker disease will be concentrated in the hazard-importing countries; they will not be evenly distributed around the world.

We are at a crossroads. At this time, some manufacturers are trying to hold on to established markets and develop improved technologies. Other manufacturers have pulled out of certain hazardous businesses because they cannot compete with plants using hazardous technologies in nonregulating countries. Still others have essentially gone into the hazard export business, recognizing that there is money to be made by exploiting the disparity in pollution and worker health regulations around the world. Meanwhile, developing nations are seeking ways to utilize their resources and choose technologies that will provide their people with needed goods, employment, education, and a healthful environment. The class of problems subsumed in hazard export constitutes a growing threat to the world environment, health, and international relations (99).

The United States is in a good position to provide conditions for the development of safe, clean technologies. The U.S. can improve its import-export and securities record-keeping so that hazard export components of its economy can be monitored. Further, the U.S. can see to it that its direct foreign assistance programs do not export workplace and environmental hazards to other nations. Through its representatives, the United States can insist that thorough environmental assessments be made by international organizations that finance development projects with U.S. aid, although development financing institutions have a long way to go in terms of giving competent evaluations of environmental impact (100). Sanctions can be provided to make the hazard export business less attractive to the directors of the U.S.-based firms. The United States can also play a leading role in setting up a world information service on hazard export and in seeking international solutions such as the one suggested 14 years ago by Dr. Case.

U.S. Secretary of Labor Ray Marshall has recently proposed that the relative workplace health and safety standards of nations be used as a factor in negotiating international trade agreements (101). However, it would take much more information than is available today to develop the terms for trade agreements.

REFERENCES

1. Castleman, B. Hazard export. In *Dust and Disease.* Society for Occupational and Environmental Health, Washington, D.C., 1979.
2. Selikoff, I. J. Cancer Risk of Asbestos Exposure. Abstract of paper presented at meeting on Origins of Human Cancer, Cold Spring Harbor, N.Y., September 1976.
3. Curtis, R. A., and Bierbaum, P. J. Technological feasibility of the 2 fibers/cc asbestos standard in asbestos textile facilities. *Amer. Ind. Hyg. Assoc. J.* 36: 115-125, 1975.
4. Jones, F. R. Occupational disease compensation. *Indust. Med.* 5: 179-183, 1936.
5. Hoffman, F. L. *Mortality from Respiratory Diseases in Dusty Trades (Inorganic Dusts),* pp. 172-180. United States Bureau of Labor Statistics Bulletin 231, Washington, D.C., June 1918.
6. Brodeur, P. *Expendable Americans.* Viking Press, New York, 1974.
7. Seidman, H., Lillis, R., and Selikoff, I. J. Short-term Asbestos Exposure and Delayed Cancer Risk. Paper presented at the Third International Symposium on Detection and Prevention of Cancer, New York, April-May 1976.
8. Wagner, J. D., Sleggs, C. A., and Marchand, P. Diffuse pleural mesothelioma and asbestos exposure. *Br. J. Ind. Med.* 17: 260-271, 1960.
9. Mancuso, T. F., and Coulter, E. J. Methodology in industrial health studies. *Arch. Environ. Health* 6: 210-226, 1963.
10. Newhouse, M. L., and Thompson, H. Mesothelioma of pleura and peritoneum following exposure to asbestos in the London area. *Br. J. Ind. Med.* 22: 261-269, 1965.
11. United States Department of Labor. Standard for exposure to asbestos dust. *Federal Register* 37(110): 11318, June 7, 1972.
12. United States Department of Labor. Occupational exposure to asbestos/notice of proposed rulemaking. *Federal Register* 40(197): 47652, October 9, 1975.
13. Finklea, J. Memorandum to M. Corn (Assistant Secretary of Labor for Occupational Safety and Health) and support document. *Re-examination and Update of Information on the Health Effects of Occupational Exposure to Asbestos.* National Institute for Occupational Safety and Health, December 15, 1976.
14. Daly, A. R., Zupko, A. J., and Hebb, J. L. *Technological Feasibility and Economic Impact of OSHA Proposed Revision to the Asbestos Standard.* Weston Consultants, West Chester, Pa., March 29, 1976.
15. *1976 Annual Report,* p. 3. Raybestos-Manhattan, Inc., Trumbull, Ct., 1977.
16. Putting the brake on asbestos. *Science for People,* No. 36. British Society for Social Responsibility in Science, London, 1977.
17. Hunt, G., and Dill, J. Materials from annual reports and project files. Overseas Private Investment Corporation, September 1977.
18. United States Department of Commerce. Records for import commodity, TSUSA No. 518.2100.
19. Year of closing inferred from advertisements in *Asbestos* and letter head in the company's correspondence with OSHA in 1973. *Asbestos,* August 1967.
20. Yoakum, G. Workers inhale deadly asbestos. *Arizona Daily Star,* March 27, 1977.
21. United States Customs Service data.
22. Yoakum, G. Asbestos pressure dwindles. *Arizona Daily Star,* May 30, 1977.
23. Sweeney, P. Juarez plant a "runaway" firm? *El Paso Times,* April 4, 1978.
24. Open Letter to California Employees (Subject: Occupational Carcinogens Control Act). California State Department of Health, May 1977.

25. Occupational Safety and Health Act of 1970, Sec. 17.
26. United States Department of Labor. Inorganic arsenic/proposed exposure standard. *Federal Register* 40(14): 3392, January 21, 1975.
27. National Institute for Occupational Safety and Health. *Criteria for a Recommended Standard. ... Occupational Exposure to Inorganic Arsenic/New Criteria–1975.* United States Government Printing Office, Washington, D.C., 1975.
28. *Inflationary Impact Statement/Inorganic Arsenic.* United States Department of Labor, Washington, D.C., 1976.
29. Asarco says OSHA arsenic rule would force closure of its Tacoma plant. *Job Safety and Health Report,* p. 241, September 13, 1976.
30. Blot, W. J., and Fraumeni, J. F. Arsenical air pollution and lung cancer. *Lancet* 2: 142-144, 1975.
31. Lee, A. M., and Fraumeni, J. F. Arsenic and respiratory cancer in man: An occupational study. *J. Nat. Cancer Inst.* 42: 1045-1052, 1969.
32. Ott, M. G., Holder, B. B., and Gordon, H. L. Respiratory cancer and occupational exposure to arsenicals. *Arch. Environ. Health* 29: 250-255, 1974.
33. Milham, S., and Strong, T. Human arsenic exposure in relation to a copper smelter. *Envir. Research* 7: 176-182, 1974.
34. Greenspoon, G. N. Arsenic. In *Mineral Facts and Problems.* United States Bureau of Mines, Washington, D.C., 1975.
35. *World Mining* 28(10): 78, September 1975.
36. United States Department of Commerce. Figures for import commodity, TSUSA No. 417.6200.
37. Greenspoon, G. N. Minor metals. *1975 Bureau of Mines Minerals Yearbook.* United States Government Printing Office, Washington, D.C., 1975.
38. *The Effects of Pollution Abatement on International Trade–III,* pp. B-1 to B-52. United States Department of Commerce, Washington, D.C., April 1975.
39. *Annual Report 1976,* p. 10. Kennecott Copper Corporation and Peabody Coal Company, New York, 1977.
40. Shroeder, H. J. Copper. In *Mineral Facts and Problems.* United States Bureau of Mines, Washington, D.C., 1975.
41. Shroeder, H. J. Mineral industry surveys for copper in 1976. United States Bureau of Mines, Washington, D.C., 1976.
42. *1974-1976 Annual Reports.* Amax, Inc., Greenwich, Ct.
43. Cammarota, V. A. Mercury. *1973 Bureau of Mines Minerals Yearbook* and *1974 Bureau of Mines Minerals Yearbook.* United States Government Printing Office, Washington, D.C. Also mineral industry surveys on mercury, United States Bureau of Mines, Washington, D.C., 1975, 1976.
44. Cammarota, V. A. Mercury. In *Mineral Facts and Problems.* United States Government Printing Office, Washington, D.C., 1975.
45. Cassady, M. E., and Larsen, L. B. *Progress Report/Environmenal Phase Bunker Hill Study.* National Institute for Occupational Safety and Health, Cincinnati, Ohio, 1975.
46. *Lead Disease Among Workers in Secondary Lead Smelters.* Environmental Sciences Laboratory, Mount Sinai School of Medicine, New York, May 15, 1976.
47. United States Center for Disease Control. Lead poisoning in children of battery plant employees–North Carolina. *Morbidity and Mortality Weekly Report* 26(39), September 30, 1977.
48. Weinstein, H. A battery plant and lead poisoning. *New York Times,* June 6, 1976.
49. United States Department of Labor. Lead occupational exposure, proposed standard. *Federal Register* 40(193): 45934, October 3, 1975.
50. *Documentation of the Threshold Limit Values for Substances in Workroom Air,* Ed. 3, pp. 143-145. American Conference of Governmental Industrial Hygienists, Cincinnati, Ohio, 1971.
51. Statement of George Becker, Safety and Health Representative, United Steelworkers of America (includes summary critique of the proposed OSHA standard on lead, by S. S. Epstein). *Hearings before the Subcommittee on Manpower, Compensation, and Health and Safety of the Committee on Education and Labor of the House of Representatives,* Part 2, pp. 435-452. United States Government Printing Office, Washington, D.C., March 24, 1976.
52. *Air Pollution Assessment Report on Arsenic,* pp. 35, 43. United States Environmental Protection Agency, Research Triangle Park, N.C., July 1976.

53. Landrigan, P. J., et al. Neuropsychological dysfunction in children with chronic low-level lead absorption. *Lancet* 1: 708-712, 1975.
54. *Annual Report 1975,* pp. 6-16. Asarco, Inc., New York, 1976.
55. Cammarota, V. A., Babitzke, H. R., and Hague, J. M. Zinc. In *Mineral Facts and Problems.* United States Bureau of Mines, Washington, D.C., 1975.
56. Cammarota, V. A. Zinc. In *1974-1976 Bureau of Mines Minerals Yearbooks,* United States Government Printing Office, Washington, D.C., 1974-1976.
57. Bosson, R., and Varon, B. *The Mining Industry and the Developing Countries* (published for the World Bank). Oxford University Press, New York, 1977.
58. Bray, T. J. Chemical firm's story underscores problems of cleaning up plants. *Wall Street Journal,* December 2, 1975.
59. Kiernan, L. A. Key kepone case figure pleads guilty. *Washington Post,* August 11, 1976.
60. Coping with kepone (editorial). *Washington Post,* July 16, 1976.
61. Virginia bans fishing in James River because of kepone contamination. *Toxic Materials News,* January 1, 1976.
62. Kiernan, L. A. Kepone indictments cite 1096 violations. *Washington Post,* May 8, 1976.
63. Paying the cost of kepone (editorial). *Washington Post,* February 4, 1977.
64. Report of Carcinogenesis Bioassay of Technical Grade Chlordecone (Kepone), National Cancer Institute, March 1976.
65. Milius, P. Articles in the *Washington Post,* December 1, 2, 3, 4, 8, 9, 14 and 26, 1976.
66. Curry, B. U.S. is changing emphasis in aid to developing nations for pesticides. *Washington Post,* May 14, 1977.
67. Peterson, B., and Shinoff, P. Dow recalling pesticide DBCP. *Washington Post,* August 26, 1977.
68. Dewar, H. Agencies announce steps to restrict a pesticide. *Washington Post,* September 9, 1977.
69. Peterson, B., and Shinoff, P. Firms had sterility data on pesticide. *Washington Post,* August 23, 1977.
70. Wider sterility problem with pesticide is found. *Washington Post,* August 25, 1977.
71. Taylor, R. B. Production of highly toxic pesticide shifts to Mexico. *Los Angeles Times,* September 9, 1978.
72. Mexico shuts down DBCP production. *Toxic Materials News,* December 13, 1978.
73. Dewar, H. Job health agency plans new pesticide standards. *Washington Post,* September 7, 1977.
74. EPA Proposes That 23 Pesticides Be Restricted to Trained Users, Asks for Comment on 38 Others. EPA Press Release, September 2, 1977.
75. *IARC Monographs on the Evaluation of Carcinogenic Risk of Chemicals to Man,* Vol. 1, pp. 80-86. International Agency for Research on Cancer, Lyon, France, 1972.
76. Goldwater, L. J., Russo, A. J., and Kleinfield, M. Bladder tumors in a coal tar dye plant. *Arch. Environ. Health* 11: 814, 1965.
77. Five Italians jailed after deaths at "cancer factory." *Los Angeles Times,* June 21, 1977.
78. Case, R. A. M. Tumours of the urinary tract as occupational disease in several industries. *Ann. Royal Coll. Surg. Eng.* 39: 213-235, 1966.
79. Clayson, D. B. Case study 2: Benzidine and 2-naphthylamine—Voluntary substitution or technological alternatives? *Ann. N.Y. Acad. Sci.* 271: 170-175, 1976.
80. Dawson, D. H. Statement before the Trade Policy Staff Committee on Multilateral Trade Negotiations and the Generalized System of Preferences, representing Manufacturing Chemists Associations et al. July 23, 1975.
81. Benzidine derived dyes. *NIOSH-NCI Current Intelligence Bulletin* 24, National Institute for Occupational Safety and Health, April 17, 1978.
82. Lobo-Mendonca, R. Prevention of bladder cancer in the dye industry. *Indian J. Occup. Health* 20(9)i: 172-177, September 1977.
83. Rattner, S. Did industry cry wolf? *New York Times,* December 28, 1975.
84. United States Department of Transportation. Environmental and health effects materials. *Federal Register* 41: 53824, December 9, 1975.
85. PVC rolls out of jeopardy, into jubilation. *Chemical Week,* September 15, 1976.
86. Redmond, C. K., et al. Long-term mortality study of steelworkers. *J. Occup. Med.* 14: 621-629, 1972.
87. United States Department of Labor. Exposure to coke oven emissions/occupational safety and health standards. *Federal Register* 41(206): 46742, October 22, 1976.

88. Reno, H. T. Iron and Steel. In *1973 Bureau of Mines Minerals Yearbook*. United States Government Printing Office, Washington, D.C., 1973.
89. Salvatierra, W. Kawasaki Steel: The giant abroad. Also Etsuko, K. Kawasaki Steel: The giant at home. *AMPO: Japan-Asia Quarterly Review* 7(4), Series No. 26, October-December, 1975.
90. Kido Junko, Philippines: Kawasaki Steel Corporation and sinter plant in Mindanao. Free trade zones and industrialization of Asia. *AMPO: Japan-Asia Quarterly Review*, Special issue, Tokyo, 1977.
91. Walsh, J. Seveso: The questions persist where dioxin created a wasteland. *Science* 197: 1064-1067, 1977.
92. Whiteside, T. The pendulum and the toxic cloud. *The New Yorker*, July 25, 1977.
93. Sullen, E., and Parks, M. *The Chemical Cloud that Fell on Seveso. Review and Selected Translations from the Italian Press, July 10, 1976 through September 10, 1976.* Rachel Carson Trust for the Living Environment, 1976.
94. Kirayama, T. Exporting pollution. *Kogai—The Newsletter from Polluted Japan*, No. 2, Winter 1974.
95. Action Committee to Stop Toyama Kagaku's Pollution Export. The development of the chromium pollution struggle: The voices of the people of Japan and South Korea encircle Nihon Kagaku. *AMPO: Japan-Asia Quarterly Review* 7(4), Series No. 26, October-December 1975.
96. *Kogai—The Newsletter from Polluted Japan*, No. 7, Spring 1975.
97. Bommarito, P. Concluding remarks at International Conference on Occupational Health. In *The New Multinational Health Hazards*, edited by C. Levinson. ICF, Geneva, 1975.
98. International Metalworkers' Federation. General statement at IMF World Conference on Health and Safety in the Metal Industry (Oslo), Geneva, August 16-19, 1976. Resolution adopted by International Conference of the IFBWW on health hazards in the painting trades. In *Occupational Health Hazards in the Painting Trade International Federation of Building and Woodworkers*, edited by G. K. Busch. Geneva, 1977.
99. *Report on Export of Products Banned by U.S. Regulatory Agencies.* United States House of Representatives Committee on Government Operations, Washington, D.C., 1978.
100. International Institute for Environment and Development. *Multilateral Aid and the Environment/A Study of the Environmental Procedures and Practices of Nine Development Financing Agencies.* Washington, D.C., 1977.
101. Dewar, H. Labor standards urged as lever in trade talks. *Washington Post*, January 11, 1978.

APPENDIX

Information Service on Hazard Export

There is an urgent need for systematic appraisal by a reputable agency of the world-wide movements of hazardous industries. Such an information service would be of value the world over.

The service would have to identify target industries, and break these into at least two classes: presumed runaways and suspected ones. For each of the presumed runaways, regular monitoring would be in effect. For suspect industries, investigations would be carried out to see if there is any basis for real concern. After a time on the suspected list, an industry could be moved into the presumed category. Actual retrospective evidence of flight from regulation need not be a prerequisite for listing an industry in the presumed category; in some cases, a health hazard may be detected in a major industry suddenly, whereupon that industry would become a top priority for study.

In investigating an industry to see if there is evidence of flight from national regulation, several major variables and many lesser economic variables should be considered. First, it is necessary to assess the preregulated posture of the industry globally. The locations of raw materials, manufacturing and refining centers, and major markets in the 1960s and early 1970s must be recorded and understood from an economic viewpoint. If there have been patterns of change (e.g. erection of smelters nearer to mines, with corresponding closures of smelters near markets for the refined metals), these should be thoroughly examined for their basis in political terms and in terms of ordinary marketplace economics.

The flight from regulation, or the decline of a regulated industry under the pressure of imports from nonregulating countries, occurs plant-by-plant. Though the closing of plants sometimes will coincide with the implementation date of new regulations, there may also be evidence of a shift in centers of production even before the new regulations take effect. This was the case with the workplace standard for asbestos implemented in July 1976, a standard whose implementation had been scheduled back in June 1972. In some cases, the announcement of a newly discovered health hazard in an industry may be sufficient to cause firms to abandon plans for expansion in the United States, even before any regulations are promulgated. In all this, the fundamental units are the individual plants that are beset with workplace and pollution problems.

It is therefore essential to map the world industry output country-by-country and plant-by-plant to the fullest extent possible. Plant closings, openings and expansions, announced new ventures, and new constructions all must be monitored. The owner- ship of all plants should be noted and kept up-to-date, as the sources of investment capital and the identity of vested interests play a crucial role in the political and economic decisions to move production around the world.

Import and export records are an important gross indicator of industry movement into or out of a country. These must be combined with domestic production figures, in order to assess the significance of shifts in annual import and export figures. The era of regulations began at different times for various industries and has not yet begun for others. However, milestone dates to be recorded include: a) date of *proposal* of regulations in the United States or other nations (especially the Scandinavian countries); b) date of announcement of discovery of a severe health hazard in an industry, especially if it is shown that the effects can be caused by levels of exposure well below those allowed by existing workplace standards; and c) date of promulga- tion of final rules by individual countries for control of workplace exposure, air pollution, and water pollution. It is to be expected that members of the industry would be aware at the earliest indication that they will have to face increased regulation. In some cases, health hazards are first recognized by the companies themselves, as they observe an unusual pattern of morbidity or mortality among their workers. Previously announced plans to expand the industry in the United States and other regulating countries could be swiftly reversed ("postponed"). The construction of new plants and expansion of existing ones in nonregulating countries might occur within a couple of years of the scientific discovery of an industrial hazard.

In assessing the effects on industry of proposed and promulgated regulations, it is useful to consider the industry's cost estimates of the regulations that are presented at rule-making hearings in industrial nations. Government documents are also helpful in computing the effect of regulations applied to plants whose design varies little around the world. The OSHA Economic Impact Statements issued for proposed workplace regulations contain some useful data. Similarly, the EPA usually publishes economic impact figures associated with its major rule making. It is crucial to determine as accurately as possible the incremental cost increase that manufacturers would incur from regulations. All regulations on the horizon should be considered separately and together. (One must be careful in integrating separate cost impacts of workplace and pollution rules, since there is some overlap. Separate cost estimates cannot simply be added, or overestimation will result.) Industry and government sources should be consulted for estimates of overall historic and projected industry capital outlays so that pollution control costs may be seen in perspective.

Price history of the products of target hazardous industries is a major variable, and one readily available. In cases where the product of a hazardous industry is also quite dangerous, the recognition of hazards may be accompanied by local or world-wide decline in demand and price. This was the case with mercury. On the subject of price, an important question is, "Will manufacturers have to absorb the costs of health regulations, or can these costs be passed on as price increases?" In order to answer this, it is necessary to assess the competitive position of the hazardous industry in the marketplace for all major sectors of demand for its product(s). The asbestos-cement pipe industry competes with cast iron, clay, concrete, and plastic pipe; as a result, cost increases for protecting workers will have to be largely absorbed, since a rise in price would favor competitive products and reduce sales of asbestos-cement pipe.

On the other hand, even a product in high demand for which price increases could be passed on is not secure in a regulating country, as long as transportation costs are small enough compared to control regulation costs to favor imports from nonregulating countries (e.g. asbestos textiles). It may, for instance, be profitable to make asbestos-cement building panels in Colombia for export to the United States, but not worthwhile to make the panels as far away as Taiwan. Thus, it will be necessary to develop the best possible information on added transportation costs that would be incurred by manufacturing for export in various nonregulating countries.

Of course, the attractiveness of relocating to nonregulating countries will vary depending on the state of technology in each industry. The marginal plants most likely to close rather than clean up are usually quite old. Technological advancements, especially in these times, lead toward less wasteful (thus less polluting) processes. Often the polluter's choice is not simply between moving the old plant, closing it, or building a new one like it with a lot of ventilation equipment. An information service that evaluates flight of hazardous industries to avoid regulation will have to be well informed about technological advances being made anywhere in the world in those industries—including new processes that have not been developed on a commercial scale.

Specific national restrictions, such as a ban on the use of a chemical in the work-place, should always prompt some investigation for evidence of hazard export. A number of countries have banned well-known deadly dye intermediates, yet they may freely import textiles with dyes made from these compounds, and even import the dyes themselves. Sometimes one country has such a bad experience with a chemical problem that the most advanced regulations issue from that country (e.g. Japan on mercury pollution). It is therefore advisable to look to particularly afflicted countries for the most stringent regulations, the most advanced technology, and for an increase in imports of a particular product (e.g. mercury-cell caustic for the Japanese rayon industry).

It will be necessary to consult with experts on target industries and governments around the world to take account of myriad factors such as changes in political climate, strikes, natural disasters, and changes in the market that are essential to understanding trends in import and export figures. Understanding the status of the medical literature on toxic substances is similarly vital in appraising the outlook for regulations not yet proposed but likely to come out over the next decade. Major centers of government and private research on toxic substances should be monitored to assure that the most current information is obtained, even before it is formally published in medical journals.

For industries targeted for ongoing surveillance, a compendium should be maintained of international treaties and agreements to control hazard export to developing nations, as well as national laws and regulations around the world. The pollution and workplace problems of each target industry should be well explained in a form available for distribution upon request. There should be a report on each industry that deals frankly with the problem of hazard export, naming the parties involved. This, too, should be available to anyone upon request.

The information service will have to reach out to the "corners of the world" to properly perform its function of gathering and disseminating information. A regular mailing of a newsletter to interested parties and contacts may be the best way to maintain their active participation.

Though its focus would be exported hazardous industries, the information service should also compile other evidence of hazard export to developing nations, such as the export from a country of foods, drugs, pesticides, and consumer products that have been banned in that country.

CONTRIBUTORS TO THE VOLUME

GIORGIO ASSENNATO is assistant professor of occupational medicine at the University of Bari, Italy. He also serves as consultant to the Italian Federation of Metal Workers. He is currently a doctoral student at the Johns Hopkins University School of Hygiene and Public Health.

DEAN BAKER is currently working for the National Institute of Occupational Safety and Health (NIOSH) in New York. He recently completed a residency in Family Medicine at Montefiore Hospital in New York. He received an M.D. from the University of California at San Diego and an M.P.H. from the University of California at Berkeley, where he specialized in epidemiology. He is a consultant at Columbia University on a NIOSH grant concerning job stress and coronary heart disease. Dr. Baker is a member of the New York Committee on Occupational Safety and Health, and has worked with unions in the New York area on noise and occupational stress.

DANIEL M. BERMAN, as Director of the Occupational Health Project of the Medical Committee for Human Rights, helped organize a number of grassroots committees for occupational safety and health ("COSH" groups) in the United States over the past decade. He has worked for the Oil, Chemical and Atomic Workers International Union and is the author of the book *Death On the Job*. Dr. Berman is the Research Director of Asbestos Victims of America and resides at 893 Rhode Island Street, San Francisco, California 94107.

BARRY I. CASTLEMAN is an environmental consultant who has worked for U.S. regulatory agencies and environmental groups and served as an expert witness in litigation involving asbestos disease. He holds a master's degree in environmental engineering from the Johns Hopkins University.

DAVID COBURN is an associate professor in the Department of Behavioural Science, Faculty of Medicine, University of Toronto. He received his Ph.D. in sociology from the same University in 1973. Among his publications in the work-health area are "Job-Worker Incongruence: Consequences for Health" (*Journal of Health and Social Behavior*, 1975) and articles on work and health, social stress, and stratification. Dr. Coburn is a founding member of the Patients' Rights Association of Ontario. His current research interests are comparisons of the health and education systems in Ontario and the political economy of British Columbia.

R. CHARLES CLUTTERBUCK is a lecturer in health and safety at the Trades Union Studies Center of Blackburn College of Technology, England. He received a B.Sc. degree from Newcastle University, an M.Sc. in agricultural sciences from London University, and a Ph.D. in agricultural ecology, also from London University. He previously lectured on the social implications of science at North East London Polytechnic, and worked for the British Society for Social Responsibility in Science where he was involved in establishing the *Hazards Bulletin*. His particular research interest is pesticide toxicity.

HANS-URICH DEPPE is professor and head of the medical sociology section at the Johann Wolfgang Goethe University of Frankfurt, Federal Republic of Germany. Dr. Deppe received his M.D. in 1965 from the University of Würzburg, after which he studied sociology at the University of Marburg/Lahn. His main research interests are the political economy of health, the social aspects of occupational health, and labor movements and health care.

ASA CRISTINA LAURELL has served since 1977 as professor and researcher in the postgraduate studies program of social medicine at the Metropolitan University in Xochimilco in Mexico City, and has coordinated a project on work and health. She graduated as a Licenciate of Medicine from the University of Lund, Sweden, in 1971, and earned an M.P.H. degree from the University of California at Berkeley, specializing in epidemiology. From 1972 to 1974 she served as a coordinator of sociomedical research on the Faculty of Medicine at the National Autonomous University of Mexico. In 1975 and 1976 Dr. Laurell conducted research on socio-economic and health problems in slum areas of Mexico City. She is presently completing her doctoral studies in sociology.

VICENTE NAVARRO is Professor of Health Policy in The Johns Hopkins University School of Hygiene and Public Health. He is president of the International Association for the Advanced Study of the Political Economy of Health and Advisor to the United Nations, to the World Health Organization and to many governments, political forces and labor unions on occupational health policy and social policy. He is the Editor-in-Chief of the *International Journal of Health Services*.

BARBARA ELLEN SMITH is currently director of an educational program on women's occupational health, funded by the National Science Foundation. Her previous employment experience includes public school teaching in southern West Virginia and organizing for the Black Lung Association. She received a B.A. in political science from Antioch College, an M.A. in sociology from Brandeis University, and a Ph.D. in sociology from Brandeis. Her research interests include stress as an occupational disease and the role of law in maintaining labor discipline in the Appalachian coalfields.

THEODOR D. STERLING is a professor at Simon Fraser University, British Columbia, and president of the Canadian Computer Science Association. He served for many years as a consultant to the Food and Drug Administration's Division of Radiological Health and has taught biostatistics and computing at Princeton University and the Universities of Alabama, Cincinnati, and Washington. Since 1960, he has investigated and published on the health effects of ionizing radiation and uses of radiation for therapy. He is the author of eight books and over 150 scientific articles.

MANUEL J. VERA VERA is an attorney for Servicios Legales de Puerto Rico in Aguadilla.

J. V. VILANILAM, a journalist and communications researcher, has six years of experience in occupational safety and health documentation. Before coming to the United States, he was on the management staff of the Madras Rubber Factory, India, for ten years. His experiences in the tire industry aroused his interest in industrial health and safety issues. He received an M.S. in communications from Temple University in 1973 and a Ph.D. from Sussex College of Technology in 1976. In addition to hundreds of freelance articles to English and Malayalam newspapers and magazines, he has contributed to professional journals in communications. He is the author of *National Development and Communication Education in Six South Asian Countries*, and is currently writing a book on occupational safety and health in India.